Antimicrobial Resistance and Therapy in Intensive Care Unit

Antimicrobial Resistance and Therapy in Intensive Care Unit

Guest Editors

Pablo Vidal-Cortés
Borja Suberviola-Cañas
David Andaluz-Ojeda

MDPI

Basel • Beijing • Wuhan • Barcelona • Belgrade • Novi Sad • Cluj • Manchester

Guest Editors
Pablo Vidal-Cortés
Intensive Care Unit Department
Hospital Universitario de Ourense
Ourense
Spain

Borja Suberviola-Cañas
Intensive Care Department
Hospital Universitario Marqués de Valdecilla
Santander
Spain

David Andaluz-Ojeda
Intensive Care Department
Complejo Universitario Asistencial de Palencia
Palencia
Spain

Editorial Office
MDPI AG
Grosspeteranlage 5
4052 Basel, Switzerland

This is a reprint of the Special Issue, published open access by the journal *Antibiotics* (ISSN 2079-6382), freely accessible at: https://www.mdpi.com/journal/antibiotics/special_issues/266QJC8E33.

For citation purposes, cite each article independently as indicated on the article page online and as indicated below:

Lastname, A.A.; Lastname, B.B. Article Title. *Journal Name* **Year**, *Volume Number*, Page Range.

ISBN 978-3-7258-6310-5 (Hbk)
ISBN 978-3-7258-6311-2 (PDF)
https://doi.org/10.3390/books978-3-7258-6311-2

Contents

About the Editors

Pablo Vidal-Cortés

Pablo Vidal-Cortés is an intensivist at the Intensive Care Unit of Complexo Hospitalario Universitario de Ourense, Spain. His main research interests focus on sepsis, antimicrobial resistance, and optimization of antimicrobial therapy in critically ill patients. He has participated in multiple national and international clinical studies exploring infection management and prognostic biomarkers in intensive care medicine. Dr. Vidal-Cortés has also contributed to collaborative projects on antimicrobial stewardship and precision medicine in the ICU, promoting the integration of clinical, microbiological, and pharmacological data into daily practice. He has authored numerous peer-reviewed publications, book chapters, and educational materials for critical care professionals and regularly participates in national forums on infection in critically ill patients.

Borja Suberviola-Cañas

Borja Suberviola-Cañas is an intensivist at the Hospital Universitario Marqués de Valdecilla in Santander, Spain. His main fields of interest include sepsis, severe pneumonia, antimicrobial resistance, and the development of prognostic models for critically ill patients. He has been a principal investigator and co-investigator in numerous observational and interventional studies focused on infection management in the ICU. Dr. Suberviola is an active contributor to national and international critical care research initiatives and has published extensively in peer-reviewed journals. His academic work reflects a commitment to advancing clinical knowledge and improving therapeutic strategies for patients with life-threatening infections.

David Andaluz-Ojeda

David Andaluz-Ojeda is a specialist in Intensive Care Medicine at the Complejo Asistencial Universitario de Palencia, Spain, with extensive experience in sepsis research and immunological response in critically ill patients. His scientific activity centers on the identification of immune dysfunction patterns and their prognostic relevance in severe infections. He has coordinated and participated in multicenter studies on host response biomarkers and novel therapeutic strategies against sepsis and septic shock. Dr. Andaluz-Ojeda has published widely in leading critical care journals and serves as a reviewer and collaborator in national research networks dedicated to improving outcomes in severe infection and organ failure.

Preface

Antimicrobial resistance has become one of the most critical threats to global health, particularly within Intensive Care Units (ICUs), where vulnerable patients and high antibiotic exposure create a perfect environment for the emergence and spread of multidrug-resistant pathogens. This Reprint, "Antimicrobial Resistance and Therapy in the Intensive Care Unit", was conceived to provide an updated, evidence-based overview of the mechanisms, epidemiology, and clinical management of multidrug-resistant infections in critically ill patients. It gathers original research and expert reviews exploring diagnostic innovation, optimization of antimicrobial pharmacokinetics and pharmacodynamics, and stewardship strategies specifically adapted to the ICU setting. The Reprint aims to guide clinicians, microbiologists, and researchers in translating scientific progress into improved bedside practice, encouraging a balanced approach between effective treatment and resistance containment. Our motivation stems from the urgent need to integrate surveillance data, precision diagnostics, and rational therapeutic use into daily critical-care decision-making. By combining multidisciplinary perspectives, this collection seeks to inspire collaboration and continuous learning in the fight against antimicrobial resistance in intensive care.

Pablo Vidal-Cortés, Borja Suberviola-Cañas, and David Andaluz-Ojeda
Guest Editors

antibiotics

Editorial

Antimicrobial Resistance and Therapy in the Intensive Care Unit

Pablo Vidal-Cortés [1], Borja Suberviola-Cañas [2] and David Andaluz-Ojeda [3,*]

1 Intensive Care Department, Complejo Hospitalario Universitario de Ourense, 32003 Ourense, Spain; pablo.vidal.cortes@sergas.es
2 Intensive Care Department, Hospital Universitario Marqués de Valdecilla, 39008 Santander, Spain; borja.suberviola@scsalud.es
3 Intensive Care Department, Complejo Universitario Asistencial de Palencia, 34005 Palencia, Spain
* Correspondence: dandaluz@saludcastillayleon.es; Tel.: +34-979-16-70-00

Antimicrobial resistance (AMR) has emerged as one of the greatest public health challenges in the last decades. Despite considerable investment and scientific effort, bacteria continue to develop new resistance mechanisms soon after the introduction of novel antibiotics. Critically ill patients are particularly vulnerable to infections caused by multidrug-resistant (MDR) microorganisms due to their severe underlying conditions, frequent exposure to invasive procedures, and high utilization of broad-spectrum antimicrobials. When infection occurs in such patients, timely and appropriate treatment becomes a race against time, with therapeutic success or failure often determined within the first hours of clinical management.

In this context, clinicians are confronted with the need to be familiar with local epidemiology, novel microbiological diagnostic tools, and the pharmacological properties of both traditional agents and newer antibiotics. The current antimicrobial arsenal is more diverse than ever before, with agents differing not only in their spectrum and mechanisms of action, but also in their safety profiles and pharmacokinetic/pharmacodynamic (PK/PD) properties, which can significantly influence outcomes.

This Special Issue of Antibiotics brings together ten original studies and reviews that comprehensively address the epidemiology, therapeutic strategies, and optimization of antimicrobial use against key MDR pathogens in ICU settings.

The issue opens with the large epidemiologic multicentre study by Kilinc et al. [1], which examines the burden of AMR in critically ill patients and its profound impact on mortality. Their findings underscore the critical importance of rapid, targeted therapy, particularly in infections caused by *Acinetobacter baumannii* and *Pseudomonas aeruginosa*, two pathogens notorious for their resistance profiles and poor clinical outcomes.

This provides a natural segue into the work of Rodríguez-Aguirregabiria et al. [2], who evaluate cefiderocol as a therapeutic option against carbapenem-resistant *A. baumannii* (CRAB) infections in ICU patients. Their results support the role of cefiderocol as a valuable alternative, while also identifying concerning resistance in approximately 20% of isolates, notably those harbouring blaNDM-1 carbapenemase and mutations in the AmpC gene. The discussion on difficult-to-treat pathogens continues with the review by Vidal-Cortés et al. [3] on *P. aeruginosa*. They present a comprehensive review covering epidemiology, resistance mechanisms, risk factors as well as future therapeutic options. In addition, the authors explore strategies for optimizing treatment, including the integration of PK/PD principles and combination therapy approaches to improve outcomes in this challenging clinical context.

Attention then shifts to *Stenotrophomonas maltophilia*, an emergent significant MDR pathogen in ICUs. One review and a research article address the treatment of this increasingly prevalent resistant microorganism in many ICUs. Carbonell et al. [4] provide valuable insights into its management, discussing antimicrobial susceptibility patterns and the importance of tailored therapeutic strategies. Complementing this, Barrasa et al. [5] apply Monte Carlo simulations to evaluate PK/PD target attainment in the optimization of antibiotic therapy for *S. maltophilia* infections in critically ill patients, offering a practical framework for dose adjustment in complex scenarios.

Another impactful contribution in this Special Issue is the meta-analysis by Risco-Risco et al. [6], which assesses the efficacy of cefiderocol for severe MDR Gram-negative infections in ICU patients. Their pooled analysis suggests adequate safety profile and significant benefits, including improved survival especially in CRAB infections, reinforcing cefiderocol's role in the therapeutic arsenal against these challenging infections.

Beyond the choice of the right drug, administration strategy is a crucial determinant of clinical success. Continuous and extended infusions of β-lactams have gained prominence, with emerging evidence linking these approaches to improved clinical cure and even survival rates in severe infections. In this context, Hyun et al. [7] compare extended versus intermittent meropenem infusion in ICU patients with severe MDR infections, finding a reduction in mortality with extended infusion, supporting the broader adoption of optimised dosing strategies. In this sense, Therapeutic Drug Monitoring (TDM) is further explored by Gatti et al. [8], who investigate meropenem administration in continuous infusion in critically ill patients receiving continuous renal replacement therapy (CRRT). Their findings are particularly noteworthy: more than 80% of patients required dose adjustment after the first drug level measurement, and with this innovative technique for optimizing antibiotic treatment over 90% ultimately survived—figures exceeding expected survival rates in such critically ill populations.

Finally, looking beyond systemic antimicrobial therapy, innovative therapeutic approaches in severe infections treatment are presented in this issue. Ruiz-Rodríguez et al. [9] describe individualized, phenotype-driven management in a case series of streptococcal toxic shock syndrome using adjuvant therapies as hemoadsorptive techniques or immunoglobulins infusion in selected patients, while Hajska et al. [10] evaluate the antimicrobial efficacy of impregnated human acellular dermal substitutes in burn wound models. These pioneering studies open new avenues for adjunctive or alternative therapies, aiming to improve outcomes in the most complex and fragile ICU patients.

Collectively, the contributions in this Special Issue provide a comprehensive and clinically relevant overview of the multifaceted challenge posed by MDR pathogens in ICUs. From large-scale epidemiological analyses to detailed PK/PD optimisation studies and novel therapeutic strategies, these works highlight both the progress made and the hurdles that remain. The evidence presented here will undoubtedly serve as a valuable reference for intensivists, infectious disease specialists, and clinical microbiologists striving to improve outcomes in this high-risk patient population.

Conflicts of Interest: The authors declare no conflict of interest.

References

1. Kilinc, M. Antibiotic Resistance and Mortality in ICU Patients: A Retrospective Analysis of First Culture Growth Results. *Antibiotics* **2025**, *14*, 290. [CrossRef] [PubMed]
2. Rodríguez-Aguirregabiria, M.; Lázaro-Perona, F.; Cacho-Calvo, J.B.; Arellano-Serrano, M.S.; Ramos-Ramos, J.C.; Rubio-Mora, E.; Díaz-Almirón, M.; Asensio-Martín, M.J. Challenges Facing Two Outbreaks of Carbapenem-Resistant *Acinetobacter baumannii*:

From Cefiderocol Susceptibility Testing to the Emergence of Cefiderocol-Resistant Mutants. *Antibiotics* **2024**, *13*, 784. [CrossRef] [PubMed]
3. Vidal-Cortés, P.; Campos-Fernández, S.; Cuenca-Fito, E.; del Río-Carbajo, L.; Fernández-Ugidos, P.; López-Ciudad, V.J.; Nieto-Del Olmo, J.; Rodríguez-Vázquez, A.; Tizón-Varela, A.I. Difficult-to-Treat *Pseudomonas aeruginosa* Infections in Critically Ill Patients: A Comprehensive Review and Treatment Proposal. *Antibiotics* **2025**, *14*, 178. [CrossRef] [PubMed]
4. Carbonell, N.; Oltra, M.R.; Clari, M.A. *Stenotrophomonas maltophilia*: The Landscape in Critically Ill Patients and Optimising Management Approaches. *Antibiotics* **2024**, *13*, 577. [CrossRef] [PubMed]
5. Barrasa, H.; Morán, M.A.; Fernández-Ciriza, L.; Isla, A.; Solinís, M.A.; Canut-Blasco, A.; Rodríguez-Gascón, A. Optimizing Antibiotic Therapy for *Stenotrophomonas maltophilia* Infections in Critically Ill Patients: A Pharmacokinetic/Pharmacodynamic Approach. *Antibiotics* **2024**, *13*, 553. [CrossRef] [PubMed]
6. Risco-Risco, C.; Henriquez-Camacho, C.; Herrera-Rueda, M.; Barberán, J.; Andaluz-Ojeda, D. Cefiderocol versus Best Available Therapy in the Treatment of Critically Ill Patients with Severe Infections Due to Resistant Gram-Negative Bacteria: A Systematic Review and Meta-Analysis. *Antibiotics* **2024**, *13*, 1048. [CrossRef] [PubMed]
7. Hyun, D.G.; Seo, J.; Lee, S.Y.; Ahn, J.H.; Hong, S.B.; Lim, C.M.; Koh, Y.; Huh, J.W. Extended versus Intermittent Meropenem Infusion in the Treatment of Nosocomial Pneumonia: A Retrospective Single-Center Study. *Antibiotics* **2023**, *12*, 1542. [CrossRef] [PubMed]
8. Gatti, M.; Rinaldi, M.; Tonetti, T.; Siniscalchi, A.; Viale, P.; Pea, F. Real-Time TDM-Based Expert Clinical Pharmacological Advice Program for Attaining Aggressive Pharmacokinetic/Pharmacodynamic Target of Continuous Infusion Meropenem in the Treatment of Critically Ill Patients with Documented Gram-Negative Infections Undergoing Continuous Veno-Venous Hemodiafiltration. *Antibiotics* **2023**, *12*, 1524. [CrossRef]
9. Ruiz-Rodríguez, J.C.; Chiscano-Camón, L.; Maldonado, C.; Ruiz-Sanmartin, A.; Martin, L.; Bajaña, I.; Bastidas, J.; Lopez-Martinez, R.; Franco-Jarava, C.; González-López, J.J.; et al. Catastrophic *Streptococcus pyogenes* Disease: A Personalized Approach Based on Phenotypes and Treatable Traits. *Antibiotics* **2024**, *13*, 187. [CrossRef] [PubMed]
10. Hajská, M.; Kurin, E.; Bittner Fialová, S.; Vidiščák, M.; Panyko, A. Antimicrobial Efficacy of Impregnated Human Acellular Dermal Substitutes in Burn Wound Models. *Antibiotics* **2025**, *14*, 707. [CrossRef] [PubMed]

antibiotics

MDPI

Article

Antibiotic Resistance and Mortality in ICU Patients: A Retrospective Analysis of First Culture Growth Results

Metin Kilinc

Department of Anesthesiology and Reanimation, Faculty of Medicine, Mardin Artuklu University, Mardin 47200, Turkey; metinkilinc@artuklu.edu.tr; Tel.: +90-532-456-37-03

Abstract: Objectives: This study aimed to analyze the antibiotic resistance patterns of microorganisms isolated from intensive care unit (ICU) patients and evaluate their impact on mortality and length of ICU stay. Given the increasing prevalence of multidrug-resistant (MDR) pathogens in critically ill patients, understanding their resistance profiles is crucial for optimizing empirical antibiotic therapy and improving patient outcomes. Methods: This retrospective study included 237 ICU patients admitted between 1 July 2022, and 1 January 2024. The initial culture growth results from blood and urine samples were analyzed. Microorganism identification was performed using VITEK 2 Compact and conventional bacteriological methods, while antibiotic susceptibility testing followed CLSI 2022 and EUCAST 2022 guidelines. Results: A total of 237 ICU patients were included in this study. The most frequently isolated microorganisms were *Escherichia coli* (*E. coli*) (44.3%), *Klebsiella pneumoniae* (*K. pneumoniae*) (35.0%), and *Pseudomonas aeruginosa* (*P. aeruginosa*) (25.3%), *with Acinetobacter baumannii* (*A. baumannii*) (31.2%) being the most resistant pathogen. Among Gram-positive bacteria, *methicillin-resistant Staphylococcus aureus* (*MRSA*) (12.2%) and vancomycin-resistant enterococci (*VRE*) (21.5%) were the most frequently identified multidrug-resistant (MDR) pathogens. Regarding antimicrobial resistance, carbapenem resistance was highest in *A. baumannii* (55%), followed by *P. aeruginosa* (40%) and *K. pneumoniae* (30%). Additionally, ESBL-producing *E. coli* (43.2%) and *K. pneumoniae* (38.5%), as well as carbapenemase-producing *K. pneumoniae* (18.6%) and *E. coli* (9.2%), were identified as key resistance mechanisms impacting clinical outcomes. Patients with MDR infections had significantly longer ICU stays ($p < 0.05$) and higher mortality rates. The Kaplan–Meier survival analysis revealed that *A. baumannii* infections were associated with the highest mortality risk (HR: 4.6, $p < 0.001$), followed by *MRSA* (HR: 3.5, $p = 0.005$) and *P. aeruginosa* (HR: 2.8, $p = 0.01$). Among laboratory biomarkers, elevated procalcitonin (≥2 ng/mL, OR: 2.8, $p = 0.008$) and CRP (≥100 mg/L, OR: 2.2, $p = 0.01$) were significantly associated with ICU mortality. Additionally, patients who remained in the ICU for more than seven days had a 1.4-fold increased risk of mortality ($p = 0.02$), further emphasizing the impact of prolonged hospitalization on adverse outcomes. Conclusions: MDR pathogens, particularly *A. baumannii*, *MRSA*, *P. aeruginosa*, and *K. pneumoniae*, are associated with longer ICU stays and higher mortality rates. Carbapenem, cephalosporin, fluoroquinolone, and aminoglycoside resistance significantly impact clinical outcomes, emphasizing the urgent need for antimicrobial stewardship programs. ESBL, p-AmpC, and carbapenemase-producing *Enterobacterales* further worsen patient outcomes, highlighting the need for early infection control strategies and optimized empirical antibiotic selection. Biomarkers such as procalcitonin and CRP, alongside clinical severity scores, serve as valuable prognostic tools for ICU mortality.

Keywords: ICU infections; antibiotic resistance; multidrug-resistant pathogens; mortality

https://doi.org/10.3390/antibiotics14030290

1. Introduction

Intensive care units (ICUs) are specialized departments that provide high-level medical care for critically ill patients. Patients admitted to these units are highly susceptible to infections due to various factors such as immunosuppression, prolonged hospital stays, invasive procedures, and the widespread empirical use of broad-spectrum antibiotics [1]. In particular, infections caused by multidrug-resistant (MDR) microorganisms are among the most significant causes of hospital-acquired infections, contributing to increased morbidity and mortality rates in ICU patients [2,3]. The rising prevalence of antibiotic resistance in critically ill patients today limits effective empirical treatment options and complicates treatment processes [4].

Multidrug-resistant (MDR) bacteria are a significant global health concern, particularly in ICU settings, where infections caused by these pathogens contribute to increased morbidity and mortality rates. Among Gram-negative bacteria, *K. pneumoniae* and *E. coli* are frequently associated with extended-spectrum beta-lactamase (ESBL) and carbapenemase production, limiting treatment options and often requiring the use of last-resort antibiotics such as colistin or tigecycline [5]. In addition to extended-spectrum beta-lactamases (ESBLs) and carbapenemases, AmpC beta-lactamases—both chromosomal and plasmid-mediated—contribute to resistance against expanded-spectrum cephalosporins, cephamycins, and beta-lactam inhibitor combinations, further limiting treatment options in ICU settings [5]. *P. aeruginosa* and *A. baumannii* also exhibit high levels of resistance, particularly to carbapenems, making them difficult to eradicate and increasing the likelihood of adverse clinical outcomes [6]. Among Gram-positive bacteria, *MRSA* and *VRE* remain prevalent in hospital-acquired infections, further complicating empirical antibiotic selection [7]. The clinical relevance of these resistance traits lies in their direct impact on patient outcomes, as infections caused by MDR pathogens are associated with prolonged ICU stays, higher rates of septic shock, and increased mortality [8]. Therefore, continuous surveillance of resistance patterns and the implementation of effective antimicrobial stewardship programs are critical in reducing the burden of MDR infections in critically ill patients [9].

Early diagnosis and appropriate management of sepsis are crucial in reducing in-hospital mortality. The timely initiation of effective empirical antibiotic therapy in the early hours can improve patient prognosis, whereas inappropriate or inadequate treatment increases mortality risk [10]. However, the pathogens responsible for infections in ICU patients and their antibiotic susceptibility profiles vary between hospitals and even among different departments within the same hospital [11]. Therefore, obtaining up-to-date microbiological data to guide empirical treatment in ICU patients is of paramount importance.

The distribution of bacterial pathogens and their antibiotic resistance profiles can change over time. To detect these changes and optimize effective antibiotic treatment in ICU patients, each hospital and even individual ICUs should regularly analyze their microbiological data and update empirical treatment protocols accordingly [12]. The increasing resistance of Gram-negative bacteria to carbapenems and broad-spectrum cephalosporins further limits treatment options and complicates infection management [13]. Similarly, among Gram-positive bacteria, *MRSA* and *VRE* pose significant resistance challenges [7].

This study aims to compare antibiotic resistance profiles based on the initial culture growth results of newly admitted ICU patients, evaluating the distribution of infectious microorganisms and antimicrobial resistance patterns. The findings obtained from this study will contribute to more effective empirical antibiotic selection in ICU patients, supporting the development of strategies to control antibiotic resistance.

2. Results

The socio-demographic and clinical characteristics of 237 patients admitted to the ICU are presented in Table 1. The mean age of the patients was 69.5 ± 18.5 years, with the majority belonging to the elderly age group. In terms of gender distribution, 54.9% of the patients were male, while 45.1% were female, suggesting that male patients may have a higher ICU admission rate.

Table 1. Socio-demographic and clinical characteristics of ICU patients.

Parameters	Patients (N = 237)
Age (Mean ± SD)	69.5 ± 18.5 years
Gender	
- Male	130 (54.9%)
- Female	107 (45.1%)
Admission Complaints	
- Respiratory Distress	115 (48.5%)
- Altered Consciousness	60 (25.3%)
- Impaired Oral Intake	20 (8.4%)
- Femur Fracture	10 (4.2%)
- Gastrointestinal Bleeding	8 (3.4%)
- Post-CPR	6 (2.5%)
- Nausea–Vomiting	5 (2.1%)
- Speech Disorder	4 (1.7%)
- Epilepsy	3 (1.3%)
- Traffic Accident	3 (1.3%)
- Gunshot Injury	2 (0.8%)
- Headache	1 (0.4%)
- Fever	1 (0.4%)
- Diarrhea	1 (0.4%)
- Myocardial Infarction	1 (0.4%)
Comorbidities	
- Hypertension (HT)	100 (42.2%)
- Diabetes Mellitus (DM)	80 (33.8%)
- Coronary Artery Disease (CAD)	60 (25.3%)
- Heart Failure (HF)	50 (21.1%)
- Chronic Obstructive Pulmonary Disease (COPD)	45 (19.0%)
- Chronic Kidney Disease (CKD)	30 (12.7%)
- Asthma	20 (8.4%)
Neurological Diseases	
- Stroke (CVA)	50 (21.1%)
- Dementia (including Alzheimer's Disease)	55 (23.2%)
- Epilepsy	15 (6.3%)
- Parkinson's Disease	10 (4.2%)
Malignancy Status	40 (16.9%)
APACHE II Score (Mean ± SD)	12.5 ± 6.2
Charlson Comorbidity Index (Mean ± SD)	4.0 ± 2.0
ICU Length of Stay (Mean ± SD)	7.3 ± 4.2 days
Survival Status	
- Survived	180 (75.9%)
- Deceased	57 (24.1%)

Regarding admission complaints, the most common reason for ICU admission was respiratory distress (48.5%), followed by altered consciousness (25.3%) and impaired oral intake (8.4%). Other frequently observed reasons included gastrointestinal bleeding, post-cardiopulmonary resuscitation (post-CPR) care, and neurological symptoms. These findings indicate that respiratory failure, altered mental status, and critical illness syndromes are among the leading causes of ICU admissions.

An analysis of comorbidities revealed that the most prevalent conditions were hypertension (42.2%) and diabetes mellitus (33.8%), followed by coronary artery disease (25.3%), heart failure (21.1%), and chronic obstructive pulmonary disease (COPD) (19.0%). Furthermore, chronic kidney disease (CKD) (12.7%) was also found to be a significant comorbidity among ICU patients. In terms of neurological diseases, the most common conditions were stroke (21.1%) and dementia (including Alzheimer's disease) (23.2%).

The clinical status of patients was assessed using scoring systems, where the APACHE II score was 12.5 ± 6.2, indicating that ICU patients generally had severe clinical conditions. The Charlson Comorbidity Index (4.0 ± 2.0) further confirmed that most patients had a high comorbidity burden. The average ICU length of stay was 7.3 ± 4.2 days, and the mortality rate was 24.1% (57 patients). These findings demonstrate that ICU patients often have significant comorbidities and that ICU mortality remains substantial.

In summary, most ICU patients are elderly, with multiple comorbidities and severe clinical conditions. Respiratory distress, altered consciousness, and postoperative monitoring were the most common reasons for ICU admission, with cardiovascular and pulmonary diseases being highly prevalent. The high ICU mortality rate (24.1%) highlights the importance of implementing optimized treatment strategies for critically ill patients (Table 1).

The laboratory findings of ICU patients are presented in Table 2. The mean hemoglobin level was 10.5 ± 2.0 g/dL, reflecting the common presence of anemia in ICU patients. The white blood cell (WBC) count was 9.85 ± 4.83 × $10^3/\mu L$, suggesting that inflammatory or infectious processes were active in many patients. Platelet count was measured as 220 ± 90 × $10^3/\mu L$, highlighting its importance in evaluating coagulation status.

Table 2. Laboratory Findings of ICU Patients.

Parameters (Units)	Mean ± SD
Hemoglobin (g/dL)	10.5 ± 2.0
White Blood Cell Count (×$10^3/\mu L$)	9.85 ± 4.83
Platelet Count (×$10^3/\mu L$)	220 ± 90
Sodium (mmol/L)	140 ± 5
Potassium (mmol/L)	4.0 ± 0.5
Chloride (mmol/L)	103 ± 5
Bicarbonate (mmol/L)	22 ± 4
Blood Urea Nitrogen (mg/dL)	25 ± 15
Creatinine (mg/dL)	1.2 ± 0.6
Glucose (mg/dL)	150 ± 60
Calcium (mg/dL)	8.5 ± 1.0
Magnesium (mEq/L)	1.9 ± 0.4
Phosphorus (mg/dL)	3.8 ± 1.2
Albumin (g/dL)	2.8 ± 0.7
Total Bilirubin (mg/dL)	1.5 ± 0.8
Alkaline Phosphatase (U/L)	100 ± 50
Alanine Aminotransferase (U/L)	45 ± 20
Aspartate Aminotransferase (U/L)	50 ± 25
Lactate Dehydrogenase (U/L)	250 ± 100
C-Reactive Protein (mg/L)	100 ± 70
Troponin (ng/mL)	0.804 ± 0.048
D-dimer (mg/L)	5.06 ± 8.79
Procalcitonin (ng/mL)	1.76 ± 5.33

Regarding electrolyte levels, sodium (140 ± 5 mmol/L), potassium (4.0 ± 0.5 mmol/L), and bicarbonate (22 ± 4 mmol/L) were within the generally accepted ranges for ICU patients.

However, blood urea nitrogen (BUN) (25 ± 15 mg/dL) and creatinine (1.2 ± 0.6 mg/dL) were slightly elevated, indicating possible renal impairment. The glucose level of 150 ± 60 mg/dL supports the frequent occurrence of stress-induced hyperglycemia in ICU patients.

Liver function tests revealed total bilirubin at 1.5 ± 0.8 mg/dL, alkaline phosphatase at 100 ± 50 U/L, alanine aminotransferase (ALT) at 45 ± 20 U/L, and aspartate aminotransferase (AST) at 50 ± 25 U/L. These findings suggest that some patients may have hepatic dysfunction or liver failure. Lactate dehydrogenase (LDH) was 250 ± 100 U/L, which may serve as an indicator of cellular damage or hypoxia-related metabolic alterations.

Among inflammatory markers, CRP was 100 ± 70 mg/L, suggesting ongoing systemic inflammation or sepsis in most patients. Troponin levels were 0.804 ± 0.048 ng/mL, which may indicate cardiac injury in some cases. D-dimer levels were 5.06 ± 8.79 mg/L, reflecting a high risk of coagulopathy and thromboembolic events. Procalcitonin levels were measured at 1.76 ± 5.33 ng/mL, highlighting its role as a key biomarker for bacterial infections and sepsis in ICU patients.

In summary, the laboratory findings of ICU patients indicate frequent hematological, biochemical, and inflammatory alterations, which are commonly encountered in critical care settings. These findings provide valuable insights into early diagnosis, appropriate treatment planning, and prognostic assessment in ICU patients (Table 2).

The microorganisms isolated from blood and urine of ICU patients are presented in Table 3. The most frequently isolated microorganism was *E. coli* (44.3%), predominantly found in urine cultures (35.9%). This finding confirms that *E. coli* is the most common causative agent of urinary tract infections in ICU patients.

Table 3. Microorganisms Isolated from Blood and Urine Cultures in ICU Patients.

Isolated Microorganism	Blood *n* (%)	Urine *n* (%)	Total *n* (%)
E. coli	12 (5.1%)	85 (35.9%)	105 (44.3%)
K. pneumoniae	18 (7.6%)	50 (21.1%)	83 (35.0%)
P. aeruginosa	10 (4.2%)	20 (8.4%)	60 (25.3%)
MRSA	22 (9.3%)	5 (2.1%)	29 (12.2%)
VRE	8 (3.4%)	40 (16.9%)	51 (21.5%)
A. baumannii	14 (5.9%)	10 (4.2%)	74 (31.2%)
C. albicans	7 (3.0%)	5 (2.1%)	14 (5.9%)

The second most frequently isolated microorganism was *K. pneumoniae* (35.0%), which was found in urine cultures (21.1%) and blood cultures (7.6%). *P. aeruginosa* (25.3%) was frequently associated with respiratory infections, which was found in urine cultures (8.4%) and blood cultures (4.2%).

Among blood cultures, *MRSA* (12.2%) was one of the most commonly isolated pathogens, with a significant proportion (9.3%) being identified as a bloodstream infection pathogen. *VRE* (21.5%) was predominantly found in urine cultures (16.9%), emphasizing its role as a significant multidrug-resistant pathogen in urinary tract infections.

As one of the multidrug-resistant pathogens, *A. baumannii* (31.2%) was most commonly isolated from blood cultures (5.9%). *Candida albicans* (*C. albicans*) (5.9%) was most frequently detected in blood (3.0%) and urine cultures (2.1%), suggesting that invasive fungal infections should also be considered in ICU patients.

In summary, the most frequently isolated pathogens in ICU patients were *E. coli*, *K. pneumoniae*, and *P. aeruginosa*. Gram-negative bacteria were dominant in urinary tract and respiratory infections, whereas resistant Gram-positive bacteria such as *MRSA* and *VRE* played a significant role in bloodstream and urinary tract infections. *A. baumannii*, a highly resistant pathogen, was particularly associated with respiratory infections. These findings highlight the importance of infection control strategies and empirical antibiotic selection in ICU settings (Table 3).

The antibiotic resistance rates of microorganisms isolated from ICU patients are presented in Table 4. Carbapenem resistance was detected at high rates in *K. pneumoniae* (30%) and *P. aeruginosa* (40%). In contrast, *E. coli* exhibited a lower carbapenem resistance rate (12%) compared to other Gram-negative bacteria. *A. baumannii* displayed the highest carbapenem resistance rate (55%), indicating a critical resistance problem for this pathogen.

Table 4. Antibiotic resistance rates of microorganisms isolated from ICU Patients.

Antimicrobial Agent	*E. Coli* (n = 105)	*Klebsiella* spp. (n = 83)	*Pseudomonas* spp. (n = 60)	*MRSA* (n = 29)	*VRE* (n = 51)	*Acinetobacter* spp. (n = 74)	*Candida* spp. (n = 14)
Carbapenems	12%	30%	40%	-	-	55%	-
Cephalosporins	35%	60%	20%	-	-	50%	-
Fluoroquinolones	45%	55%	35%	-	-	48%	-
Aminoglycosides	20%	40%	50%	-	-	35%	-
Vancomycin	-	-	-	100%	85%	-	-
Colistin	-	-	10%	-	-	20%	-
Fluconazole	-	-	-	-	-	-	25%
ESBL	43.2%	38.5%	-	-	-	-	-
p-AmpC	12.8%	16.4%	-	-	-	-	-
Carbapenemase	9.2%	18.6%	-	-	-	-	-

ESBL: extended-spectrum beta-lactamase; p-AmpC: plasmid-mediated AmpC beta-lactamase.

Cephalosporin resistance was found to be particularly high in *K. pneumoniae* (60%). Lower resistance rates were observed in *E. coli* (35%) and *P. aeruginosa* (20%). However, *A. baumannii* also exhibited a cephalosporin resistance rate of 50%, suggesting that cephalosporins have become largely ineffective against this pathogen.

Fluoroquinolone resistance was high among all Gram-negative bacteria. Resistance rates were 45% in *E. coli*, 55% in *K. pneumoniae*, and 35% in *P. aeruginosa*. *A. baumannii* exhibited a fluoroquinolone resistance rate of 48%, raising concerns about the decreasing efficacy of this antibiotic class against multidrug-resistant pathogens.

Aminoglycoside resistance was notably high in *P. aeruginosa* (50%) and *K. pneumoniae* (40%). *E. coli* had a lower aminoglycoside resistance rate (20%) compared to other Gram-negative bacteria. *A. baumannii* exhibited a resistance rate of 35%, reinforcing the challenge of treating infections caused by this opportunistic pathogen.

Among Gram-positive bacteria, *MRSA* isolates were fully susceptible to vancomycin (100%), while *VRE* isolates exhibited a high vancomycin resistance rate (85%). This finding underscores the need for alternative agents in treating ICU-associated VRE infections.

Regarding polymyxin group antibiotics, colistin resistance was detected in *P. aeruginosa* (10%) and *A. baumannii* (20%). These relatively low resistance rates suggest that colistin remains partially effective against multidrug-resistant pathogens.

For fungal infections, *C. albicans* exhibited a fluconazole resistance rate of 25%, indicating that amphotericin B or echinocandin antifungals may be preferred for severe candidiasis cases in the ICU.

ESBL-producing *E. coli* was detected in 43.2% of isolates, while ESBL-producing *K. pneumoniae* was found in 38.5% of cases. p-AmpC-producing *E. coli* was observed in 12.8%, and p-AmpC-producing *K. pneumoniae* in 16.4% of isolates. Carbapenemase-producing *K. pneumoniae* was detected in 18.6%, while carbapenemase-producing *E. coli* was found in 9.2% of cases (Table 4).

The effect of microorganism growth on the length of stay in the ICU is presented in Table 5. Overall, patients with culture-positive infections had a significantly longer ICU stay compared to those without infections ($p < 0.05$).

Table 5. Impact of Microorganism Growth on ICU Length of Stay.

Isolated Microorganism	Length of Stay in the ICU (Days)		*p* Value
	Growth (+)	Growth (−)	
E. coli	10.5 ± 3.2	6.8 ± 2.5	0.02
K. pneumoniae	12.1 ± 4.5	7.3 ± 2.8	0.01
P. aeruginosa	14.0 ± 5.1	8.0 ± 3.0	0.005
MRSA	13.2 ± 4.8	7.5 ± 2.7	0.009
VRE	11.8 ± 4.2	7.0 ± 2.6	0.015
A. baumannii	15.5 ± 5.7	8.3 ± 3.2	0.003
C. albicans	9.8 ± 3.6	6.5 ± 2.3	0.04
ESBL-producing *Enterobacterales*	11.4 ± 3.8	7.2 ± 3.1	0.004
p-AmpC-producing *Enterobacterales*	12.1 ± 4.3	7.5 ± 3.2	0.01
Carbapenemase-producing *Enterobacterales*	14.8 ± 5.2	7.9 ± 3.5	<0.001

For *E. coli*-positive patients, the mean ICU length of stay was 10.5 ± 3.2 days, which was significantly longer than in culture-negative patients (6.8 ± 2.5 days, $p = 0.02$). Similarly, patients infected with *K. pneumoniae* had a mean ICU stay of 12.1 ± 4.5 days, which was markedly longer compared to culture-negative patients (7.3 ± 2.8 days, $p = 0.01$).

Among ICU patients, those infected with *P. aeruginosa* had one of the longest ICU stays, with a mean duration of 14.0 ± 5.1 days. In contrast, culture-negative patients had a significantly shorter ICU stay of 8.0 ± 3.0 days ($p = 0.005$). Similarly, *MRSA*-positive patients had a prolonged ICU stay of 13.2 ± 4.8 days, compared to 7.5 ± 2.7 days in culture-negative patients ($p = 0.009$).

VRE-positive patients also had a significantly longer ICU stay (11.8 ± 4.2 days) compared to those without infection (7.0 ± 2.6 days, $p = 0.015$). However, *A. baumannii* infections were associated with the longest ICU stays, with an average of 15.5 ± 5.7 days, which was significantly longer than in culture-negative patients (8.3 ± 3.2 days, $p = 0.003$).

For *C. albicans*-positive patients, the mean ICU length of stay was 9.8 ± 3.6 days, which was significantly longer than in culture-negative patients (6.5 ± 2.3 days, $p = 0.04$).

Patients infected with ESBL-producing *Enterobacterales* had a significantly longer ICU stay (11.4 ± 3.8 days) compared to non-ESBL infections (7.2 ± 3.1 days, $p = 0.004$). p-AmpC-producing infections were associated with an ICU stay of 12.1 ± 4.3 days, significantly longer than non-p-AmpC cases (7.5 ± 3.2 days, $p = 0.01$). Carbapenemase-producing *Enterobacterales* resulted in the longest ICU stays (14.8 ± 5.2 days) compared to non-carbapenemase cases (7.9 ± 3.5 days, $p < 0.001$) (Table 5).

The relationship between microorganism growth and mortality in ICU patients is presented in Table 6. The findings indicate that certain multidrug-resistant microorganisms significantly increase ICU mortality rates ($p < 0.05$). Among patients with *E. coli* infections, the survival rate was 76.2%, while the mortality rate was 23.8% ($p = 0.04$). Similarly, patients infected with *K. pneumoniae* had a mortality rate of 27.7%, showing a significant association between this microorganism and ICU mortality ($p = 0.03$).

P. aeruginosa infections were associated with a mortality rate of 33.3%, indicating a strong correlation between the presence of this microorganism in cultures and ICU mortality ($p = 0.02$). *MRSA*-positive patients had a high mortality rate of 48.3%, with only 51.7% surviving, confirming the significant impact of *MRSA* infections on ICU mortality ($p = 0.006$). VRE infections were associated with a mortality rate of 41.2%, suggesting a substantial impact on ICU mortality ($p = 0.008$). *A. baumannii*-infected patients had the highest mortality rate (73.0%), with only 27.0% surviving, making it the most lethal pathogen in ICU settings ($p < 0.001$). *C. albicans* infections were linked to a mortality rate of 28.6%, indicating that fungal infections also play a role in ICU mortality ($p = 0.05$).

Table 6. Relationship Between Microorganism Growth and Mortality in ICU Patients.

Isolated Microorganism	Survived *n* (%)	Deceased *n* (%)	*p* Value
E. coli	80 (76.2%)	25 (23.8%)	0.04
K. pneumoniae	60 (72.3%)	23 (27.7%)	0.03
P. aeruginosa	40 (66.7%)	20 (33.3%)	0.02
MRSA	15 (51.7%)	14 (48.3%)	0.006
VRE	30 (58.8%)	21 (41.2%)	0.008
A. baumannii	20 (27.0%)	54 (73.0%)	<0.001
C. albicans	10 (71.4%)	4 (28.6%)	0.05
ESBL positive Enterobacterales	43 (66.3%)	22 (33.7%)	0.02
p-AmpC positive Enterobacterales	27 (61.8%)	17 (38.2%)	0.01
Carbapenemase positive Enterobacterales	18 (52.5%)	18 (47.5%)	<0.001

The mortality rate in ESBL-producing *Enterobacterales* infections was 33.7%, significantly higher than in non-ESBL cases (18.5%, $p = 0.02$). p-AmpC-producing infections showed a mortality rate of 38.2%, compared to 19.3% in non-p-AmpC patients ($p = 0.01$). Carbapenemase-producing *Enterobacterales* infections had the highest mortality rate at 47.5%, nearly doubling the mortality risk compared to non-carbapenemase cases (24.8%, $p < 0.001$) (Table 6).

The multivariate logistic regression analysis of factors influencing ICU mortality is presented in Table 7. The results indicate that certain microorganisms and laboratory parameters are significantly associated with ICU mortality ($p < 0.05$).

Table 7. Multivariate logistic regression analysis of factors affecting mortality in ICU Patients.

Variables	Odds Ratio	95% CI	*p* Value
E. coli (+)	1.5	1.1–2.1	0.04
K. pneumoniae (+)	2.2	1.4–3.3	0.02
P. aeruginosa (+)	2.8	1.6–4.5	0.01
MRSA (+)	3.5	1.8–6.7	0.005
VRE (+)	2.7	1.5–4.8	0.007
A. baumannii (+)	4.6	2.5–7.9	<0.001
C. albicans (+)	1.9	1.1–3.2	0.05
Carbapenems Resistance	3.1	1.8–5.4	0.003
Cephalosporins Resistance	1.8	1.1–2.8	0.03
Fluoroquinolones Resistance	2.5	1.6–4.0	0.01
Aminoglycosides Resistance	2.0	1.2–3.5	0.03
ESBL-*Enterobacterales*	1.8	1.2–2.9	0.02
p-AmpC-*Enterobacterales*	2.4	1.5–4.1	0.008
Carbapenemase-*Enterobacterales*	3.9	2.2–6.7	<0.001
Vancomycin Resistance	2.9	1.7–4.6	0.005
Colistin Resistance	3.7	2.1–6.3	0.004
Fluconazole Resistance	1.5	1.0–2.5	0.05
Procalcitonin (≥2 ng/mL)	2.8	1.5–4.9	0.008
C-Reactive Protein (CRP) (≥100 mg/L)	2.2	1.3–3.6	0.01
Charlson Comorbidity Index (CCI) (≥4)	3.2	1.9–5.4	0.003
APACHE II score (≥15)	4.1	2.6–6.8	<0.001
NLR (Neutrophil-to-Lymphocyte Ratio) (≥5)	2.6	1.4–4.1	0.01
Hospital Stay (days) (≥7)	1.4	1.1–1.9	0.02

Among the identified microorganisms, *A. baumannii* infection was associated with the highest mortality risk (OR: 4.6, 95% CI: 2.5–7.9, $p < 0.001$). Other multidrug-resistant organisms (MDROs), including *MRSA* (OR: 3.5, $p = 0.005$), *P. aeruginosa* (OR: 2.8, $p = 0.01$), and *K. pneumoniae* (OR: 2.2, $p = 0.02$), were also significantly associated with ICU mortality. Additionally, *VRE* infection (OR: 2.7, $p = 0.007$) was identified as a notable risk factor for mortality. *C. albicans* infection was associated with a 1.9-fold increase in mortality risk ($p = 0.05$), indicating that fungal infections may contribute to ICU mortality.

Among antibiotic resistance patterns, carbapenem resistance (OR: 3.1, $p = 0.003$), fluoroquinolone resistance (OR: 2.5, $p = 0.01$), and aminoglycoside resistance (OR: 2.0, $p = 0.03$) were significantly associated with ICU mortality. Vancomycin resistance (OR: 2.9, $p = 0.005$) and colistin resistance (OR: 3.7, $p = 0.004$) were also identified as key contributors to increased mortality risk in ICU patients.

Carbapenemase production was an independent predictor of mortality (OR: 3.9, 95% CI: 2.2–6.7, $p < 0.001$). p-AmpC production was associated with a 2.4-fold increased mortality risk ($p = 0.008$). ESBL production was linked to a 1.8-fold increased mortality risk ($p = 0.02$).

In terms of biochemical markers, procalcitonin levels ≥ 2 ng/mL were associated with a 2.8-fold increase in mortality risk ($p = 0.008$), highlighting sepsis as a major cause of ICU mortality. Similarly, C-reactive protein (CRP ≥ 100 mg/L) was linked to a 2.2-fold increase in mortality risk ($p = 0.01$).

Among clinical severity scores, the Charlson Comorbidity Index ($\geq$4) (OR: 3.2, $p = 0.003$) and APACHE II score ($\geq$15) (OR: 4.1, $p < 0.001$) were significant predictors of poor prognosis and higher ICU mortality risk. Furthermore, NLR ≥ 5 was associated with a 2.6-fold increase in mortality risk ($p = 0.01$), indicating the impact of systemic inflammation on ICU mortality. Patients who remained in the ICU for more than seven days had a 1.4-fold increased risk of mortality ($p = 0.02$) (Table 7).

The Kaplan–Meier survival curve for ICU patients was shown in Figure 1. *A. baumannii* shows the lowest survival probability over time, indicating it is the most lethal infection. MRSA also has a significantly reduced survival rate compared to other infections. *P. aeruginosa, K. pneumoniae,* and *E. coli* have better survival rates, but a steady decline is observed. *E. coli* patients have the highest survival probability, making it the least critical among the compared infections (Figure 1).

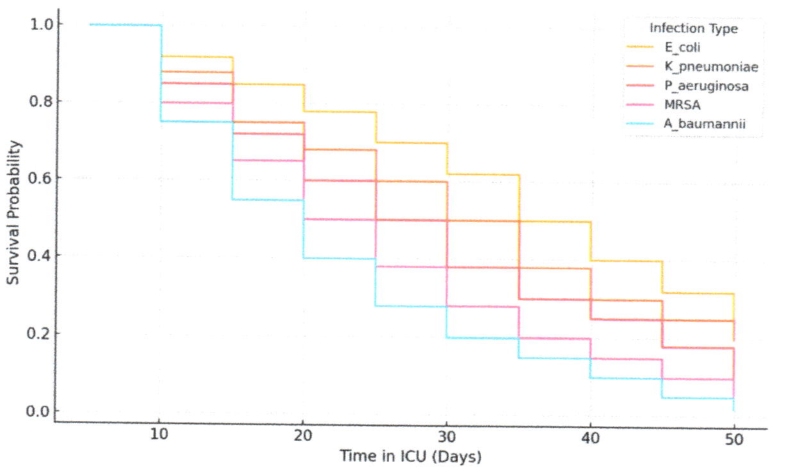

Figure 1. Kaplan–Meier survival curve for ICU patients.

For ESBL-producing Enterobacterales infections, carbapenems (meropenem/imipenem) were the most frequently used targeted therapy in 68.4% of cases. In p-AmpC-producing infections, a combination of cefepime + aminoglycosides or carbapenems was used in 52.9%

of cases. For carbapenemase-producing Enterobacterales, colistin-based regimens, often combined with tigecycline or fosfomycin, were required in 73.1% of patients due to limited treatment options. Empirical therapy was modified in 85.6% of patients with confirmed multidrug-resistant infections based on susceptibility testing.

3. Discussion

This study comprehensively analyzed the antibiotic resistance patterns of microorganisms isolated from ICU patients and their impact on patient outcomes, particularly mortality. Our findings reveal that MDR pathogens, including *A. baumannii*, MRSA, *P. aeruginosa*, and *K. pneumoniae*, remain among the most frequently isolated organisms and are strongly associated with prolonged ICU stays, increased illness severity, and higher mortality rates. Additionally, ESBL-, p-AmpC-, and carbapenemase-producing *Enterobacterales* demonstrated a significant impact on both ICU length of stay and patient survival, with carbapenemase producers showing the highest mortality risk. The strong association between carbapenem, cephalosporin, fluoroquinolone, aminoglycoside, and vancomycin resistance with adverse clinical outcomes further underscores the growing challenge of antimicrobial resistance in ICU settings. These findings highlight the urgent need for enhanced surveillance of resistance traits, targeted infection control strategies, and optimized antimicrobial stewardship programs, particularly in high-risk ICU populations.

A. baumannii infections had the highest mortality risk among ICU patients (OR: 4.6) in our study. Similarly, Wei et al. reported that MDR A. baumannii colonization in ICU patients was a significant predictor of in-hospital mortality [14]. Golli et al. observed high rates of MDR in *A. baumannii* (97.77%), *P. aeruginosa* (65%), and *K. pneumoniae* (50%), underscoring the critical impact of these pathogens on patient outcomes [3]. Other MDR pathogens, including MRSA (OR: 3.5, $p = 0.005$), *P. aeruginosa* (OR: 2.8), and *K. pneumoniae* (OR: 2.2), were also significantly associated with ICU mortality. These findings align with previous studies highlighting the impact of MDR bacteria on poor patient outcomes in critical care settings [3,11].

In our study, other MDR pathogens, including MRSA (OR: 3.5, $p = 0.005$), *P. aeruginosa* (OR: 2.8), and *K. pneumoniae* (OR: 2.2), were also significantly associated with ICU mortality. These findings are consistent with previous studies highlighting the detrimental effects of MDR bacteria on critically ill patients. For instance, Golli et al. reported that MDR *P. aeruginosa* and *K. pneumoniae* were prevalent in bloodstream infections within ICU settings, contributing to increased mortality rates [3]. Furthermore, Schinas et al. emphasized that MDR *A. baumannii* colonization significantly elevates the risk of in-hospital mortality among ICU patients, reinforcing the need for stringent infection control measures [15]. In our study, it was indicated that infections caused by MDR pathogens such as *A. baumannii*, MRSA, *P. aeruginosa*, and *K. pneumoniae* are associated with higher mortality risks in ICU patients. This underscores the imperative for effective antimicrobial stewardship and robust infection prevention strategies to mitigate the impact of these formidable pathogens.

Our study identified significant associations between specific antibiotic resistance patterns and increased ICU mortality. Notably, carbapenem resistance (OR: 3.9), ESBL production (OR: 1.8), p-AmpC production (OR: 2.4), and carbapenemase production (OR: 3.9) were strongly linked to higher mortality rates. Among antibiotic classes, fluoroquinolone resistance (OR: 2.5), aminoglycoside resistance (OR: 2.0), and cephalosporin resistance (OR: 1.8) were significantly associated with worse clinical outcomes. Additionally, vancomycin resistance (OR: 2.9) and colistin resistance (OR: 3.7) emerged as major risk factors for increased ICU mortality, particularly among multidrug-resistant *A. baumannii* and *K. pneumoniae* infections. Corona et al. emphasized that rising carbapenem and fluoroquinolone resistance has led to worse outcomes and limited treatment options in ICU patients [4]. Yoo et al. reported that patients in the ICU are particularly susceptible to *carbapenem-resistant Enterobacterales* (CRE) infections, which are associated with increased mortality rates [16]. Ebbing et al. found that fluoroquinolone resistance is an independent risk factor for mortality in patients with healthcare-acquired *E. coli* and *K. pneumoniae* infections [17]. Golli et al. observed high rates of multidrug resistance in *A. baumannii* (97.77%), *P. aeruginosa* (65%), and *K. pneumoniae* (50%), underscoring the critical impact of these pathogens on patient outcomes [3]. In our study, we demonstrated that infections caused by multidrug-resistant (MDR) pathogens, including *A. baumannii*, MRSA, *P. aeruginosa*, and *K. pneumoniae*, are significantly associated with increased mortality risks in ICU patients. Additionally, we found that ESBL-, p-AmpC-, and carbapenemase-producing *Enterobacterales* further exacerbate clinical outcomes, contributing to prolonged ICU stays and higher mortality rates. These findings emphasize the critical need for enhanced antimicrobial stewardship, routine surveillance of resistance mechanisms, and stringent infection prevention strategies to mitigate the impact of MDR pathogens and improve patient outcomes in ICU settings.

It was showed that significant associations between elevated inflammatory markers and increased ICU mortality in our study. Specifically, PCT levels $\geq$ 2 ng/mL were linked to a 2.8-fold increase in mortality risk, underscoring the role of sepsis as a critical determinant of poor prognosis. Similarly, CRP levels $\geq$ 100 mg/L were associated with a 2.2-fold increase in mortality risk. Silvestre et al. found that while CRP levels did not correlate with sepsis severity, higher CRP concentrations were not associated with increased ICU mortality [18]. In contrast, Schupp et al. reported that patients with CRP levels exceeding 100 mg/L had a higher risk of mortality, aligning with our observations [19].

Regarding clinical severity scores, we found that a CCI score $\geq$ 4 was a significant predictor of poor prognosis and higher ICU mortality risk (OR: 3.2). Similarly, an APACHE II score $\geq$ 15 was associated with increased mortality risk (OR: 4.1, $p < 0.001$). Quach et al. compared the predictive abilities of the CCI and APACHE II scores, concluding that while the CCI is useful, the APACHE II score performs better in predicting hospital mortality in ICU patients [20]. Furthermore, our analysis revealed that an NLR $\geq$ 5 was associated with a 2.6-fold increase in mortality risk, highlighting the impact of systemic inflammation on ICU outcomes. This finding is supported by studies demonstrating that elevated NLR is a significant predictor of mortality in critically ill patients [7,10].

In our study, we found that patients who remained in the ICU for more than seven days had a 1.4-fold increased risk of mortality. Gaudet et al. reported that prolonged ICU stays are associated with an increased risk of nosocomial infections, which, in turn, contribute to higher mortality rates. Their study found that each additional day in the ICU increased the risk of acquiring an infection, highlighting the importance of minimizing ICU length of stay when possible [21]. Bardi et al. observed that patients with extended ICU stays had a higher incidence of multidrug-resistant bacterial colonization, which was associated with increased mortality. Their findings underscore the need for stringent infection control measures to prevent the spread of MDR bacteria in ICU settings [22]. Collectively, these studies align with our findings, indicating that prolonged ICU stays are associated with increased mortality, primarily due to the heightened risk of nosocomial infections and MDR bacterial colonization. These insights emphasize the importance of strategies aimed at reducing ICU length of stay and implementing robust infection prevention protocols to improve patient outcomes.

Our study contributes to the existing literature by providing a comprehensive analysis of MDR bacterial infections in ICU patients, with a focus on regional resistance patterns, biomarker-based prognostic assessments, and clinical severity scores. Unlike previous studies, which primarily report MDR prevalence and associated mortality rates, this study emphasizes the prognostic role of procalcitonin and CRP levels in MDR infections, identifies a critical ICU stay duration threshold (≥7 days) for increased mortality risk, and highlights the predictive value of CCI and APACHE II scores. These findings underscore the need for early identification of high-risk ICU patients, targeted antimicrobial stewardship programs, and enhanced infection control strategies.

Limitations of the Study

This study provides important insights into antibiotic resistance patterns and ICU mortality, but certain limitations should be noted. The single-center retrospective design may limit generalizability, and the retrospective nature poses a risk of information bias and incomplete data on prior antibiotic exposure and comorbidities. Additionally, the lack of molecular resistance analysis prevents identification of specific genetic mechanisms driving resistance. The heterogeneous ICU population may introduce confounding factors, and fungal/viral co-infections were not extensively analyzed.

Despite these limitations, the study has notable strengths. It provides real-world data on antibiotic resistance trends, includes a relatively large sample size, and uses standardized clinical scoring systems (APACHE II, Charlson Comorbidity Index). By demonstrating the impact of MDR pathogens on ICU mortality, it highlights the need for improved infection control and antimicrobial stewardship programs.

4. Materials and Methods

4.1. Study Design and Study Population

This study was approved by the Clinical Research Ethics Committee of Mardin Training and Research Hospital (Date: 7 May 2024, No: 2024/5-2). The study was designed as a retrospective analysis of the initial culture growth results of patients admitted to the intensive care unit (ICU) of Mardin Training and Research Hospital between 1 July 2022, and 1 January 2024. The distribution of microorganisms isolated from clinical specimens collected from newly admitted ICU patients and their antibiotic resistance profiles were evaluated.

The primary hypothesis of this study is to determine the distribution of microorganisms isolated from the initial cultures of ICU patients and analyze their antibiotic resistance profiles. In this way, this study aims to contribute to the selection of empirical antibiotic therapy for newly admitted ICU patients.

Patients aged 18 years and older who were admitted to the ICU were included in the study. However, patients who became hemodynamically unstable and deceased within the first six hours of ICU admission and those younger than 18 years of age were excluded. The data were obtained retrospectively through the hospital information management system (HIMS) of Mardin Training and Research Hospital. The clinical specimens analyzed in the study included blood culture and urine culture. Endotracheal aspirate (ETA) samples were excluded as they are primarily used for surveillance rather than clinical diagnosis. In addition to microbiological data, demographic characteristics, length of ICU stay, and treatment protocols applied during the ICU stay were also evaluated.

Microorganism identification was performed using automated bacterial identification systems (VITEK 2 Compact, bioMérieux, Lyon, France) and conventional bacteriological methods [23]. Antibiotic susceptibility testing was conducted according to the Clinical and Laboratory Standards Institute (CLSI) 2022 or European Committee on Antimicrobial Susceptibility Testing (EUCAST) 2022 guidelines [24].

For Gram-negative bacteria, resistance to carbapenems, extended-spectrum beta-lactamase (ESBL) production, and colistin susceptibility were analyzed. For Gram-positive bacteria, resistance mechanisms such as methicillin resistance in *MRSA* and *VRE* were examined. Extended-spectrum beta-lactamase (ESBL) production was detected using the combination disk test (CDT) with cefotaxime, ceftazidime, and cefepime, both alone and in combination with clavulanic acid, following CLSI 2022 guidelines. A $\geq$5 mm increase in zone diameter in the presence of clavulanic acid was considered indicative of ESBL production. Plasmid-mediated AmpC beta-lactamase (p-AmpC) detection was performed using the AmpC disk test with cefoxitin and a boronic acid inhibitor. A significant increase in the inhibition zone in the presence of the inhibitor was considered a positive result for p-AmpC production. Carbapenemase production was assessed using the modified carbapenem inactivation method (mCIM) and the EDTA-based carbapenemase inhibition test (eCIM) to differentiate metallo-beta-lactamases from serine carbapenemases, in accordance with EUCAST 2022 recommendations [24].

We have specified that empirical antibiotic therapy was initiated based on local antibiogram data, commonly including piperacillin-tazobactam, cefepime, meropenem, and vancomycin for broad-spectrum coverage. Targeted therapy was adjusted based on culture and susceptibility results, following CLSI and EUCAST guidelines.

4.2. Statistical Analysis

All statistical analyses were performed using SPSS Statistics Version 27.0 (IBM Corp., Armonk, NY, ABD). The descriptive statistics were presented as mean $\pm$ standard deviation (SD) for continuous variables and frequency (percentage) for categorical variables. To compare continuous variables, we used the independent samples t-test for normally distributed data and the Mann–Whitney U test for non-normally distributed data. The Kolmogorov–Smirnov test and Shapiro–Wilk test were applied to assess normality. The categorical variables were compared using the chi-square test (χ^2) or Fisher's exact test, where appropriate. To evaluate the association between microorganism type, antibiotic resistance, and ICU mortality, we conducted univariate and multivariate logistic regression analyses. Variables with a p-value < 0.10 in univariate analysis were included in the multivariate model, using a stepwise forward selection method. Adjusted odds ratios (ORs) with 95% confidence intervals (CIs) were calculated to determine risk factors for ICU mortality. A Kaplan–Meier survival analysis was performed to compare ICU survival rates based on infection type and resistance profile, with differences assessed using the log-rank test. Additionally, a Cox proportional hazards regression model was used to estimate the hazard ratios (HRs) for mortality among ICU patients. A p-value < 0.05 was considered statistically significant.

5. Conclusions

The increasing threat of antibiotic resistance in ICU settings remains a significant challenge in modern medicine. Our study highlights the critical impact of MDR pathogens, particularly *A. baumannii*, MRSA, *P. aeruginosa*, and *K. pneumoniae*, on ICU mortality and prolonged hospitalization. Additionally, infections caused by ESBL-, p-AmpC-, and carbapenemase-producing Enterobacterales were associated with worse clinical outcomes, emphasizing the growing burden of resistance mechanisms in critically ill patients. The strong correlation between carbapenem, cephalosporin, fluoroquinolone, aminoglycoside, and vancomycin resistance with increased mortality underscores the urgent need for enhanced antimicrobial stewardship and infection control strategies.

Beyond bacterial resistance, biomarkers such as procalcitonin, CRP, and NLR, along with clinical severity scores (APACHE II, Charlson Comorbidity Index), serve as valuable prognostic tools for identifying high-risk ICU patients. Our findings emphasize that early detection, optimized empirical antibiotic selection, and stringent infection prevention measures are essential to improving ICU survival rates.

As the global burden of antimicrobial resistance continues to rise, a multidisciplinary approach integrating microbiological surveillance, rapid diagnostics, and precision-guided antibiotic therapy is essential. Future research should focus on molecular resistance mechanisms and novel therapeutic interventions to address the increasing crisis of drug-resistant infections in critically ill patients. The fight against MDR pathogens is not just about reducing mortality—it is about shaping the future of critical care medicine.

Funding: This research received no external funding.

Institutional Review Board Statement: This study was approved by the Ethics Committee of Mardin Artuklu University. The Declaration of Helsinki protocol was followed in the research protocol (Approval: 2024/5-2, Date: 7 May 2024).

Informed Consent Statement: Informed consent was obtained from all subjects involved in the study.

Data Availability Statement: The original contributions presented in the study are included in the article; further inquiries can be directed to the corresponding authors.

Conflicts of Interest: The author declares no conflicts of interest.

References

1. Segmen, F.; Aydemir, S.; Kucuk, O.; Dogu, C.; Dokuyucu, R. Comparison of Oxidative Stress Markers with Clinical Data in Patients Requiring Anesthesia in an Intensive Care Unit. *J. Clin. Med.* **2024**, *13*, 6979. [CrossRef]
2. Eygi, E.; Kucuk, O.; Aydemir, S.; Atilgan, M.; Dokuyucu, R.; Erbas, O. Hydroxychloroquine Mitigates Cytokine Storm and Prevents Critical Illness Neuromyopathy in a Rat Sepsis Model. *Medicina* **2024**, *60*, 1791. [CrossRef] [PubMed]
3. Golli, A.L.; Cristea, O.M.; Zlatian, O.; Glodeanu, A.D.; Balasoiu, A.T.; Ionescu, M.; Popa, S. Prevalence of Multidrug-Resistant Pathogens Causing Bloodstream Infections in an Intensive Care Unit. *Infect. Drug Resist.* **2022**, *15*, 5981–5992. [CrossRef] [PubMed]
4. Corona, A.; De Santis, V.; Agarossi, A.; Prete, A.; Cattaneo, D.; Tomasini, G.; Bonetti, G.; Patroni, A.; Latronico, N. Antibiotic Therapy Strategies for Treating Gram-Negative Severe Infections in the Critically Ill: A Narrative Review. *Antibiotics* **2023**, *12*, 1262. [CrossRef] [PubMed]
5. Bassetti, M.; Peghin, M.; Vena, A.; Giacobbe, D.R. Treatment of Infections Due to MDR Gram-Negative Bacteria. *Front. Med.* **2019**, *6*, 74. [CrossRef]
6. Tacconelli, E.; Carrara, E.; Savoldi, A.; Harbarth, S.; Mendelson, M.; Monnet, D.L.; Pulcini, C.; Kahlmeter, G.; Kluytmans, J.; Carmeli, Y.; et al. Discovery, research, and development of new antibiotics: The WHO priority list of antibiotic-resistant bacteria and tuberculosis. *Lancet Infect. Dis.* **2018**, *18*, 318–327. [CrossRef]
7. Turner, A.M.; Lee, J.Y.H.; Gorrie, C.L.; Howden, B.P.; Carter, G.P. Genomic Insights Into Last-Line Antimicrobial Resistance in Multidrug-Resistant *Staphylococcus* and Vancomycin-Resistant *Enterococcus*. *Front. Microbiol.* **2021**, *12*, 637656. [CrossRef]
8. Peleg, A.Y.; Hooper, D.C. Hospital-acquired infections due to gram-negative bacteria. *N. Engl. J. Med.* **2010**, *362*, 1804–1813. [CrossRef]
9. Magiorakos, A.P.; Srinivasan, A.; Carey, R.B.; Carmeli, Y.; Falagas, M.E.; Giske, C.G.; Harbarth, S.; Hindler, J.F.; Kahlmeter, G.; Olsson-Liljequist, B.; et al. Multidrug-resistant, extensively drug-resistant and pandrug-resistant bacteria: An international expert proposal for interim standard definitions for acquired resistance. *Clin. Microbiol. Infect.* **2012**, *18*, 268–281. [CrossRef]
10. Segmen, F.; Aydemir, S.; Kucuk, O.; Dokuyucu, R. The Roles of Vitamin D Levels, Gla-Rich Protein (GRP) and Matrix Gla Protein (MGP), and Inflammatory Markers in Predicting Mortality in Intensive Care Patients: A New Biomarker Link? *Metabolites* **2024**, *14*, 620. [CrossRef]
11. Gong, Y.; Peng, Y.; Luo, X.; Zhang, C.; Shi, Y.; Zhang, Y.; Deng, J.; Peng, Y.; Luo, G.; Li, H. Different Infection Profiles and Antimicrobial Resistance Patterns Between Burn ICU and Common Wards. *Front. Cell Infect. Microbiol.* **2021**, *11*, 681731. [CrossRef] [PubMed]
12. Calvo, M.; Stefani, S.; Migliorisi, G. Bacterial Infections in Intensive Care Units: Epidemiological and Microbiological Aspects. *Antibiotics* **2024**, *13*, 238. [CrossRef] [PubMed]
13. Bassetti, M.; Garau, J. Current and future perspectives in the treatment of multidrug-resistant Gram-negative infections. *J. Antimicrob. Chemother.* **2021**, *76*, iv23–iv37. [CrossRef]
14. Wei, Z.; Zhou, S.; Zhang, Y.; Zheng, L.; Zhao, L.; Cui, Y.; Xie, K. Microbiological characteristics and risk factors on prognosis associated with *Acinetobacter baumannii* bacteremia in general hospital: A single-center retrospective study. *Front. Microbiol.* **2022**, *13*, 1051364. [CrossRef] [PubMed]

15. Schinas, G.; Polyzou, E.; Spernovasilis, N.; Gogos, C.; Dimopoulos, G.; Akinosoglou, K. Preventing Multidrug-Resistant Bacterial Transmission in the Intensive Care Unit with a Comprehensive Approach: A Policymaking Manual. *Antibiotics* **2023**, *12*, 1255. [CrossRef]
16. Yoo, E.H.; Hong, H.-L.; Kim, E.J. Epidemiology and Mortality Analysis Related to *Carbapenem-Resistant Enterobacterales* in Patients After Admission to Intensive Care Units: An Observational Study. *Infect. Drug Resist.* **2023**, *16*, 189–200. [CrossRef]
17. Ebbing, L.; Metlay, J.P.; Bilker, W.B.; Edelstein, P.H.; Fishman, N.O. Association between Fluoroquinolone Resistance and Mortality in *Escherichia coli* and *Klebsiella pneumoniae* Infections: The Role of Inadequate Empirical Antimicrobial Therapy. *Clin. Infect. Dis.* **2005**, *41*, 923–929. [CrossRef]
18. Silvestre, J.; Póvoa, P.; Coelho, L.; Almeida, E.; Moreira, P.; Fernandes, A.; Mealha, R.; Sabino, H. Is C-reactive protein a good prognostic marker in septic patients? *Intensive Care Med.* **2009**, *35*, 909–913. [CrossRef]
19. Schupp, T.; Weidner, K.; Rusnak, J.; Jawhar, S.; Forner, J.; Dulatahu, F.; Dudda, J.; Brück, L.M.; Hoffmann, U.; Bertsch, T.; et al. C-reactive protein and procalcitonin during course of sepsis and septic shock. *Ir. J. Med. Sci. (1971-)* **2023**, *193*, 457–468. [CrossRef]
20. Quach, S.; Hennessy, D.A.; Faris, P.; Fong, A.; Quan, H.; Doig, C. A comparison between the APACHE II and Charlson Index Score for predicting hospital mortality in critically ill patients. *BMC Health Serv. Res.* **2009**, *9*, 129. [CrossRef]
21. Gaudet, A.; Kreitmann, L.; Nseir, S. ICU-Acquired Colonization and Infection Related to Multidrug-Resistant Bacteria in COVID-19 Patients: A Narrative Review. *Antibiotics* **2023**, *12*, 1464. [CrossRef] [PubMed]
22. Bardi, T.; Pintado, V.; Gomez-Rojo, M.; Escudero-Sanchez, R.; Azzam Lopez, A.; Diez-Remesal, Y.; Martinez Castro, N.; Ruiz-Garbajosa, P.; Pestaña, D. Nosocomial infections associated to COVID-19 in the intensive care unit: Clinical characteristics and outcome. *Eur. J. Clin. Microbiol. Infect. Dis.* **2021**, *40*, 495–502. [CrossRef] [PubMed]
23. Papadomanolaki, A.; Siopi, M.; Karakosta, P.; Vourli, S.; Pournaras, S. Comparative Evaluation of Vitek 2 and Etest versus Broth Microdilution for Ceftazidime/Avibactam and Ceftolozane/Tazobactam Susceptibility Testing of *Enterobacterales* and *Pseudomonas aeruginosa*. *Antibiotics* **2022**, *11*, 865. [CrossRef]
24. Edmondson, R.; Saeed, K.; Green, S.; O'Dwyer, M. Improving Turnaround Times for Routine Antimicrobial Sensitivity Testing Following European Committee on Antimicrobial Susceptibility Testing Methodology in Patients with Bacteraemia. *Antibiotics* **2024**, *13*, 1094. [CrossRef] [PubMed]

antibiotics

MDPI

Article

Extended Versus Intermittent Meropenem Infusion in the Treatment of Nosocomial Pneumonia: A Retrospective Single-Center Study

Dong-gon Hyun [1], Jarim Seo [2], Su Yeon Lee [1], Jee Hwan Ahn [1], Sang-Bum Hong [1], Chae-Man Lim [1], Younsuck Koh [1] and Jin Won Huh [1,*]

1 Department of Pulmonary and Critical Care Medicine, Asan Medical Centre, University of Ulsan College of Medicine, Seoul 05505, Republic of Korea; dghyun@amc.seoul.kr (D.-g.H.)
2 Department of Pharmacy, Asan Medical Centre, Seoul 05505, Republic of Korea
* Correspondence: jwhuh@amc.seoul.kr; Tel.: +82-2-3010-3985; Fax: +82-8-3010-6677

Abstract: The efficacy of extended meropenem infusions in patients with nosocomial pneumonia is not well defined. Therefore, we compared the clinical outcomes of extended versus intermittent meropenem infusions in the treatment of nosocomial pneumonia. We performed a retrospective analysis of extended versus intermittent meropenem infusions in adult patients who had been treated for nosocomial pneumonia at a medical ICU between 1 May 2018 and 30 April 2020. The primary outcome was mortality at 14 days. Overall, 64 patients who underwent an extended infusion and 97 with an intermittent infusion were included in this study. At 14 days, 10 (15.6%) patients in the extended group and 22 (22.7%) in the intermittent group had died (adjusted hazard ratio (HR), 0.55; 95% confidence interval (CI): 0.23–1.31; $p = 0.174$). In the subgroup analysis, significant differences in mortality at day 14 were observed in patients following empirical treatment with meropenem (adjusted HR, 0.17; 95% CI: 0.03–0.96; $p = 0.045$) and in Gram-negative pathogens identified by blood or sputum cultures (adjusted HR, 0.01; 95% CI: 0.01–0.83; $p = 0.033$). Extended infusion of meropenem compared with intermittent infusion as a treatment option for nosocomial pneumonia may have a potential advantage in specific populations.

Keywords: meropenem; intensive care unit; pneumonia; ventilator-associated pneumonia; intravenous infusion

1. Introduction

Nosocomial pneumonia represents one of the most common hospital-acquired infections and is a global public health concern associated with high mortality rates [1–3]. Causative pathogens of nosocomial pneumonia include Gram-negative bacteria and an increasing number of antimicrobial-resistant pathogens, such as carbapenem-resistant *Acinetobacter baumannii* (CRAB) and carbapenem-resistant *Pseudomonas aeruginosa* (CRPA) [4–6]. The surge in drug resistance and the scarcity of new antibacterial drugs have caused efforts to be focused on optimizing antibiotic dosing [7,8]. The antibacterial activity of beta-lactam antibiotics depends on the duration of its concentration above the minimal inhibitory concentration (MIC) of the causative bacteria [9]. However, critically ill patients often undergo changes in antibiotic pharmacokinetic profiles, leading to insufficient drug concentrations [10–12]. Since inadequate antibiotic exposure reduces antibacterial susceptibility in patients with sepsis, the optimization of antibacterial concentrations is warranted [13,14]. Attaining the target concentration through extended or continuous infusion of beta-lactam antibiotics has been associated with lower mortality rates in patients with sepsis or severe infections [15–17].

Antibiotics administered intravenously must diffuse across the structurally complex blood–alveolar barrier into the lungs [18]. As a result, the intrapulmonary concentration, represented as the epithelial lining fluid (ELF), is substantially lower than the serum concentration [19]. To achieve a higher exposure in the ELF compared with intermittent infusions, the administering of an extended infusion (EI) of meropenem has been introduced for critically ill patients with nosocomial pneumonia [20–22]. However, the efficacy of meropenem EIs compared to nosocomial pneumonia remains controversial [23,24]. Therefore, we aimed to compare clinical outcomes between the EI of meropenem and intermittent infusion in patients with nosocomial pneumonia.

2. Results

We assessed 687 patients who had undergone meropenem treatments for inclusion (Figure 1); among them, 526 patients were excluded because they did not receive meropenem in the ICU for more than 48 h, were not diagnosed with nosocomial pneumonia, or had received meropenem treatment before enrollment. Thus, 161 patients—64 undergoing extended infusion and 97 undergoing intermittent infusion—were included in this study.

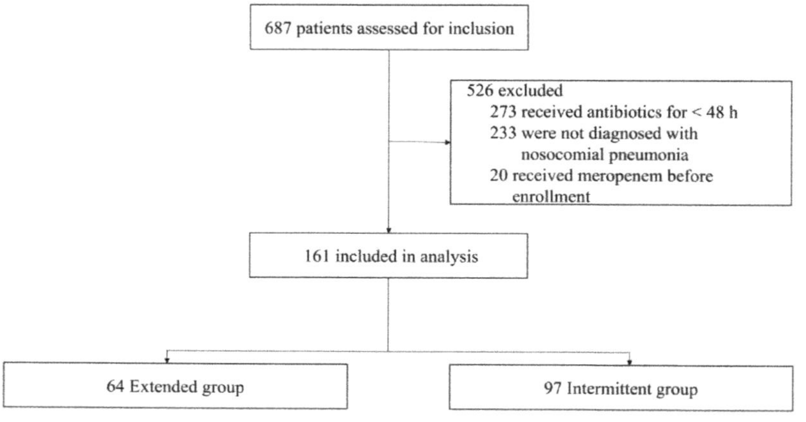

Figure 1. Flowchart of patient population and analysis.

2.1. Baseline Characteristics

The baseline characteristics were generally balanced between the two groups (Table 1). The mean age of all the patients was 63.8 ± 12.9, and over two-thirds of all participants were male. Being immunocompromised was the most common condition amongst participants in the extended group (34.4%), while diabetes mellitus (32.0%) was the most common in the intermittent group. The SOFA score and PaO_2/FiO_2 ratio were similar between the two groups. A total of 26 (40.6%) and 38 (39.2%) patients in the extended and intermittent groups, respectively, were diagnosed with ventilator-associated pneumonia (VAP). Antibiotic use revealed no difference in the median duration between the two groups (9.0 days in the EI group vs. 7.0 days in the II group, $p = 0.165$). Most patients (66.4%) discontinued meropenem treatment during their ICU stay due to the de-escalation or cessation of antibiotics. There were no differences between the previous use of antibiotics and the concomitant use of antibiotics across the two groups. Before meropenem treatment, the most commonly prescribed class of antibiotics was beta-lactam, followed by quinolone and glycopeptide. In addition, the two groups showed no significant difference in laboratory variables or organ support proportions at the baseline.

Table 1. Baseline characteristics according to the type of meropenem infusion.

Variable	Extended (n = 64)	Intermittent (n = 97)	p-Value
Age, y	62.4 ± 14.1	64.7 ± 12.0	0.255
Sex, male	42 (65.6)	75 (77.3)	0.103
BMI, kg/m^2	22.9 (19.9–24.8)	22.1 (19.2–24.5)	0.111
Comorbidity			
Diabetes mellitus	17 (26.6)	31 (32.0)	0.464
Solid cancer	13 (20.3)	26 (26.8)	0.347
Hematologic malignancy	16 (25.0)	17 (17.5)	0.250
Congestive heart failure	8 (12.5)	5 (5.2)	0.094
Respiratory failure	17 (26.6)	20 (20.6)	0.380
Chronic liver disease	7 (10.9)	14 (14.4)	0.519
End-stage renal disease	9 (14.1)	12 (12.4)	0.755
Immunocompromised	22 (34.4)	25 (25.8)	0.240
Severity of pneumonia			
SOFA score	10.0 (6.3–12.0)	10.0 (8.0–13.0)	0.237
Sepsis	61 (95.3)	92 (94.8)	1.000
Septic shock	12 (18.8)	33 (34.0)	0.035
PaO_2/FiO_2 ratio, mmHg (n = 157)	212.3 ± 98.5	201.2 ± 133.2	0.573
Type of nosocomial pneumonia			0.854
Hospital-acquired pneumonia	38 (59.4)	59 (60.8)	
Ventilator-associated pneumonia	26 (40.6)	38 (39.2)	
Parameters of antibiotics			
Duration of meropenem, days	9.0 (5.3–13.0)	7.0 (5.0–11.0)	0.165
Duration of antibiotic, days	17.0 (8.3–22.0)	13.0 (7.0–23.5)	0.357
Discontinuation during ICU stay (n = 143)			0.135
De-escalation or cessation	42 (73.7)	53 (61.6)	
Escalation or death	15 (26.3)	33 (38.4)	
Previous antibiotics			
Class of beta-lactam	36 (56.3)	66 (68.0)	0.137
Class of quinolone	18 (28.1)	32 (33.0)	0.514
Class of glycopeptide	11 (17.2)	21 (21.6)	0.487
Concomitant antibiotics			
Use of colistin	8 (12.5)	13 (13.4)	0.868
Use of quinolone	24 (37.5)	40 (41.2)	0.742
Use of others *	5 (7.8)	7 (7.2)	1.000
Coverage for MRSA	43 (67.2)	64 (66.0)	0.874
Laboratory variables			
White cell count, $\times 10^3$/L	10.9 ± 8.7	13.2 ± 9.3	0.112
C-reactive protein, mg/dL (n = 158)	10.5 ± 8.4	12.4 ± 8.8	0.182
Organ support at baseline			
Mechanical ventilation	57 (89.1)	90 (92.8)	0.412
Renal replacement therapy	17 (26.6)	19 (19.6)	0.299
Extracorporeal membrane oxygenation	9 (14.1)	12 (12.4)	0.755
Vasopressors	41 (64.1)	59 (60.8)	0.679

Abbreviations: BMI, body mass index; SOFA, sequential organ failure assessment; PaO_2, partial oxygen pressure in arterial blood; FiO_2, fraction of inspired oxygen; MRSA, methicillin-resistant *Staphylococcus aureus*. Data are reported as n (%), mean ± standard deviation, or median (interquartile range). * Others included aminoglycoside, tigecycline, ampicillin/sulbactam, cefoperazone/sulbactam, and trimethoprim-sulfamethoxazole.

2.2. Microbiological Data

The microbiological profiles showed a similar pattern across the two groups (Table 2). Here, 8 (12.5%) of the 64 patients in the EI group and 5 (5.2%) of the 97 patients in the II group had bacteremia documented from blood cultures (p = 0.094). Furthermore, one patient (12.5%) in the EI group and five patients (100.0%) in the II group had the same bacteria cultured from both blood and sputum, while three patients (37.5%) in the EI group had different bacteria at each culture site. The identification of pathogens in the sputum culture totaled 37 (57.8%) and 59 (60.8%) in the EI and II groups, respectively (p = 0.744). One patient (2.7%) in the EI group had both *Staphylococcus aureus* and *Klebsiella pneumoniae*. Two patients (3.4%) in the II group had *Stenotrophomonas maltophilia* alongside other pathogens, such as *Klebsiella pneumonia* and *Pseudomonas aeruginosa*. From the multi-drug resistance (MDR) pathogens in the sputum culture, CRAB was isolated in 7 (10.9%) specimens taken from the EI group and in 21 (21.6%) from the II group (p = 0.092). Each patient in the EI (2.7%) and II groups (1.7%) possessed *Klebsiella pneumonia* and *Stenotrophomonas maltophilia*, alongside CRAB. Six patients (9.4%) in the EI group and four (4.1%) in the II group had CRPA (p = 0197). Only four patients (4.1%) in the II group had Carbapenemase-producing Enterobacteriaceae (CPE; p = 0.152). No difference was observed for any other pathogens between the two groups (p = 0.104).

Table 2. Microbiological profile of nosocomial pneumonia according to the type of meropenem infusion.

Variable	Extended (n = 64)	Intermittent (n = 97)	p-Value
Bacteremia	8 (12.5)	5 (5.2)	0.094
Staphylococcus aureus	3 (37.5)	0 (0.0)	
Enterococcus faecium	3 (37.5)	0 (0.0)	
Klebsiella pneumoniae	2 (25.0)	0 (0.0)	
Pseudomonas aeruginosa	0 (0.0)	1 (20.0)	
Acinetobacter baumanii	0 (0.0)	4 (80.0)	
Pathogen of sputum culture	37 (57.8)	59 (60.8)	0.744
Gram(+) pathogen	4 (6.3)	6 (6.2)	1.000
Staphylococcus aureus	3 (75.0)	3 (50.0)	
Staphylococcus haemolyticus	1 (25.0)	0 (0.0)	
Corynebacterium striatum	0 (0.0)	3 (50.0)	
Gram(−) pathogen	25 (39.1)	45 (46.4)	0.418
Escherichia coli	1 (4.0)	1 (2.2)	
Klebsiella pneumoniae or *oxytica*	7 (28.0)	10 (22.2)	
Pseudomonas aeruginosa	7 (28.0)	11 (24.4)	
Acinetobacter baumannii or iwoffii	10 (40.0)	21 (46.7)	
Stenotrophomonas maltophilia	1 (4.0)	5 (11.1)	
Serratia marcescens	0 (0.0)	1 (2.2)	
CRE	13 (20.3)	28 (28.9)	0.223
CRAB	7 (10.9)	21 (21.6)	0.092
CRPA	6 (9.4)	4 (4.1)	0.197
CPE	0 (0.0)	4 (4.1) *	0.152
MIC distribution ofmeropenem (n = 70)			0.796
≤1 mg/L	10 (40.0)	15 (33.3)	
2–4 mg/L	2 (8.0)	3 (6.7)	
>4 mg/L	13 (52.0)	27 (60.0)	
Other pathogens **	9 (14.1)	6 (6.2)	0.104

Abbreviations: CRE, carbapenem-resistant Enterobacterales; CRAB, carbapenem-resistant *Acinetobacter baumannii*; CRPA, carbapenem-resistant *Pseudomonas aeruginosa*; CPE, carbapenemase-producing Enterobacteriaceae; MIC, minimum inhibitory concentration. * One patient was positive for both CRPA and CPE in the sputum culture. ** Other pathogens indicate virus or fungus as the etiology of pneumonia. Data are reported as n (%).

2.3. Outcomes

Mortality occurred at 14 days for 10 patients (15.6%) in the EI group and for 22 (22.7%, p = 0.272) in the II group (Table 3). The clinical and microbiological outcomes were generally similar between both groups. There was no difference in the proportion of CRP level improvement between the two groups (65.1% in the EI group vs. 64.2% in the II group, p = 1.000). Further, 24.4% of the patients in the EI group presented with carbapenem resistance, while 26.9% possessed it in the II group (p = 0.829). Even after adjusting for covariables, including solid cancer, chronic liver disease, SOFA scores, septic shock, VAP, previous use of quinolone and glycopeptide, and bacteremia (Supplementary Materials Table S1), there was no significant difference between the two groups (adjusted HR, 0.55; 95% CI: 0.23–1.31, p = 0.174; Figure 2). In addition, the two groups had similar rates of ventilator liberation (adjusted HR for PaO_2/FiO_2 ratio, use of colistin, and lactate level, 0.93; 95% CI: 0.51–1.68, p = 0.80) and rate of discharge from the ICU (adjusted HR for solid cancer, hematologic malignancy, respiratory failure, mechanical ventilator, and use of colistin, previous use of quinolone, 0.77; 95% CI 0.44–1.35, p = 0.36) at day 14 (Supplementary Materials Tables S2 and S3).

Table 3. Clinical outcomes according to the type of meropenem infusion.

Outcome Measure	Extended (n = 64)	Intermittent (n = 97)	p-Value
Mortality			
14-day mortality	10 (15.6)	22 (22.7)	0.272
28-day mortality	16 (25.0)	29 (29.9)	0.498
ICU mortality	21 (32.8)	40 (41.2)	0.281
LOS, median (IQR)			
Hospital days	79.9 ± 76.8	81.3 ± 71.7	0.906
ICU days	26.5 ± 35.6	20.5 ± 18.2	0.223
Ventilator days (n = 146)	24.8 ± 37.7	18.5 ± 17.3	0.243
Improvement of CRP level (n = 158)	41 (65.1)	61 (64.2)	1.000
Occurrence of carbapenem resistance (n = 112)	11 (24.4)	18 (26.9)	0.829

Abbreviations: ICU, intensive care unit; LOS, length of stay; IQR, interquartile range; CRP, C-reactive protein. Data are reported as n (%) or mean ± standard deviation.

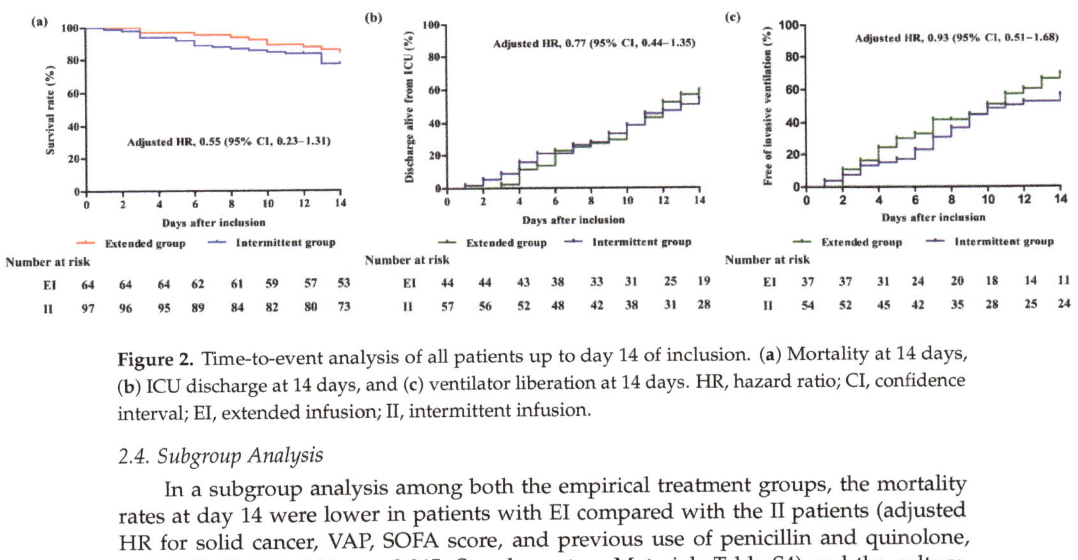

Figure 2. Time-to-event analysis of all patients up to day 14 of inclusion. (**a**) Mortality at 14 days, (**b**) ICU discharge at 14 days, and (**c**) ventilator liberation at 14 days. HR, hazard ratio; CI, confidence interval; EI, extended infusion; II, intermittent infusion.

2.4. Subgroup Analysis

In a subgroup analysis among both the empirical treatment groups, the mortality rates at day 14 were lower in patients with EI compared with the II patients (adjusted HR for solid cancer, VAP, SOFA score, and previous use of penicillin and quinolone, 0.17; 95% CI: 0.03–0.96, p = 0.045; Supplementary Materials Table S4) and the culture-proven group (adjusted HR for liver cirrhosis, bacteremia, SOFA score, septic shock, Gram-positive pathogen, and previous use of quinolone, 0.01; 95% CI: 0.01–0.83, p = 0.033; Figure 3 and Supplementary Materials Table S5). Moreover, lower morbidity at 14 days was observed among patients with CRE—including CRAB and CRPA—in the EI group (0.0%) compared to those in the II group (25.0%), although these differences were not statistically significant (p = 0.056; Supplementary Materials Figure S1). Additionally, the baseline characteristics, absolute standardized mean differences, and results of the primary outcome in the propensity-matched cohort and the subgroup of patients with concurrent bacteremia are shown in Table S6, Figure S2, Figure S3 and Table S7, Figure S4, respectively.

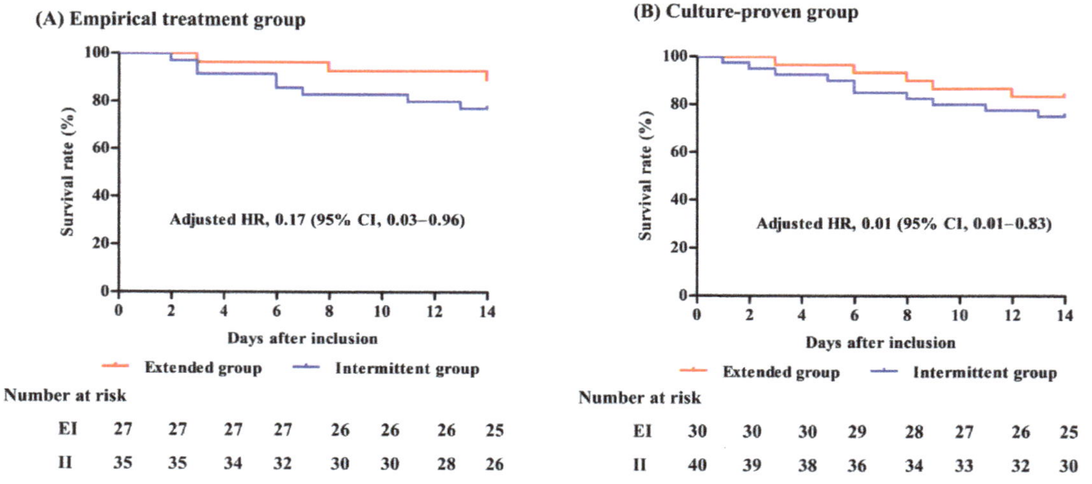

Figure 3. Subgroup mortalities on day 14. (**A**) Empirical treatment group and (**B**) culture-proven group. HR, hazard ratio; CI, confidence interval, EI, extended infusion; II, intermittent infusion.

3. Discussion

This single-center study was retrospectively conducted to compare clinical outcomes between patients undergoing EI and II of meropenem. Our results showed that EI provided no additional survival benefits compared to II in the treatment of nosocomial pneumonia, even after controlling for any covariates. The incidence of carbapenem resistance following EI was similar to that after II. In the subgroups, EI of meropenem resulted in lower 14-day mortality rates than in patients receiving II, who were empirically treated for nosocomial pneumonia or had culture-proven pathogens. Although there were no differences in the clinical outcomes according to the type of infusion across all patients, EI of meropenem may confer a survival advantage over II in a specific population of patients with nosocomial pneumonia.

Several novel antibiotics, including ceftazidime–avibactam, ceftolozane–tazobactam, and cefiderocol, have been developed to target nosocomial pneumonia caused by Gram-negative pathogens [25]. Although these drugs have shown an efficacious and tolerable profile for the treatment of nosocomial pneumonia, their clinical outcomes are not superior to those of meropenem [26–28]. In addition, reports of resistance to novel beta-lactam/beta-lactamase inhibitor combination agents, such as ceftolozane–tazobactam, have recently emerged [29,30]. Several efforts, including antimicrobial stewardship programs, have been introduced to reverse the large burden associated with antimicrobial resistance and to preserve antimicrobial armamentariums in the ICU [8]. Optimizing the appropriate initial antibiotic therapy for critically ill patients is a key component of these interventions [31]. This strategy improves patient outcomes and reduces the emergence of resistance, while also avoiding the use of unnecessary antibiotics [7]. Although no statistically significant differences were observed, patients who received EI also had a lower mortality rate at 14 days than those in the II group, according to our subgroup analysis of patients with CRE. Therefore, attempts to optimize antibiotic concentrations in critically ill patients in the ICU are important.

The clinical outcomes of our study were consistent with those of previous studies. Indeed, a randomized-controlled, single-center study in China presented 28-day survival rates of 18.4% and 40.0% in patients with hospital-acquired pneumonia undergoing treatment with 1 g meropenem via 3 h infusions and 30 min infusions, respectively [32]. In another study comparing the efficacy of ceftolozane–tazobactam with meropenem for the treatment of nosocomial pneumonia, a mortality rate of 25.3% was observed at 28 days in patients who received meropenem (1 g by 30 min infusion every 8 h), which was similar to the II group in our results (29.9%) [27]. Recently, there was a randomized clinical trial for patients with sepsis or septic shock who received 1 g meropenem by either continuous or intermittent infusion [33]. No statistically significant difference was observed in 28-day mortality rates between the two groups (30% versus 33%), which were similar rates to those observed in our study (25.0% versus 29.9%). In addition, the rate of emerging drug resistance (24.3%) in this study was consistent with our study (25.9%). These similarities between the data presented in our study to those in other studies help support the reliability of our results.

The optimal dosage and duration of meropenem infusion remains elusive [34]. Thus, to determine the optimal meropenem concentration in patients, both its efficacy and safety should be considered. Since drug concentrations at the site of infection influence efficacy, the probability of attaining drug concentrations above the MIC for over 40% of the time between doses (% T > MIC) in the ELF is considered the best marker of bacterial activity for extracellular respiratory tract pathogens [20]. Several studies analyzing the concentration of meropenem on the epithelial lining fluid, according to dosage or duration, showed that a meropenem dosage of 2 g or its prolonged infusion—more than 3 h—could achieve higher exposure in the ELF [21,23]. However, the risk of toxicity—such as neurotoxicity—also increases as the concentration of meropenem increases [35]. A recent study considering both target attainment and potential toxicity reported that the optimal dose regimens were either to administer 2 g every 8 h with 3 h prolonged infusions, or 4 g per day by continuous infusion [36]. Considering these results, administering 1 g of meropenem by 3 h infusion may have provided an insufficient concentration in the ELF against these pathogens—especially those with an MIC > 4 mg/L [21]. Therefore, a randomized, controlled trial of meropenem of 2 g by 3 h infusion or 4 g per day by continuous infusion is needed to evaluate the proper efficacy of extended infusion in patients with pneumonia, including pathogens with an MIC above 4 mg/L.

Our study has several limitations: First, the results of our study are limited by its small sample size and low statistical power, which is a common limitation in retrospective studies. However, it is worth noting that this study included a representative population similar to real-world patients with nosocomial pneumonia. Additionally, due to the retrospective nature of the study, it was not possible to determine the reasons why the medical staff chose a particular method of meropenem infusion. Second, we did not monitor the meropenem antibiotic concentration. Therefore, it is unclear whether the failure to attain target levels by an improper regimen of meropenem caused any differences in clinical outcomes between the two groups. Third, adverse event data were not collected in our study. To optimize the meropenem drug concentration, further studies should investigate its adverse effects—especially in patients who receive high doses of meropenem. Finally, although subgroup analyses may have shown the potential benefits of EI, the results should be interpreted with caution. Large prospective studies are required to confirm the potential advantage of EI over II in these specific subgroups.

4. Materials and Methods

4.1. Study Design and Patients

We retrospectively collected data from patients treated for nosocomial pneumonia at the medical intensive care unit (ICU) of Asan Medical Center between May 2018 and April 2020, to investigate the efficacy of EI of meropenem compared to intermittent infusion. Eligible patients were aged 18 years or older, were treated for nosocomial pneumonia at the medical ICU, and received meropenem infusion for at least 48 h during their ICU stay. Nosocomial pneumonia was defined as the onset of pneumonia occurring at least 48 h after admission or less than 7 days after discharge from the hospital. Pneumonia occurring within 48 h in patients who stayed for 48 h or longer at another hospital immediately before admission was considered nosocomial pneumonia. Diagnosis of pneumonia was based on clinical assessment by attending physicians, including laboratory and radiologic tests and respiratory signs on electronic medical records. VAP was diagnosed as pneumonia that develops in patients who received mechanical ventilation for over 48 h. Patients were excluded if they did not receive at least 48 h of meropenem treatment in the ICU, had meropenem therapy within 48 h before inclusion, or were simultaneously treated by other beta-lactam antibiotics.

4.2. *Infusion of Meropenem*

Patients received meropenem by EI (EI group) or intermittent infusion (II group). Patients in the EI group received 1 g of meropenem in 100 mL of normal saline over 3 h of intravenous infusion every 8 h, and immediately after, a loading dose of 1 g in 100 mL of normal saline by intravenous line over 30 min; meanwhile, those in the II group received 1 g meropenem in 100 mL of normal saline by 30 min intravenous infusion every 8 h. Meropenem dosages were adjusted for creatinine clearance across both groups. Drug–drug compatibility was considered during the EI of meropenem. Infusion type, treatment duration, and other antibacterial drugs were determined at the discretion of the medical staff. All patients received standard intensive care from an intensivist throughout their stay in the ICU.

4.3. *Data Collection and Outcomes*

We collected data from electronic medical records, including information on demographics, Sequential Organ Failure Assessment (SOFA) scores, and partial oxygen pressure in arterial blood ((PaO_2)/fraction of inspired oxygen (FiO_2) ratio) within 24 h of inclusion. The parameters of the antibiotics, laboratory variables, and organ support at baseline were also recorded. Pathogens from appropriate respiratory specimens collected by bronchoalveolar lavage, endotracheal aspirate, or expectorated sputum and blood samples 48 h before and after the first dose of meropenem were considered as causative species. The pharmacokinetics of meropenem, such as concentrations, were not evaluated.

The primary outcome was a difference in all-cause mortality on day 14 between the two groups. Subgroup analyses for all-cause mortality at day 14 were conducted in patients with empirical treatment and culture-proven Gram-negative pathogens. Patients in the empirical treatment group received meropenem without any previous antibiotics within 48 h or 24 h after initiating antibiotic therapy; they may have also received other antibiotics after starting meropenem, depending on the microbiologic results or the clinical status of the patient. Patients with Gram-negative bacterial pathogens in blood or sputum cultures were considered the culture-proven group. The key secondary outcomes were 28-day mortality, ventilator liberation, and discharge from the ICU on day 14. Other secondary outcomes included clinical response to the improvement of serum C-reactive protein (CRP) levels—which was defined as a decrease in the level at the end of treatment—and the occurrence of carbapenem resistance, which was defined according to Clinical and Laboratory Standards Institute breakpoints (MIC $\geq$ 4 mg/L for CRPA, $\geq$4 mg/L for CRAB, and $\geq$2 mg/L for carbapenem-resistant Enterobacterales (CRE)) [37].

4.4. *Statistical Analysis*

Categorical variables are reported as numbers with percentages, and continuous variables are presented as the mean plus standard deviation (SD) or median with interquartile range (IQR). To compare the variables between the two groups, the Chi-squared test or Fisher's exact test was used for categorical variables, whereas the Student's *t*-test or Mann–Whitney U test was used for continuous variables with a normal or non-normal distribution, respectively. The Kaplan–Meier method was used for time-to-event analysis. Time-to-event analysis was right-censored at 14 days. Modeling of the association between time-to-event and variables was estimated by Cox proportional hazards regression analysis. Covariables with statistical differences in comparison between groups or p-values < 0.10 in the univariable analysis were selected, considering the collinearity problem. A final model was constructed using a stepwise method for the covariables. The results are presented as hazard ratios (HRs) with 95% confidence intervals (CIs). During the analysis of the ventilator liberation and ICU discharge on day 14, patients who died were assigned 0 days for both. The proportional hazards assumption was assessed through the inspection of Schoenfeld residuals. Two-sided p-values of <0.05 were used to indicate significance. All analyses were performed using R software version 4.1.2 accessed on 6 April 2023 (R Core Team).

5. Conclusions

In this study, an extended infusion of meropenem for the treatment of nosocomial pneumonia did produce better clinical outcomes than intermittent infusion. However, our results suggest a potential advantage of EI in critically ill, empirically treated or culture-proven nosocomial pneumonia patients with CRE. A large, randomized controlled trial is needed to confirm our findings in specific subgroups.

Supplementary Materials: The following supporting information can be downloaded at: https://www.mdpi.com/article/10.3390/antibiotics12101542/s1, Figure S1: Mortality in subgroups at 14 days; Figure S2: Absolute standardized mean differences between the extended infusion group and intermittent infusion group before and after propensity-score matching; Figure S3: Time-to-event analysis after inclusion to day 14 in the propensity-score matched cohort; Figure S4: Time-to-event analysis after inclusion to day 14 in patients with concurrent bacteremia; Table S1: Cox proportional hazards model of factors associated with mortality in all patients at 14 days; Table S2: Cox proportional hazards model of factors associated with ICU discharge in all patients at 14 days; Table S3: Cox proportional hazards model of factors associated with ventilator liberation in all patients at 14 days; Table S4: Cox proportional hazards model of factors associated with mortality at 14 days in the subgroup with empirical treatment; Table S5: Cox proportional hazards model of factors associated with mortality at 14 days in the subgroup of culture-proven patients; Table S6: Baseline characteristics of the propensity-score matched cohorts; Table S7: Baseline characteristics of patients with concurrent bacteremia according to the type of meropenem infusion.

Author Contributions: All authors have contributed significantly. D.-g.H., J.S., S.Y.L., J.H.A., S.-B.H., C.-M.L., Y.K. and J.W.H. conceived the study. D.-g.H., J.S. and S.Y.L. managed the data. J.H.A., S.-B.H., C.-M.L. and Y.K. provided statistical advice on study design and analyzed the data. D.-g.H. drafted the article, and all authors contributed substantially to its revision. All authors take responsibility for the paper as a whole and agree with the manuscript's content. All authors have read and agreed to the published version of the manuscript.

Funding: This research received no external funding.

Institutional Review Board Statement: This study was approved by the Institutional Review Board of Asan Medical Center (IRB No. 2021-0879).

Informed Consent Statement: The requirement for informed consent was waived because of the retrospective nature of this study. This study was conducted per the Guidelines for Good Clinical Practice and the 1964 Declaration of Helsinki.

Data Availability Statement: Not applicable.

Acknowledgments: This study was supported by the University of Ulsan College of Medicine. Editorial support in the form of writing assistance, collation of the authors' comments, and grammatical editing was provided by the Scientific Publications Team of Asan Medical Centre.

Conflicts of Interest: The authors declare no conflict of interest.

References

1. Magill, S.S.; Edwards, J.R.; Bamberg, W.; Beldavs, Z.G.; Dumyati, G.; Kainer, M.A.; Lynfield, R.; Maloney, M.; McAllister-Hollod, L.; Nadle, J.; et al. Multistate point-prevalence survey of health care-associated infections. *N. Engl. J. Med.* **2014**, *370*, 1198–1208. [CrossRef] [PubMed]
2. Bassetti, M.; Welte, T.; Wunderink, R.G. Treatment of Gram-negative pneumonia in the critical care setting: Is the beta-lactam antibiotic backbone broken beyond repair? *Crit. Care.* **2016**, *20*, 19. [CrossRef] [PubMed]

3. Koulenti, D.; Tsigou, E.; Rello, J. Nosocomial pneumonia in 27 ICUs in Europe: Perspectives from the EU-VAP/CAP study. *Eur. J. Clin. Microbiol. Infect. Dis.* **2017**, *36*, 1999–2006. [CrossRef] [PubMed]
4. Chung, D.R.; Song, J.H.; Kim, S.H.; Thamlikitkul, V.; Huang, S.G.; Wang, H.; So, T.M.-K.; Yasin, R.M.D.; Hsueh, P.-R.; Carlos, C.C.; et al. High prevalence of multidrug-resistant nonfermenters in hospital-acquired pneumonia in Asia. *Am. J. Respir. Crit. Care Med.* **2011**, *184*, 1409–1417. [CrossRef] [PubMed]
5. Ko, R.E.; Min, K.H.; Hong, S.B.; Baek, A.R.; Lee, H.K.; Cho, W.H.; Kim, C.; Chang, Y.; Lee, S.-S.; Oh, J.Y.; et al. Characteristics, Management, and Clinical Outcomes of Patients with Hospital-Acquired and Ventilator-Associated Pneumonia: A Multicenter Cohort Study in Korea. *Tuberc. Respir. Dis.* **2021**, *84*, 317–325. [CrossRef] [PubMed]
6. Bassetti, M.; Poulakou, G.; Ruppe, E.; Bouza, E.; Van Hal, S.J.; Brink, A. Antimicrobial resistance in the next 30 years, humankind, bugs and drugs: A visionary approach. *Intensive Care Med.* **2017**, *43*, 1464–1475. [CrossRef] [PubMed]
7. Kollef, M.H.; Bassetti, M.; Francois, B.; Burnham, J.; Dimopoulos, G.; Garnacho-Montero, J.; Lipman, J.; Luyt, C.E.; Nicolau, D.P.; Postma, M.J.; et al. The intensive care medicine research agenda on multidrug-resistant bacteria, antibiotics, and stewardship. *Intensive Care Med.* **2017**, *43*, 1187–1197. [CrossRef]
8. Dhaese, S.A.M.; Hoste, E.A.; De Waele, J.J. Why We May Need Higher Doses of Beta-Lactam Antibiotics: Introducing the 'Maximum Tolerable Dose'. *Antibiotics* **2022**, *11*, 889. [CrossRef]
9. Póvoa, P.; Moniz, P.; Pereira, J.G.; Coelho, L. Optimizing Antimicrobial Drug Dosing in Critically Ill Patients. *Microorganisms.* **2021**, *9*, 1401. [CrossRef]
10. Blot, S.I.; Pea, F.; Lipman, J. The effect of pathophysiology on pharmacokinetics in the critically ill patient–concepts appraised by the example of antimicrobial agents. *Adv. Drug. Deliv. Rev.* **2014**, *77*, 3–11. [CrossRef]
11. Felton, T.W.; McCalman, K.; Malagon, I.; Isalska, B.; Whalley, S.; Goodwin, J.; Bentley, A.M.; Hope, W.W. Pulmonary penetration of piperacillin and tazobactam in critically ill patients. *Clin. Pharmacol. Ther.* **2014**, *96*, 438–448. [CrossRef]
12. Rodvold, K.A.; Hope, W.W.; Boyd, S.E. Considerations for effect site pharmacokinetics to estimate drug exposure: Concentrations of antibiotics in the lung. *Curr. Opin. Pharmacol.* **2017**, *36*, 114–123. [CrossRef] [PubMed]
13. Roberts, J.A.; Paul, S.K.; Akova, M.; Bassetti, M.; De Waele, J.J.; Dimopoulos, G.; Kaukonen, K.M.; Koulenti, D.; Martin, C.; Montravers, P.; et al. DALI: Defining antibiotic levels in intensive care unit patients: Are current β-lactam antibiotic doses sufficient for critically ill patients? *Clin. Infect. Dis.* **2014**, *58*, 1072–1083. [CrossRef]
14. Taccone, F.S.; Laterre, P.-F.; Dugernier, T.; Spapen, H.; Delattre, I.; Witebolle, X.; De Backer, D.; Layeux, B.; Wallemacq, P.; Vincent, J.-L.; et al. Insufficient β-lactam concentrations in the early phase of severe sepsis and septic shock. *Crit. Care.* **2010**, *14*, R126. [CrossRef] [PubMed]
15. Yu, Z.; Pang, X.; Wu, X.; Shan, C.; Jiang, S. Clinical outcomes of prolonged infusion (extended infusion or continuous infusion) versus intermittent bolus of meropenem in severe infection: A meta-analysis. *PLoS ONE* **2018**, *13*, e0201667. [CrossRef]
16. Vardakas, K.Z.; Voulgaris, G.L.; Maliaros, A.; Samonis, G.; Falagas, M.E. Prolonged versus short-term intravenous infusion of antipseudomonal β-lactams for patients with sepsis: A systematic review and meta-analysis of randomised trials. *Lancet Infect. Dis.* **2018**, *18*, 108–120. [CrossRef] [PubMed]
17. Kondo, Y.; Ota, K.; Imura, H.; Hara, N.; Shime, N. Prolonged versus intermittent β-lactam antibiotics intravenous infusion strategy in sepsis or septic shock patients: A systematic review with meta-analysis and trial sequential analysis of randomized trials. *J. Intensive Care.* **2020**, *8*, 77. [CrossRef]
18. Drwiega, E.N.; Rodvold, K.A. Penetration of Antibacterial Agents into Pulmonary Epithelial Lining Fluid: An Update. *Clin. Pharmacokinet.* **2022**, *61*, 17–46. [CrossRef]
19. Paal, M.; Scharf, C.; Denninger, A.K.; Ilia, L.; Kloft, C.; Kneidinger, N.; Liebchen, U.; Michel, S.; Schneider, C.; Schröpf, S.; et al. Target Site Pharmacokinetics of Meropenem: Measurement in Human Explanted Lung Tissue by Bronchoalveolar Lavage, Microdialysis, and Homogenized Lung Tissue. *Antimicrob. Agents Chemother.* **2021**, *65*, e0156421. [CrossRef]
20. Frippiat, F.; Musuamba, F.T.; Seidel, L.; Albert, A.; Denooz, R.; Charlier, C.; Van Bambeke, F.; Wallemacq, P.; Descy, J.; Lambermont, B.; et al. Modelled target attainment after meropenem infusion in patients with severe nosocomial pneumonia: The PROMESSE study. *J. Antimicrob Chemother.* **2015**, *70*, 207–216. [CrossRef]
21. Benítez-Cano, A.; Luque, S.; Sorlí, L.; Carazo, J.; Ramos, I.; Campillo, N.; Curull, V.; Sánchez-Font, A.; Vilaplana, C.; Horcajada, J.P.; et al. Intrapulmonary concentrations of meropenem administered by continuous infusion in critically ill patients with nosocomial pneumonia: A randomized pharmacokinetic trial. *Crit. Care.* **2020**, *24*, 55. [CrossRef] [PubMed]
22. Del Bono, V.; Giacobbe, D.R.; Marchese, A.; Parisini, A.; Fucile, C.; Coppo, E.; Marini, V.; Arena, A.; Molin, A.; Martelli, A.; et al. Meropenem for treating KPC-producing Klebsiella pneumoniae bloodstream infections: Should we get to the PK/PD root of the paradox? *Virulence* **2017**, *8*, 66–73. [PubMed]
23. Razzazzadeh, S.; Darazam, I.A.; Hajiesmaeili, M.; Salamzadeh, J.; Mahboubi, A.; Sadeghnezhad, E.; Sahraei, Z. Investigation of pharmacokinetic and clinical outcomes of various meropenem regimens in patients with ventilator-associated pneumonia and augmented renal clearance. *Eur. J. Clin. Pharmacol.* **2022**, *78*, 823–829. [CrossRef] [PubMed]
24. Carrié, C.; Chadefaux, G.; Sauvage, N.; de Courson, H.; Petit, L.; Nouette-Gaulain, K.; Pereira, B.; Biais, M. Increased β-Lactams dosing regimens improve clinical outcome in critically ill patients with augmented renal clearance treated for a first episode of hospital or ventilator-acquired pneumonia: A before and after study. *Crit. Care.* **2019**, *23*, 379. [CrossRef] [PubMed]
25. Bassetti, M.; Mularoni, A.; Giacobbe, D.R.; Castaldo, N.; Vena, A. New Antibiotics for Hospital-Acquired Pneumonia and Ventilator-Associated Pneumonia. *Semin. Respir. Crit. Care Med.* **2022**, *43*, 280–294.

26. Torres, A.; Zhong, N.; Pachl, J.; Timsit, J.F.; Kollef, M.; Chen, Z.; Song, J.; Taylor, D.; Laud, P.J.; Stone, G.G.; et al. Ceftazidime-avibactam versus meropenem in nosocomial pneumonia, including ventilator-associated pneumonia (REPROVE): A randomised, double-blind, phase 3 non-inferiority trial. *Lancet Infect. Dis.* **2018**, *18*, 285–295. [CrossRef] [PubMed]
27. Kollef, M.H.; Nováček, M.; Kivistik, Ü.; Réa-Neto, Á.; Shime, N.; Martin-Loeches, I.; Timsit, J.-F.; Wunderink, R.G.; Bruno, C.J.; Huntington, J.A.; et al. Ceftolozane-tazobactam versus meropenem for treatment of nosocomial pneumonia (ASPECT-NP): A randomised, controlled, double-blind, phase 3, non-inferiority trial. *Lancet Infect. Dis.* **2019**, *19*, 1299–1311. [PubMed]
28. Wunderink, R.G.; Matsunaga, Y.; Ariyasu, M.; Clevenbergh, P.; Echols, R.; Kaye, K.S.; Kollef, M.; Menon, A.; Pogue, J.M.; Shorr, A.F.; et al. Cefiderocol versus high-dose, extended-infusion meropenem for the treatment of Gram-negative nosocomial pneumonia (APEKS-NP): A randomised, double-blind, phase 3, non-inferiority trial. *Lancet Infect. Dis.* **2021**, *21*, 213–225. [CrossRef] [PubMed]
29. Tamma, P.D.; Beisken, S.; Bergman, Y.; Posch, A.E.; Avdic, E.; Sharara, S.L.; Cosgrove, S.E.; Simner, P.J. Modifiable Risk Factors for the Emergence of Ceftolozane-tazobactam Resistance. *Clin. Infect. Dis.* **2021**, *73*, e4599–e4606. [CrossRef]
30. Sid Ahmed, M.A.; Khan, F.A.; Hadi, H.A.; Skariah, S.; Sultan, A.A.; Salam, A.; Al Khal, A.L.; Söderquist, B.; Ibrahim, E.B.; Omrani, A.S.; et al. Association of bla(VIM-2), bla(PDC-35), bla(OXA-10), bla(OXA-488) and bla(VEB-9) β-Lactamase Genes with Resistance to Ceftazidime-Avibactam and Ceftolozane-Tazobactam in Multidrug-Resistant Pseudomonas aeruginosa. *Antibiotics* **2022**, *11*, 130.
31. Roberts, J.A.; Roger, C.; De Waele, J.J. Personalized antibiotic dosing for the critically ill. *Intensive Care Med.* **2019**, *45*, 715–718. [CrossRef] [PubMed]
32. Wang, Z.; Shan, T.; Liu, Y.; Ding, S.; Li, C.; Zhai, Q.; Du, B.; Li, Y.; Zhang, J.; Wang, H.; et al. Comparison of 3-hour and 30-minute infusion regimens for meropenem in patients with hospital acquired pneumonia in intensive care unit: A randomized controlled clinical trial. *Zhonghua Wei Zhong Bing Ji Jiu Yi Xue* **2014**, *26*, 644–649. [PubMed]
33. Giacomo, M.; Nikola, B.; Matteo, M.; Aidos, K.; Evgeny, F.; Yuki, K.; Likhvantsev, V.V.; Momesso, E.; Nogtev, P.; Lobreglio, R.; et al. Continuous vs Intermittent Meropenem Administration in Critically Ill Patients With Sepsis: The MERCY Randomized Clinical Trial. *JAMA.* **2023**, *330*, L141–L151.
34. Yang, N.; Wang, J.; Xie, Y.; Ding, J.; Wu, C.; Liu, J.; Pei, Q. External Evaluation of Population Pharmacokinetic Models to Inform Precision Dosing of Meropenem in Critically Ill Patients. *Front. Pharmacol.* **2022**, *13*, 838205. [CrossRef] [PubMed]
35. Imani, S.; Buscher, H.; Marriott, D.; Gentili, S.; Sandaradura, I. Too much of a good thing: A retrospective study of β-lactam concentration-toxicity relationships. *J. Antimicrob. Chemother.* **2017**, *72*, 2891–2897. [CrossRef] [PubMed]
36. An, G.; Creech, C.B.; Wu, N.; Nation, R.L.; Gu, K.; Nalbant, D.; Jimenez-Truque, N.; Fissell, W.; Rolsma, S.; Patel, P.C.; et al. Evaluation of Empirical Dosing Regimens for Meropenem in Intensive Care Unit Patients Using Population Pharmacokinetic Modeling and Target Attainment Analysis. *Antimicrob. Agents Chemother.* **2023**, *67*, e0131222. [CrossRef]
37. Iovleva, A.; Doi, Y. Carbapenem-Resistant Enterobacteriaceae. *Clin. Lab. Med.* **2017**, *37*, 303–315. [CrossRef]

antibiotics

Review

Difficult-to-Treat *Pseudomonas aeruginosa* Infections in Critically Ill Patients: A Comprehensive Review and Treatment Proposal

Pablo Vidal-Cortés [1,*], Sandra Campos-Fernández [1], Elena Cuenca-Fito [1], Lorena del Río-Carbajo [1], Paula Fernández-Ugidos [1], Víctor J. López-Ciudad [1], Jorge Nieto-del Olmo [1], Ana Rodríguez-Vázquez [2] and Ana I. Tizón-Varela [1]

1 Intensive Care Unit, Complexo Hospitalario Universitario de Ourense, 32003 Ourense, Spain; sandra.campos.fernandez@sergas.es (S.C.-F.); elena.cuenca.fito@sergas.es (E.C.-F.); lorena.del.rio.carbajo@sergas.es (L.d.R.-C.); paula.fernandez.ugidos@sergas.es (P.F.-U.); victor.jose.lopez.ciudad@sergas.es (V.J.L.-C.); jorge.nieto.del.olmo@sergas.es (J.N.-d.O.); ana.isabel.tizon.varela@sergas.es (A.I.T.-V.)

2 Hospital Pharmacy, Complexo Hospitalario Universitario de Ourense, 32003 Ourense, Spain; ana.rodriguez.vazquez2@sergas.es

* Correspondence: pablo.vidal.cortes@sergas.es

Abstract: The management of infections caused by difficult-to-treat *Pseudomonas aeruginosa* in critically ill patients poses a significant challenge. Optimal antibiotic therapy is crucial for patient prognosis, yet the numerous resistance mechanisms of *P. aeruginosa*, which may even combine, complicate the selection of an appropriate antibiotic. In this review, we examine the epidemiology, resistance mechanisms, risk factors, and available and future therapeutic options, as well as strategies for treatment optimization. Finally, we propose a treatment algorithm to facilitate decision making based on the resistance patterns specific to each Intensive Care Unit.

Keywords: *Pseudomonas aeruginosa*; critically ill patient; ceftolozane–tazobactam; ceftazidime–avibactam; imipenem–relebactam; cefiderocol; ventilator-associated pneumonia

1. Introduction

Pseudomonas aeruginosa is a non-fermenting, aerobic Gram-negative bacilli (GNB), first isolated in 1882. It is ubiquitous in the environment, with a particular affinity for water. *P. aeruginosa* is considered an opportunistic bacterium and has been classically associated with patients suffering from chronic structural lung diseases, burns, and neutropenia [1]. It is not part of the normal microbiota in healthy humans [2,3]; however, under conditions of high exposure pressure, such as in an Intensive Care Unit (ICU), colonization can occur in as little as 3–5 days [3].

In a 2017 World Health Organization (WHO) expert meeting held in Geneva, *P. aeruginosa* resistant to carbapenems was classified as a top priority pathogen for research [4]. This classification was updated in 2024, maintaining carbapenem-resistant *P. aeruginosa* (CR-PA) in the high-priority group [5]. The importance of *P. aeruginosa* lies in two main factors. Firstly, it is one of the leading causes of healthcare-associated infections (HAIs) [6,7], particularly in critically ill patients [8,9]. Secondly, *P. aeruginosa* exhibits intrinsic and acquired resistance to several first-line antibiotics, making treatment complex and challenging.

In this review, we summarize the epidemiology, resistance mechanisms, and therapeutic options for DTR *P. aeruginosa* in critically ill patients.

 https://doi.org/10.3390/antibiotics14020178

2. Epidemiology

2.1. Healthcare-Associated Infections (HAIs)

Globally, *P. aeruginosa* is the third most frequently isolated GNB among patients hospitalized in Intensive Care Units (ICUs) [8].

2.1.1. Nosocomial Pneumonia

P. aeruginosa is, along with *S. aureus*, the leading cause of bacterial pneumonia among hospitalized patients, being the most frequently identified GNB in nosocomial pneumonia. A U.S. study reported *P. aeruginosa* in 11% of all nosocomial pneumonia cases. Ventilator-associated pneumonia (VAP) is the most severe HAI acquired in ICUs. Data from the SMART registry, comprising 7171 respiratory samples from 209 ICUs across 56 countries, identified *P. aeruginosa* in 25% of VAP cases [6,10–13].

A notable scenario involves the SARS-CoV-2 pandemic, where patients requiring mechanical ventilation (MV) exhibited a high risk of VAP. In numerous published series, *P. aeruginosa* was identified as the primary etiologic agent [14,15].

Geographic differences influence HAI etiology. In the U.S., *P. aeruginosa* ranks second as a cause of VAP [7], while it holds the top position in Europe [16] and Spain, where it accounts for 20.7% of VAP cases according to the National Nosocomial Infection Surveillance Study (ENVIN) [9].

2.1.2. Other Healthcare-Associated Infections

While respiratory infections are the primary focus for *P. aeruginosa*, it is also frequently implicated in other sites, such as catheter-associated urinary tract infections (CAUTIs) [6,17], catheter-related bloodstream infections (CRBSIs), and surgical site infections (SSIs) [18].

The EUROBACT-2 study reported *P. aeruginosa* as responsible for 14.3% of CRBSIs in ICU patients, following *Klebsiella* spp., *Acinetobacter* spp., and *E. coli* [19]. Additionally, it caused 4% of CRBSIs in critically ill COVID-19 patients [20]. *P. aeruginosa* is the fourth leading cause of CRBSIs in Europe, the fifth in Spain, and the eleventh in the U.S. [7,9,16].

For CAUTIs, *P. aeruginosa* ranks as the third most common cause in the U.S. and Europe [7,16] and the second in Spain [9]. It is also the fifth most common pathogen responsible for SSIs in the U.S. [7].

2.2. Community-Acquired Infections

Although primarily a nosocomial pathogen, *P. aeruginosa* has been implicated in community-acquired infections, including folliculitis and other skin and soft tissue infections (SSTIs), especially those involving water exposure. It has also been associated with osteomyelitis and endocarditis in intravenous drug users and peritonitis in patients undergoing peritoneal dialysis. *P. aeruginosa* accounts for 1% of community-acquired bloodstream infections [21] and up to 5% of severe community-acquired pneumonia (CAP) [22,23].

2.3. Patients at Risk

Until 1980, *P. aeruginosa* was responsible for nearly half of infections in neutropenic and burn patients. Although its incidence in these populations has declined, it remains a significant cause of bacteremia [24], likely due to the use of empiric treatments with antipseudomonal activity.

A similar trend is observed in cystic fibrosis (CF) patients. The incidence of *P. aeruginosa* infections has decreased in recent years, likely due to improved acute infection treatments and prophylaxis [25]. However, *P. aeruginosa* remains the leading cause of respiratory infections in CF [26–28]. Data from the European CF Society registry indicate a prevalence of

30%, with half of CF patients over 40 years old presenting at least one positive culture for *P. aeruginosa* [29]. Once *P. aeruginosa* colonizes the lungs, eradication is nearly impossible [28].

A similar phenomenon occurs in patients with non-CF bronchiectasis, where *P. aeruginosa* is associated with worsening functional status and increased mortality [6,30]. *P. aeruginosa* exhibits reduced virulence in these chronic infections, but resistance becomes a significant concern [31].

Lastly, *P. aeruginosa*'s ability to persist on various materials and surfaces, especially in water-rich environments, has led to hospital outbreaks linked to inadequate medical equipment disinfection or cross-contamination of surfaces and water sources [32]. Some outbreaks have reported mortality rates of up to 30% [33].

3. Antimicrobial Resistance

In addition to possessing numerous virulence factors and a remarkable ability to survive in adverse environments, this organism has another critical feature that significantly complicates its treatment: resistance to multiple antimicrobials. It is intrinsically resistant to multiple antibiotics and has a high capacity to acquire new resistance mechanisms [34–36]. Over 40 chromosomal genes are implicated in its resistance mechanisms [37], including 8.4% regulatory genes [34], which enable it to mutate and adapt to its environment. The coexistence of combined resistance mechanisms is frequently observed [38,39].

3.1. Antimicrobial Resistance Mechanisms

Intrinsic resistance arises from the expression of efflux pumps that expel antibiotics from the cell, the production of enzymes that inactivate or hydrolyze antibiotics (e.g., extended-spectrum beta-lactamases, ESBLs, AmpC beta-lactamases, or carbapenemases), and the low permeability of its outer membrane. Particularly significant is the downregulation of the outer membrane protein OprD, which decreases membrane permeability to certain antibiotics and is often responsible for carbapenem resistance.

The inducible expression of chromosomal AmpC beta-lactamases is primarily responsible for *P. aeruginosa's* natural resistance to most penicillins and cephalosporins [3,31,40]. Constitutive production of the MexAB-OprM efflux pump contributes to reduced susceptibility to beta-lactams, while the inducible production of MexXY partially accounts for decreased susceptibility to aminoglycosides [3].

Acquired resistance can occur through horizontal gene transfer (via plasmids, transposons, integrons, and prophages, from the same or different bacterial species) or mutational changes. These can confer advantages such as reduced antimicrobial uptake, modification of the antibiotic target, efflux pump overexpression, or the emergence of antibiotic-inactivating enzymes.

Adaptive resistance enhances bacterial survival in response to environmental stimuli and is reversible when the stimulus ceases. In *P. aeruginosa*, adaptive resistance often involves biofilm formation [41,42].

Based on consensus definitions by the European Centre for Disease Prevention and Control (ECDC) and the Centers for Disease Control and Prevention (CDC) [43], *P. aeruginosa* can be categorized as multidrug resistant (MDR-PA) if it is non-susceptible to at least one antimicrobial agent in three or more classes active against *P. aeruginosa*. Extensively drug-resistant *P. aeruginosa* (XDR-PA) is defined as non-susceptible to all but two or fewer antimicrobial classes, while pan-drug-resistant *P. aeruginosa* (PDR-PA) is non-susceptible to all antimicrobial agents. The term "non-susceptible" is used, despite its less reader-friendly nature, as it encompasses both resistant and susceptible with increased exposure concepts.

The concept of difficult-to-treat resistance *P. aeruginosa* (DTR-PA) has also been proposed, including strains non-susceptible to piperacillin–tazobactam, ceftazidime, cefepime, aztreonam, meropenem, imipenem–cilastatin, ciprofloxacin, and levofloxacin [44,45] (Table 1).

Table 1. Classification of *P. aeruginosa* based on antimicrobial resistance (combining Magiorakos's [43] and Kadri's [44] definitions).

Concept	Definition
Multidrug-resistant *P. aeruginosa* (MDR-PA)	Non-susceptible to at least one antimicrobial agent in three or more antimicrobial classes active against *P. aeruginosa*.
Extensively drug-resistant *P. aeruginosa* (XDR-PA)	Non-susceptible to at least one agent in all but two or fewer antimicrobial classes.
Pandrug-resistant *P. aeruginosa* (PDR-PA)	Non-susceptible to any antimicrobial agent.
Difficult-to-treat *P. aeruginosa* (DTR-PA)	Non-susceptible to piperacillin–tazobactam, ceftazidime, cefepime, aztreonam, meropenem, imipenem–cilastatin, ciprofloxacin, and levofloxacin.

MDR-PA or DTR-PA usually result from the combination of multiple resistance mechanisms. Resistance to carbapenems often arises from the interplay of several mechanisms rather than carbapenemase production alone; however, carbapenemase production accounts for up to 20% of CR-PA cases [45], with metallo-beta-lactamases (MBLs) being the most prevalent carbapenemase group globally in *P. aeruginosa* [46,47].

3.2. Antimicrobial Resistance Prevalence

In 2020, the International Nosocomial Infection Control Consortium reported resistance rates of *P. aeruginosa* to major antibiotics in device-associated infections. In VAP, resistance rates to carbapenems, quinolones, piperacillin–tazobactam, and cefepime were 39.4%, 34.6%, 39.2%, and 40.5%, respectively. For CAUTIs, rates reached 39.3%, 40.2%, 38.2%, and 48.1% in the same order, while BSIs showed rates of 43.5%, 20%, 33%, and 41.7%. Amikacin was the only antibiotic with resistance rates below 30%: 24.7% in VAP, 26.8% in CAUTIs, and 21.4% in BSIs [48].

Fortunately, in recent years new antibiotics with activity against *P. aeruginosa* have been marketed.

European studies indicate that 95.5% of *P. aeruginosa* isolates are susceptible to ceftazidime–avibactam (CAZ-AVI), 94.3% to imipenem–relebactam (IMI-REL), 93.3% to ceftolozane–tazobactam (CFT-TAZ), and 88.7% to meropenem–vaborbactam (MER-VAB) [49]. Similarly, 73.4% and 71.0% of XDR-PA isolates remain susceptible to CFT-TAZ and CAZ-AVI, respectively. Resistance to both antibiotics was observed in only 3.9% of isolates, mainly due to carbapenemase production but also mutant AmpC presence [47,50–53].

A study of strains isolated between 2013 and 2018 across 24 European countries showed that 99.7% of *P. aeruginosa* isolates were susceptible to cefiderocol, including 97.5% of carbapenem-resistant isolates. In this study, only 43.2% and 44.1% of CR-PA maintained susceptibility to CAZ-AVI and CFT-TAZ, respectively [54]. Similar findings were observed in another study analyzing CR-PA isolates from 44 Spanish hospitals. Up to 30.6% were carbapenemase producers, primarily MBL of the VIM type, and 26.7% were susceptible only to colistin [55].

Studies also highlight that AmpC-AmpR region mutations associated with resistance to CFT-TAZ and CAZ-AVI during treatment reduce cefiderocol activity but seem to enhance IMI-REL susceptibility [56].

Patterns of resistance vary geographically and over time. For example, in Asia, almost 40% of isolates are MDR or carbapenem resistant, while in the U.S., resistance rates to cephalosporins and carbapenems range from 22 to 28%, with approximately 20% of isolates being MDR-PA [12,57–61]. A study in Spain from 2022 reported a decrease in XDR-PA prevalence from 15% to 6% over five years, with an even sharper decline in ICU settings [62]. This favorable trend has also been described in other regions of the world [16,45,60].

These findings underscore the importance of ongoing surveillance, the knowledge of local microbiological profiles, and tailored therapeutic strategies to address the challenge of resistant *P. aeruginosa*.

4. Risk Factors

Classic risk factors for *P. aeruginosa* infection include advanced age, structural lung diseases (e.g., cystic fibrosis, bronchiectasis), hematologic malignancies (particularly those associated with neutropenia), solid organ transplantation, extensive burns, prior antibiotic treatment within 90 days, the presence of a central venous catheter (CVC) or urinary catheter (UC), renal replacement therapies, prolonged hospitalization, and mechanical ventilation. A respiratory focus of infection and presentation with septic shock are also associated with a higher risk of *P. aeruginosa*, as is prior colonization [6,34,38].

Additional factors increase the risk of *P. aeruginosa* as a causative agent of community-acquired pneumonia (CAP), including male sex, chronic pulmonary diseases, a C-reactive protein level <12.35 mg/dL, and a Pneumonia Severity Index (PSI) score of IV-V [63]. For VAP, *P. aeruginosa* should always be considered [64], with the risk increasing in patients with prior colonization and prolonged hospital stays [65].

Risk factors for MDR-PA infection include prior hospitalization, ICU admission [36,46,66–68], local epidemiology with MDR-PA prevalence over 20% [66], prior *P. aeruginosa* colonization [66,69,70], prior exposure to broad-spectrum antibiotics [36,46,66–68,70–72], the presence of CVC, UC, or tracheostomy [35,47,58,60], diabetes mellitus [66,69], septic shock [69,73], chronic kidney disease [74], and MV [36].

Identifying ICU patients at risk of MDR-PA infection remains challenging due to the overlap of these risk factors [64]. Among these, prior exposure to broad-spectrum antibiotics is the most significant, with the risk increasing with prolonged exposure and the number of antibiotics administered. Notably, for MDR-PA CAP, prior antibiotic treatment is the sole identified risk factor [63], and for VAP, it has the greatest weight [67,68,75]. Lodise et al. highlighted the number of antibiotics received during hospitalization as a predictor of the risk of infection by MDR Gram-negative bacilli, including *P. aeruginosa*, with a significant increase in risk beyond the fourth antibiotic. This study also linked MDR-PA to local *P. aeruginosa* prevalence, prior infection within three months, and infection sites, such as VAP and complicated UTIs [76].

A systematic review identified 38 risk factors for CR-PA infection. These were ranked by experts, with the most critical factors related to prior hospital contact (previous hospitalization or length of stay until infection) and prior antibiotic therapy (e.g., carbapenems, aminoglycosides, cephalosporins, or quinolones). ICU admission, disease severity (measured by SAPS II or APACHE scores), and invasive devices were considered moderately important risk factors [77].

In an effort to quantify risk, a scoring system was proposed to predict CR-PA infection, including variables such as residence in a long-term care facility, tracheostomy presence, prior CR-PA infection within 30 days, hospitalization within the past six months, and treatment with carbapenems, cephalosporins, or quinolones in the last 30 days. The area under the ROC curve (AUC) for this score was 0.81. Another score to identify infections by *P. aeruginosa* resistant to carbapenems, ceftazidime, and piperacillin–tazobactam included similar variables, with an AUC of 0.82 [78].

In general, risk factors and predictive scores show high sensitivity but low specificity, resulting in high negative predictive value but low positive predictive value. Therefore, it is crucial to understand local microbiology and resistance profiles to guide clinical decisions effectively.

5. Prognosis

P. aeruginosa can sometimes persist in the lungs of patients with chronic pulmonary diseases as an indolent colonizer. However, in other cases, it behaves aggressively, invading tissues and causing severe pneumonia, bacteremia, septic shock, and death. This aggressive behavior is attributed to its ability to produce various toxins and trigger cytokine release pathways associated with sepsis and multiorgan failure [75]. When combined with the challenges of treatment, it becomes evident that the prognosis of *P. aeruginosa* infections is grim.

Mortality from *P. aeruginosa* bacteremia is higher than that caused by other bacteria, even after adjusting for comorbidities and appropriate antibiotic therapy [79], reaching a 30-day mortality rate of 26% [80]. In neutropenic patients, *P. aeruginosa* bacteremia is associated with higher mortality and an increased likelihood of ICU admission [72,81].

Community-acquired pneumonia caused by PES pathogens (*Pseudomonas aeruginosa*, extended spectrum beta-lactamase-producing Enterobacteriaceae, and methicillin-resistant *S. aureus*) is associated with higher 30-day mortality compared to infections caused by other bacteria [82].

MDR-PA infections are linked to faster disease progression, prolonged hospital stays, higher mortality rates [73,83–87], and increased healthcare costs [88]. Compared to non-MDR PA, MDR-PA pneumonia is characterized by longer ICU stays, extended durations of MV, and higher mortality rates, reaching 44% in some studies [6,83,89]. Mortality from *P. aeruginosa* bacteremia ranges between 20% and 39% [79,90,91], with CR-PA bacteremia posing a greater risk of death than non-resistant cases [92]. Although factors related to the virulence of *P. aeruginosa* contribute to the severity of its infections [93], inadequate or second-line treatments are a significant issue. Patients with MDR, XDR, or PDR infections often received suboptimal therapies due to limited treatment options [89,94,95].

6. Therapeutical Options for DTR-PA

6.1. *Aminoglycosides*

The rise in the prevalence of nosocomial infections caused by MDR-GNB, particularly MDR, XDR, and DTR-PA, has driven the development of new antibiotics as well as the re-evaluation of "old antibiotics", including aminoglycosides (AGs) [94].

The most common mechanism of resistance to AGs is the acquisition of transferable genetic elements (plasmids, transposons, and integrons) encoding AG-inactivating enzymes (acetyltransferases, phosphotransferases, and adenyltransferases). Less frequently, resistance arises from 16S rRNA methyltransferases, which confer resistance to all AGs, including plazomicin [96]. Inducible overexpression of MexXY efflux pumps is a less common mechanism of resistance [94]. Tobramycin exhibits the highest intrinsic activity among AGs, but most *P. aeruginosa* strains with enzymes that inactivate gentamicin and tobramycin remain susceptible to amikacin [97,98].

Plazomicin is a new AG recently approved by the FDA for the treatment of pyelonephritis and complicated urinary tract infections (cUTIs) caused by Enterobacteriaceae producing class A, C, and D beta-lactamases. Although plazomicin is not affected by enzymatic inactivation, it does not exhibit greater efficacy against *P. aeruginosa* compared to other AGs [99,100]. In Europe, the pharmaceutical company that had applied for approval for its use in cUTIs withdrew the application in 2020 [101].

6.1.1. In Vitro Activity

In the ASPIRE-ICU study, the analysis of 723 samples from 402 patients across 11 European countries demonstrated *P. aeruginosa* susceptibility rates of 80% for respiratory samples and 90% for perianal samples, according to EUCAST breakpoints [37]. A U.S.-based study observed that 54.3% of MDR-PA isolates were susceptible to gentamicin and 77.6% to tobramycin, according to CLSI breakpoints [102].

Additionally, there is evidence of in vitro synergy between AGs (amikacin and tobramycin) and carbapenems (imipenem or meropenem) [103].

6.1.2. Clinical Experience

In a case series of eleven ICU patients with infections caused by MDR-PA treated with high-dose AGs (seven with amikacin, three with gentamicin, and one with tobramycin, targeting peak concentrations exceeding eight times the MIC) combined with high-flow venovenous hemofiltration (>45 mL/kg/h), a favorable clinical response was achieved at the end of treatment in seven patients (65%) [104].

In recent years, the main use of AGs has been in combination therapies, including with new antibiotics, such as CFT-TAZ or CAZ-AVI [105–107]; however, no clinical benefit has been demonstrated, and there is a higher incidence of nephrotoxicity associated with these combinations.

6.2. *Cefiderocol*

Cefiderocol is a siderophore cephalosporin composed of a cephalosporin core (with side chains similar to cefepime and ceftazidime) and a catechol functional group that acts as an iron chelator. This property provides a unique mechanism for penetrating aerobic Gram-negative bacterial cells by chelating extracellular iron and actively transporting it through ferric ion transport systems [108–111].

The drug's catechol moiety binds to extracellular trivalent iron and utilizes active transport systems to enter the periplasmic space. Once inside, it dissociates from the iron. Additionally, like other beta-lactam antibiotics, cefiderocol can reach the periplasmic space through simple diffusion via porins [108,112].

Cefiderocol's structure and cellular entry mechanism allow it to retain activity despite porin channel loss, efflux pump overexpression, and hydrolysis by many beta-lactamases (including MBL) [109–113].

Like other cephalosporins, cefiderocol inhibits cell wall synthesis by binding to penicillin-binding proteins (PBPs), specifically PBP-3.

Cefiderocol is active against MDR GNB, including carbapenem-resistant strains due to carbapenemase production. It is more stable (compared to other beta-lactams, like ceftazidime, cefepime, and meropenem) against class A, B, and D carbapenemases, such as KPC, VIM, IMP, NDM, and OXA, and is effective against *P. aeruginosa* and *Acinetobacter baumannii* [110,111,114].

Cefiderocol shows weak or no activity against Gram-positive bacteria and anaerobes [109].

The FDA has approved cefiderocol for use in cUTIs, including pyelonephritis, nosocomial pneumonia, and VAP caused by susceptible Gram-negative bacilli. The EMA has authorized its use for treating infections due to aerobic Gram-negative microorganisms in adults with limited treatment options.

6.2.1. In Vitro Activity

An in vitro study reported cefiderocol MIC90 values of 1, 2, and 0.5 mg/L for *P. aeruginosa* (including MBL-producing strains), *A. baumannii* (including carbapenem-resistant strains), and *Stenotrophomonas maltophilia*, respectively, compared to meropenem's MIC90 >16 mg/L [114].

Longshaw et al. analyzed a cohort of carbapenem-resistant Gram-negative bacilli from European patients, reporting *P. aeruginosa* susceptibility to cefiderocol at 98.3%, second only to colistin [115].

In studies of CR-PA isolates (mostly carbapenemase producers), cefiderocol susceptibility rates were 98% (CLSI) and 95% (EUCAST), surpassing CAZ-AVI, CFT-TAZ, IMI-REL, MER-VAB, and amikacin. Activity varied by carbapenemase type: 92–97% (VIM), 87–100% (IMP), 69–85% (NDM), 97–100% (GES), and 100% (KPC) [116].

In an analysis of 7700 *P. aeruginosa* clinical isolates from Europe and North America, cefiderocol susceptibility was 99.9%, 99.8%, 100%, and 99.8% for all isolates, meropenem non-susceptible, CAZ-AVI non-susceptible, and CFT-TAZ non-susceptible strains, respectively. High activity was observed against MBL-producing *P. aeruginosa*, with 97.4% having MICs ≤2 mg/L (EUCAST breakpoint) and 100% ≤4 mg/L (CLSI breakpoint) [117,118]. A separate study reported 100% susceptibility of IMI-REL-resistant *P. aeruginosa* to cefiderocol [119].

6.2.2. Clinical Evidence

In the first RCT, cefiderocol (2 g infused over 1 h every 8 h) demonstrated non-inferiority to imipenem–cilastatin in treating cUTIs caused by Gram-negative bacilli. Among 371 microbiologically evaluable patients, 23 cases involved *P. aeruginosa*, with no differences between treatment groups [120].

The APEKS-NP Trial compared cefiderocol (2 g infused over 3 h every 8 h) to meropenem (2 g infused over 3 h every 8 h) in nosocomial pneumonia, including VAP. Non-inferiority was established, with 48 *P. aeruginosa* cases showing no treatment arm differences [121].

In the CREDIBLE-CR Trial, cefiderocol was compared to the best available therapy (BAT) for carbapenem-resistant Gram-negative infections, including nosocomial pneumonia, VAP, bacteremia, and cUTIs. While clinical and microbiological efficacy was similar to BAT, higher mortality (non-significant) was observed in the cefiderocol group, associated with *A. baumannii* infections. In *P. aeruginosa* infections, mortality was higher with cefiderocol (35% vs. 17%), equalizing after adjusting for *A. baumannii* co-infections (18% vs. 18%) [122].

6.2.3. Clinical Experience

In a compassionate use program for cefiderocol in treating MDR or CR-PA infections, susceptibility was 91%. Clinical response rates were 69% for infections with MIC ≤1 μg/mL, 69% (9/13) for MIC 2–4 μg/mL, and 100% (4/4) for MIC ≥8 μg/mL. All-cause 28-day mortality rates were 23% (MIC ≤1 μg/mL), 33% (MIC 2–4 μg/mL), and 0% (MIC ≥8 μg/mL) [123].

Cefiderocol is well tolerated and has a safety profile similar to other beta-lactams [120,121]. Data support its efficacy and safety in critically ill patients [124].

6.3. *Ceftazidima–Avibactam*

Ceftazidime–avibactam (CAZ-AVI) is an antibiotic combining a third-generation cephalosporin (ceftazidime) with a non-beta-lactam beta-lactamase inhibitor (avibactam). Ceftazidime exhibits bactericidal activity by inhibiting bacterial peptidoglycan cell wall synthesis through binding to penicillin-binding proteins (PBPs), leading to cell death. Avibactam inhibits the activity of Ambler class A (e.g., ESBLs and KPC), class C (e.g., AmpC), and some class D (e.g., OXA-48) beta-lactamases but does not inhibit class B enzymes (e.g., MBLs) or other class D enzymes (e.g., OXA-23, OXA-24). Avibactam does not protect against other resistance mechanisms, such as porin mutations (e.g., OprD) or efflux pump overexpression. Consequently, CAZ-AVI is ineffective in the presence of these resistance mechanisms [1,125,126].

With this profile, CAZ-AVI is active against most carbapenem-resistant *Enterobacteriaceae* and MDR-PA, making it a potential alternative to carbapenems for severe infections caused by Gram-negative MDR bacteria [127,128].

CAZ-AVI is approved by the FDA and the EMA for treating hospital-acquired bacterial pneumonia (including VAP), cUTIs (including pyelonephritis), and complicated intra-abdominal infections (cIAIs) in combination with metronidazole. EMA also approved CAZ-AVI for infections caused by aerobic Gram-negative bacteria with limited treatment options.

6.3.1. In Vitro Activity

Studies report that 95.5–98% of *P. aeruginosa* isolates are sensitive to CAZ-AVI. For CR-PA, sensitivity ranges between 43 and 83.3%, depending on resistance mechanisms.

Candel et al. analyzed over 20,000 Gram-negative isolates from 24 European countries (2013–2018) and found 98% sensitivity of *P. aeruginosa* to CAZ-AVI across different infection sites: bloodstream infections (97.9%), nosocomial pneumonia (98%), cIAIs (99.1%), and cUTIs (98.7%). CR-PA showed 43.2% sensitivity to CAZ-AVI [54].

Sader et al. evaluated the in vitro activity of new beta-lactams (including CAZ-AVI) against *P. aeruginosa* recovered from patients with pneumonia and SSTIs, finding sensitivity rates of 95.5% for pneumonia and 98.3%, respectively. Avibactam restored sensitivity in 79.8–87.5% of ceftazidime-resistant *P. aeruginosa*. Sensitivity varied by carbapenem and geographic region, with rates of 78–92.6% for imipenem-resistant and 56–81.6% for meropenem-resistant *P. aeruginosa* [49,129].

6.3.2. Clinical Evidence

Clinical trials evaluating CAZ-AVI included limited data on infections caused by MDR/XDR *P. aeruginosa* [130–134].

The RECAPTURE Trial compared CAZ-AVI (2.5 g every 8 h) with doripenem (500 mg every 8 h) in cUTIs, including pyelonephritis. Among 810 patients with microbiological results, only 38 had *P. aeruginosa* infections. Efficacy and safety were comparable between treatments [130].

The REPRISE Trial assessed CAZ-AVI (2.5 g every 8 h, plus metronidazole for abdominal infections) versus the best available therapy (BAT, 97% carbapenems) in 333 patients with cIAIs or cUTIs caused by ceftazidime-resistant Enterobacteriaceae or *P. aeruginosa*. CAZ-AVI was a viable carbapenem alternative without differences in efficacy or safety. Only 21 *P. aeruginosa* infections were included [132].

The RECLAIM Trial compared CAZ-AVI (2.5 g every 8 h, with metronidazole) to meropenem (1 g every 8 h) in 1066 patients with cIAIs, including 66 with *P. aeruginosa* infections. Both treatment arms showed similar efficacy and safety, including against ceftazidime-resistant isolates [133,134].

The REPROVE Trial, a phase 3 study in hospital-acquired pneumonia, including VAP, enrolled 879 patients randomized to CAZ-AVI (2.5 g every 8 h) or meropenem (1 g every 8 h). CAZ-AVI was non-inferior in efficacy and safety. Of the Gram-negative pathogens identified, 33.9% were *P. aeruginosa*, but carbapenem-resistant isolates were excluded [131].

Post hoc analyses confirmed CAZ-AVI's efficacy and safety in treating MDR infections caused by *P. aeruginosa* and *Enterobacteriaceae* [135,136].

6.3.3. Clinical Experience

Although high-quality evidence for CAZ-AVI in treating DTR-PA infections is limited, smaller studies suggest clinical efficacy.

Corbella et al. reviewed 61 MDR/XDR PA infections treated with CAZ-AVI. Common infection sites included pneumonia [34.4%], with 50.8% of patients meeting sepsis criteria. Clinical cure at 14 days was 54.1%, recurrence at 90 days was 12.5%, and 30-day mortality was 13.1%. Monotherapy was associated with better outcomes (14-day cure rate 63.5%, recurrence 6.5%, and mortality 6.3%) without detected resistance development [137].

Xu et al. analyzed 84 cases of severe hospital-acquired pneumonia in ventilated patients with DTR-PA (53.6%) and CR-PA isolates [46.4%]. Clinical cure was 63.1%, and 30-day mortality was 18.9%. Outcomes improved with loading doses and prolonged infusion regimens but not with combination treatment [138].

Almangour et al. compared CAZ-AVI to CFT-TAZ in 200 patients with MDR-PA, including critically ill patients (56%). Clinical cure and 30-day mortality rates were comparable between CAZ-AVI (66% cure, 23% mortality) and CFT-TAZ (61% cure, 27% mortality) [139].

6.4. *Ceftolozane–Tazobactam*

Ceftolozane–tazobactam (CFT-TAZ) is an antibiotic that combines a fourth-generation cephalosporin (ceftolozane) with a beta-lactamase inhibitor (tazobactam). Ceftolozane differs from other cephalosporins due to its potent activity against *P. aeruginosa*, achieved through modifications in its side chains at positions 3 and 7 of the dihydrothiazine ring. These modifications confer increased stability against AmpC-type chromosomal beta-lactamase-producing *P. aeruginosa* and protect it from the effects of OprD porin loss or efflux pump mutations. Tazobactam extends activity against most ESBL-producing organisms and some anaerobes (e.g., *Bacteroides* spp.) [140]. However, it lacks activity against class A beta-lactamases, such as KPC, as well as class B and class D beta-lactamases. It is also inactive against *Stenotrophomonas* spp. and *Acinetobacter* spp [141].

CFT-TAZ exhibits high activity against *P. aeruginosa*, including XDR strains, and retains activity against ESBL-producing Enterobacteriaceae and certain *Streptococcus* species. It has been approved by the FDA and EMA for the treatment of nosocomial pneumonia, including VAP, cUTIs, including pyelonephritis, and complicated intra-abdominal infection cIAIs in combination with metronidazole.

6.4.1. In Vitro Activity

CFT-TAZ demonstrates in vitro activity against 93.5–97.5% of *P. aeruginosa* isolates, with activity against carbapenem-resistant *P. aeruginosa* ranging from 44.1% to 75.4%, depending on the study. Candel et al. reported a *P. aeruginosa* sensitivity rate of 97.5% for CFT-TAZ. Sensitivity rates for different clinical sources included 96.7% in bacteremia, 97.5% in NN, 99.1% in cIAIs, and 97.6% in cUTIs. Among carbapenem-resistant *P. aeruginosa*, activity decreased to 44.1% [54].

Sader et al. reported a sensitivity rate of 93.3% for *P. aeruginosa* strains isolated from pneumonia. CFT-TAZ retained activity against 81.9% of imipenem-resistant strains and 57.1% of meropenem-resistant strains [49].

Shortridge et al. evaluated *P. aeruginosa* susceptibility to CFT-TAZ from various clinical sources globally (America, Europe, and Asia), including MDR and XDR isolates. They reported an overall sensitivity rate of 93.5%, without significant geographic differences. For MDR and XDR *P. aeruginosa* strains, sensitivity rates were 69.2% and 59.1%, respectively, with meropenem-resistant strains showing a sensitivity of 75.4% [142].

6.4.2. Clinical Evidence

In the ASPECT-cUTI Trial, CFT-TAZ was compared to levofloxacin for the treatment of cUTIs, showing superior outcomes; however, *P. aeruginosa* was detected in only 19 of 1083 patients included in the study [143].

The ASPECT-cIAI Trial included 993 patients with cIAIs, of whom 75 had *P. aeruginosa* infections. CFT-TAZ (1.5 g every 8 h) combined with metronidazole (500 mg every 8 h) was compared to meropenem (1 g every 8 h), demonstrating non-inferiority. *P. aeruginosa* isolates showed sensitivity rates of 98.6% to CFT-TAZ and 89.9% to meropenem [144].

The ASPECT-NP Trial involved 726 patients with nosocomial pneumonia (71% VAP), with *P. aeruginosa* isolated in 128 cases (39% MDR or XDR). Patients were randomized to receive CFT-TAZ (3 g every 8 h) or meropenem (1 g every 8 h). The study demonstrated the non-inferiority of CFT-TAZ compared to meropenem for nosocomial pneumonia treatment [145]. A subgroup analysis of ventilated nosocomial pneumonia patients (n = 207) showed 28-day mortality rates of 24.2% for CFT-TAZ versus 37% for meropenem (not significant); specifically, for *P. aeruginosa*-related nosocomial pneumonia, mortality rates were 11.8% and 29.4%, respectively [146].

6.4.3. Clinical Experience

Balandín et al. conducted a multicenter observational study of 95 critically ill patients treated with CFT-TAZ for severe *P. aeruginosa* infections, primarily nosocomial pneumonia (56.2%). Among these patients, 49.5% had sepsis, 45.3% had septic shock, and 36.8% had MDR-PA. Despite the severity, clinical response was favorable in 71.6% of cases, with a 30-day mortality rate of 30.5%. Monotherapy was used in 44.2% of cases, with no observed benefits of combination therapy [147].

Pogue et al. compared CFT-TAZ with polymyxins or aminoglycosides for MDR or XDR-PA infections in critically ill patients (69% ICU, 63% on MV, and 42% with septic shock). CFT-TAZ showed higher cure rates and reduced renal failure without affecting overall mortality [105].

Almangour et al. reported higher cure rates and improved safety (lower renal failure rates) with CFT-TAZ compared to colistin for MDR-PA infections, although the difference in mortality (39% vs. 49%) was not statistically significant [148].

The cohort study comparing CFT-TAZ with CAZ-AVI has been previously discussed [139].

CFT-TAZ has accumulated substantial clinical efficacy evidence, with several case series reporting favorable outcomes (cure rates between 63% and 83%) in MDR or CR-PA infections [106,149–152].

6.5. Colistin

Polymyxins are a class of antimicrobials that include five chemically distinct compounds (polymyxins A, B, C, D, and E), of which polymyxin B and colistin (polymyxin E) are the only ones currently available on the market [153–155].

Colistin was approved by the FDA in 1959 for the treatment of infections caused by Gram-negative bacteria, but its high toxicity limited its use. It is a highly nephrotoxic agent, and acute kidney injury frequently occurs at standard doses [156]. Additionally, colistin is associated with neurotoxic effects, such as dizziness, muscle weakness, facial and peripheral paresthesia, vertigo, confusion, ataxia, and neuromuscular blockade, which could lead to respiratory failure or apnea, seizures, and even coma [157]. The emergence of MDR-GNB bacteria renewed interest in colistin during the 1990s.

Colistin disrupts the bacterial membrane due to its positive charge, causing electrostatic attraction to the anionic components of magnesium and calcium that stabilize the membrane. This interaction results in the leakage of cellular contents and, ultimately, cell death Moreover, high doses of colistin reduce endotoxin and cytokine levels in sepsis [158].

The antimicrobial spectrum of colistin includes MDR and XDR GNB, regardless of the resistance mechanism, primarily *Klebsiella pneumoniae*, *Acinetobacter baumannii*, and

Pseudomonas aeruginosa. However, *Stenotrophomonas maltophilia*, *Proteus* spp., *Providencia* spp., *Serratia* spp., and *Burkholderia* are intrinsically resistant.

Colistin is active against metabolically inactive cells located in the inner layers of biofilms, which may complement the activity of antimicrobials effective only against metabolically active cells in the biofilm. This activity has been confirmed in cystic fibrosis patients using nebulized therapy [159,160].

6.5.1. In Vitro Activity

Despite decades of use, colistin retains high in vitro activity against Enterobacteriaceae and non-fermenting GNB, even in MDR bacteria. Longshaw et al. reported a sensitivity rate of 100% for *P. aeruginosa* (MDR and CR-PA), the highest among the antibiotics analyzed in their study [115]. Satlin et al. examined 46 infections caused by MDR and CR-PA and found only one resistant strain to colistin [123]. Delgado-Valverde et al. observed similar results, with 86% of 399 *P. aeruginosa* isolates resistant to imipenem being susceptible to colistin, with an MIC90 of 4 mg/L [161]. Carvalhaes et al. reported a 99.1% susceptibility of MDR-PA to colistin, with an MIC90 of 2 mg/L [162].

6.5.2. Clinical Evidence

A meta-analysis published in 2015 evaluated the treatment of respiratory infections caused by *P. aeruginosa* and *A. baumannii*. This analysis, which included nine studies (none of which were RCTs) with significant heterogeneity, suggested that the efficacy and side effects (particularly nephrotoxicity) were comparable to other available alternatives at that time [163].

However, more recent and higher-quality studies challenge this assertion. The Magic Bullet RCT compared the empirical treatment of VAP with colistin (loading dose of 4.5 million IU followed by 3 million IU every 8 h) or meropenem (2 g every 8 h), and both were combined with levofloxacin. It demonstrated that colistin was less effective than meropenem and carried a higher risk of nephrotoxicity [164].

The combination of colistin with meropenem in the treatment of infections caused by MDR GNB does not improve outcomes, reduce side effects, or prevent resistance development [165–167]. However, clinical guidelines recommend its use in combination with one or more additional antibiotics against CR-PA due to doubts about its standalone efficacy [168].

The RESTORE-IMI 1 Trial compared the combination of colistin and imipenem with imipenem–relebactam in an RCT involving infections caused by imipenem-resistant bacteria (predominantly *P. aeruginosa*). The results favored imipenem–relebactam in terms of clinical response, mortality, and nephrotoxicity [169].

6.5.3. Clinical Experience

Several case series have documented outcomes in patients with infections caused by MDR GNB treated with colistin, including *P. aeruginosa*, with cure rates of 74.6–79.1% and nephrotoxicity rates of 7.6–10% [170,171]. These results are acceptable, particularly in the absence of other therapeutic options. However, newer antibiotics with activity against MDR/XDR/DTR *P. aeruginosa* and improved safety profiles have been developed in recent years.

In a cohort study by Pogue et al., outcomes of treatments based on CFT-TAZ were compared with those based on colistin or aminoglycosides for MDR-PA infections (69% of patients in ICUs, 52% with VAP, and 42% meeting sepsis/shock criteria). The results were unfavorable for patients treated with colistin or aminoglycosides, showing lower clinical cure rates, higher risks of renal failure, and greater mortality [105]. Almangour et al. reported similar findings [148].

6.6. Fosfomycin

Fosfomycin, first marketed in 1969, is another antibiotic revived due to the emergence of MDR GNB [172].

It is a bactericidal antibiotic that inhibits the enzyme pyruvyltransferase (MurA), which is essential for the first step of peptidoglycan synthesis, making cross-resistance with other antibiotics unlikely [173]. Fosfomycin achieves high concentrations in serum and urine and penetrates well into various body compartments. Its activity may increase in acidic and anaerobic conditions, and it exhibits a post-antibiotic effect. The primary risks associated with its use are hypokalemia and sodium overload [172]. It has been used in the treatment of MDR or DTR *P. aeruginosa* infections as part of combination therapy regimens [94].

Resistance mechanisms to fosfomycin include reduced drug uptake due to mutations in transporters or alterations in biological systems regulating their expression, modifications of MurA, or the presence of fosfomycin-inactivating enzymes encoded by the fosA and fosB genes [174].

6.6.1. In Vitro Activity

The SENTRY surveillance program analyzed 141 *P. aeruginosa* isolates and found that 97.2% had an MIC ≤256 mg/L [175]. Additionally, 86.4% of *P. aeruginosa* strains evaluated in a Spanish multicenter study were susceptible, with an ECOFF of 128 mg/L [176].

A systematic review examining the role of fosfomycin in treating MDR non-fermenting GNB found that 30.2% of the 1693 MDR-PA isolates analyzed were susceptible [177]. Synergistic effects have been observed with beta-lactams, aminoglycosides, or quinolones in 53.5% of MDR-PA isolates [177], and synergy has also been demonstrated with ceftazidime–avibactam CAZ-AVI [178] and meropenem, with 100% of MDR-PA isolates showing synergy according to Albiero et al. [179].

Resistance emergence during treatment is the most feared complication and one of the reasons for recommending its use as part of a combination therapy [172].

6.6.2. Clinical Experience

A systematic review by Falagas et al. included only 33 patients with MDR-PA treated with fosfomycin (25 of them in combination therapy), reporting favorable outcomes in 90.9% of cases [177].

A study conducted in Thailand involving patients with pneumonia caused by CR-PA with intermediate sensitivity to doripenem compared two treatment regimens: high-dose doripenem in a 4 h infusion combined with fosfomycin versus colistin combined with fosfomycin in 49 patients. No differences were observed in mortality, clinical or microbiological cure, or adverse effects between the two groups [180].

Additionally, a case of meningitis caused by XDR-PA was successfully treated with high-dose CFT-TAZ and fosfomycin [181].

6.7. Imipenem–Relebactam

The most common resistance mechanisms to imipenem include the production of carbapenemases and the combination of reduced permeability due to porin alterations (OprD) with the overexpression of AmpC or ESBLs.

Relebactam is a potent non-beta-lactam beta-lactamase inhibitor. Its structure is related to that of avibactam but is distinguished by the addition of a piperidine ring to the carbonyl group at position 2. Relebactam's high reactivity, resulting from its chemical structure, leads to limited stability in the presence of bases or nucleophiles but simultaneously makes it a potent beta-lactamase inhibitor [182].

This novel combination of a beta-lactam and a beta-lactamase inhibitor has a broad spectrum of activity against Ambler class A beta-lactamases, including ESBLs and KPCs, as well as class C beta-lactamases (AmpC). However, it is ineffective against class B and class D carbapenemases [183,184].

The EMA has approved IMI-REL for hospital-acquired respiratory infections (nosocomial pneumonia and VAP), including secondary bacteremia, and infections caused by GNB when other treatments may be ineffective. The FDA has approved it for cUTI and cIAI.

6.7.1. In Vitro Activity

Adding relebactam reduces the MIC90 of imipenem-resistant *P. aeruginosa* isolates from 32 mg/L to 8 mg/L [161], restoring imipenem activity against 80% of imipenem non-susceptible *P. aeruginosa* strains [185].

IMI-REL has shown in vitro activity against 93.7% of 474 *P. aeruginosa* isolates from ICU patients in Spain and Portugal, including 94.1% of MDR-PA, 78.8% of XDR-PA, and 75% of DTR-PA [186].

It has also demonstrated high activity against *P. aeruginosa* strains resistant to CAZ-AVI or CFT-TAZ [187].

IMI-REL has demonstrated up to five times higher activity than imipenem alone against non-carbapenemase-producing CR-PA thanks to its high activity against the presence of AmpC-type beta-lactamases associated with impermeability and also against KPC-producing strain [188,189]. By adding relebactam, the proportion of CR-PA isolates (non-carbapenemase producers) susceptible to imipenem increases from 2% to 63%. Among these isolates, 98% and 80% are also susceptible to colistin and CFT-TAZ, respectively [190].

A Spanish study identified IMI-REL as the antibiotic with the highest activity against *P. aeruginosa*, with 97.3% effectiveness [191].

6.7.2. Clinical Evidence

In the RESTORE-IMI 1 Trial, IMI-REL was superior to the combination of colistin and imipenem for treating infections caused by imipenem-resistant bacteria (predominantly *P. aeruginosa*) in terms of clinical response, mortality, and nephrotoxicity [169].

The RESTORE-IMI 2 Trial demonstrated the non-inferiority of IMI-REL compared to piperacillin–tazobactam in treating nosocomial pneumonia, including VAP. Among 537 pneumonia cases included, 19% were caused by *P. aeruginosa*. In this subgroup, the all-cause mortality of patients treated with IMI-REL was 33.3%, with a favorable clinical response rate of 46.7%, compared to 12.0% and 68.0%, respectively, for infections treated with piperacillin–tazobactam [192].

6.7.3. Clinical Experience

There are limited real-world studies on the efficacy of IMI-REL. Recently, Leanza et al. published a single-center case series including five patients with DTR-PA infections treated with IMI-REL, reporting favorable outcomes [193].

6.8. Meropenem–Vaborbactam

Vaborbactam is an innovative beta-lactamase inhibitor characterized by its boron-ring structure, which provides significant activity against serine beta-lactamases, particularly KPC enzymes. This structural feature has been specifically developed to enhance the activity of carbapenems [194]. While vaborbactam lacks intrinsic antibacterial activity, its combination with meropenem significantly improves efficacy against GNB, particularly *Enterobacteriaceae* producing class A and C carbapenemases. However, this combination is ineffective against OXA-48 beta-lactamases and MBL [195].

MER-VAB has been approved by the FDA for the treatment of cUTIs and by the EMA for the treatment of cUTIs, cIAIs, and nosocomial pneumonia, including VAP. It is also indicated for infections caused by GNB when other antibiotics may not be appropriate.

6.8.1. In Vitro Activity

The contribution of vaborbactam to meropenem's activity against *Pseudomonas aeruginosa* is limited, as it does not counteract reduced permeability or increased efflux pump activity associated with meropenem resistance.

However, the overexpression of MexXY efflux pumps and AmpC enzymes may result in lower MICs for MER-VAB compared to meropenem alone [196]. In a study by Carvalhaes et al., MER-VAB was active against 59% of MDR-PA isolates recovered from pneumonia cases in U.S. hospitals, compared to 22.1% susceptibility to meropenem alone. This highlights the importance of understanding the microbiology and resistance mechanisms prevalent in specific units [162].

MER-VAB demonstrated activity against 82.1% of *P. aeruginosa* isolates (vs. 67.3% for meropenem alone) and 41.0% of MDR isolates (vs. 13.0% for meropenem alone) recovered from pneumonia (including VAP) cases in Europe [197].

6.8.2. Clinical Evidence

RCTs conducted with meropenem have not included infections caused by *P. aeruginosa* [198,199].

6.8.3. Clinical Experience

Published clinical experience with MER-VAB for *P. aeruginosa* infections is limited.

In a real-world analysis by Alosaimy et al., MER-VAB was used to treat eight MDR-PA infections, reporting a 30-day mortality rate of 0% and a 90-day mortality rate of 12.5% [200].

6.9. *New Antibiotics*

In addition to those previously described, other antibiotics have been studied and will soon be available to us [141].

6.9.1. Aztreonam–Avibactam

Aztreonam is stable against class B carbapenemases, and avibactam inhibits the action of class A, C, and D beta-lactamases. Aztreonam–avibactam is approved by the EMA for the treatment of cIAI and cUTI, nosocomial pneumonia, and infections caused by aerobic Gram-negative bacteria with limited treatment options.

The in vitro activity against *P. aeruginosa* is lower compared to other antibiotics, like CAZ-AVI, CFT-TAZ, or IMI-REL [201], but it may be useful for *P. aeruginosa* producing MBLs, like VIM or IMP [202,203].

The REVISIT Trial compared the treatment of patients with cIAI or nosocomial pneumonia/VAP with meropenem (with or without colistin) to treatment with aztreonam–avibactam. The results of both treatments were comparable, but patients with monomicrobial *P. aeruginosa* infections were excluded from this study [204].

With the data available now, treatment with aztreonam–avibactam seems a more favorable option for treating Enterobacteriaceae than for PA [205].

6.9.2. Cefepime–Enmetazobactam

Cefepime–Enmetazobactam has shown good results in an RCT when compared to piperacillin–tazobactam for the treatment of cUTIs [206]. However, the contribution of Enmetazobactam against the resistance mechanisms of *P. aeruginosa* is limited and does not enhance the spectrum of cefepime [207,208].

6.9.3. Cefepime–Taniborbactam

Taniborbactam is a potent beta-lactamase inhibitor with activity against class A, B, C, and D beta-lactamases. It has been shown to achieve 95% susceptibility against MDR-PA recovered from bacteremias in cancer patients, which is higher than its comparators (70% ceftazidime–avibactam, 65% ceftolozane–tazobactam, 65% amikacin) [209].

Cefepime–taniborbactam is active in vitro against 85.3% of meropenem-resistant *P. aeruginosa*, 79.6% of MER-VAB-resistant *P. aeruginosa*, 71.3% of CAZ-AVI-resistant *P. aeruginosa*, and 70.1% of CFT-TAZ-resistant *P. aeruginosa* [210]. It has been shown to be effective against 60% of carbapenemase-producing *P. aeruginosa* and 55.6% of MBL-producing strains, with 61.2–81.9% susceptibility to VIM and 93.3–98.8% to GES [210,211]. *P. aeruginosa's* resistance to cefepime–taniborbactam arises due to the accumulation of resistance mechanisms, such as porin mutations and PBP alterations, alongside carbapenemase production [210,212].

The CERTAIN-1 Trial showed better results (in a composite outcome of clinical and microbiological success) for patients with cUTIs treated with cefepime–taniborbactam compared to those treated with meropenem [213]. In this RCT, only twenty-three infections caused by *P. aeruginosa* were detected (sixteen in the cefepime–taniborbactam group, seven in the meropenem group), with cure rates above 80% [214]. The only patient with a *P. aeruginosa* infection caused by VIM, treated with cefepime–taniborbactam achieved clinical cure and microbiological eradication.

6.9.4. Cefepime–Zidebactam

The combination of cefepime with zidebactam, a beta-lactam enhancer, has shown efficacy in vitro against Enterobacteriaceae and *P. aeruginosa*. This combination maintains its activity in vitro in the presence of efflux pumps or the downregulation of OprD, but its MIC increases in the presence of AmpC [215]. Cefepime–zidebactam is active in vitro against a high percentage (78–97%) of CR-PA [215,216], including MBL producers [217], and against *P. aeruginosa* resistant to CAZ-AVI or CFT-TAZ [187].

Currently, there is limited clinical data on the activity of cefepime–zidebactam, mainly based on published case reports, where it is described as an effective rescue treatment for *P. aeruginosa* producing NDM [218–220].

6.9.5. Meropenem–Nacubactam

The efficacy of combining nacubactam, a non-beta-lactam beta-lactamase inhibitor, with meropenem is under investigation. Nacubactam is effective at inhibiting class A and C beta-lactamases and, to a lesser extent, class D. No clinical data are available yet, but the results from animal models are promising [221,222].

Figure 1 summarizes the activity of each antibiotic against each *P. aeruginosa* resistance mechanism.

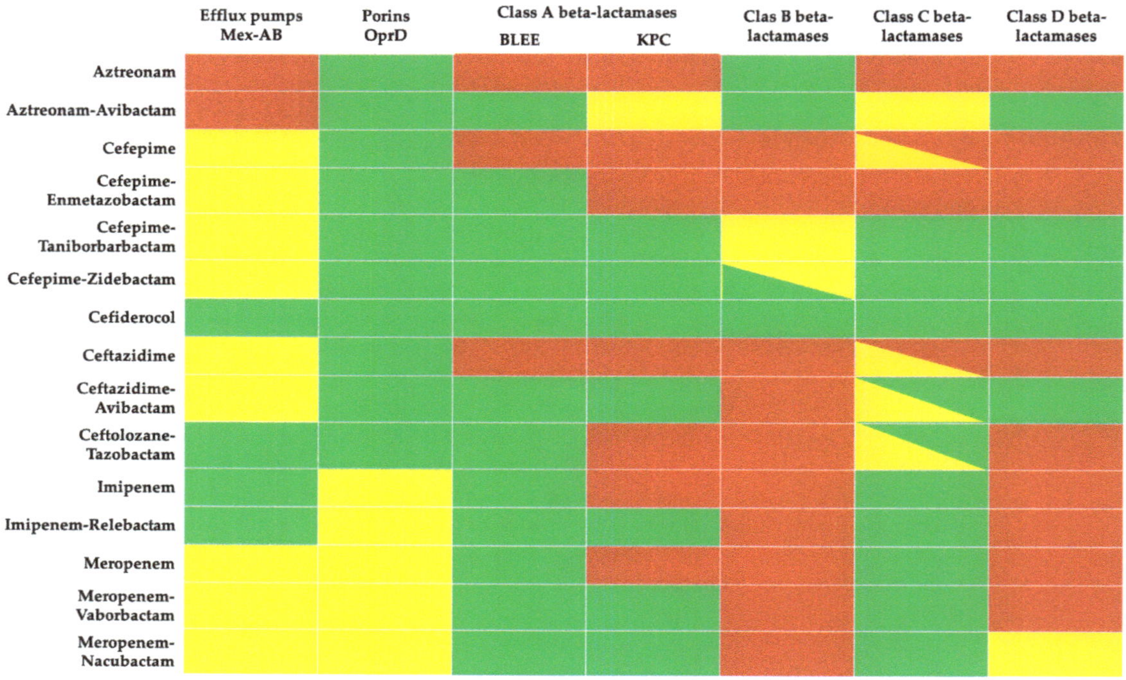

Figure 1. Antibiotic activity against *P. aeruginosa* resistance mechanisms (green: high activity, red: no activity, yellow: may be active).

7. Strategies to Optimize Antibiotic Treatment

The capacity of *P. aeruginosa* to develop antimicrobial resistance necessitates optimizing therapeutic regimens [223]. A critical factor is the accurate dosing of antibiotics. In Table 2, we can see the dosage of the reviewed antibiotics.

Table 2. Antibiotic dosage for the treatment of severe infections caused by DTR-PA.

Antibiotic	Dosage	pK/pD Target
Amikacin	25–30 mg/kg [1] (adjust according to levels)	C_{max}/MIC $\geq$ 8–10 $AUC_{0\text{-}24h}$/MIC 80–100
Aztreonam–Avibactam	0.5/0.167 g loading dose (30 min) 1.5/0.5 g (3 h infusion)/6 h	%fT > MIC
Cefepime–Enmetazobactam	2/0.5 g/8 h (2 h infusion)	$fAUC_{0\text{-}24h}$/MIC
Cefepime–Taniborbactam	2/0.5 g/8 h (2–4 h infusion)	$fAUC_{0\text{-}24h}$/MIC
Cefepime–Zidebactam	2/1 g/8 h	
Cefiderocol	2 g/8 h (2 g/6 h if GF > 120 mL/min) (3 h infusion)	%fT > 4 × MIC > 80%
Ceftazidime–Avibactam	2/0.5 g/8 h (2/0.5 g/6 h if GF > 130 mL/min) (3 h infusion)	100% fT > 4 × MIC
Ceftolozane–Tazobactam	1–2/0.5–1 g/ 8 h	100% fT > 4 × MIC
Colistin	9 MU (colistimethate), loading dose (0.5–1 h infusion) 4.5 MU/12 h (5.5 MU/12 h if GF $\geq$ 90 mL/min)	$fAUC_{0\text{-}24h}$/MIC $\geq$ 12

Table 2. *Cont.*

Antibiotic	Dosage	pK/pD Target
Fosfomycin	8 g loading dose 16–24 g as a continuous infusion/24 h	100% fT > MIC
Imipenem–Relebactam	500/250 mg/6 h (30 min infusion)	$fAUC_{0–24h}$/MIC
Meropenem–Vaborbactam	2/2 g/8 h (3 h infusion)	$fAUC_{0–24h}$/MIC
Tobramycin	6–7 mg/kg [1] (adjust according to levels)	C_{max}/MIC ≥ 8–10 $AUC_{0–24h}$/MIC 80–100

AUC: area under the curve, C_{max}: maximum concentration, MIC: Minimum Inhibitory Concentration, f: free fraction, T: time. [1] Adjusted body weight.

Additionally, various strategies have been evaluated to optimize the performance of these antibiotics, including prolonged infusion, combination therapy, and inhaled administration.

7.1. Prolonged Infusions

Prolonged, extended, and continuous infusions are strategies designed to achieve more aggressive pharmacokinetic/pharmacodynamic (pK/pD) targets for time-dependent antibiotics, such as beta-lactams. The pK/pD index that best predicts therapeutic success for these antibiotics is the percentage of time during which drug concentrations remain above the MIC (%fT > MIC). Traditionally, the target was set at 40–70% of the dosing interval (40–70% fT > MIC). However, maintaining drug concentrations at least four times above the MIC for the entirety (or most) of the dosing interval (100% T > 4 × MIC) has been shown to enhance efficacy. Some studies suggest that trough concentrations 3.5–5 times above the MIC could minimize resistance development in infections caused by Gram-negative bacteria [224–226].

Although definitive evidence linking extended infusions to reduced mortality is lacking, improved outcomes have been observed in critically ill patients and severe infections (e.g., respiratory infections or SOFA ≥ 9) [227], findings supported by several meta-analyses [228–230]. However, the MERCY Trial, published in 2023, included over 600 critically ill patients (20% with *P. aeruginosa* infections) and found no significant differences in mortality or resistance emergence between continuous and intermittent meropenem administration [231]. Prolonged infusion regimens are safe, and even reduced neurotoxicity has been reported with continuous cefepime infusion [232].

Extended infusions (3 h) of CFT-TAZ, CAZ-AVI, and cefiderocol are routinely recommended by clinical guidelines for treating severe infections with high bacterial burdens [45,233–235]. For infections caused by *P. aeruginosa* with elevated MICs or in sites with suboptimal drug penetration, prolonged infusion facilitates achieving pK/pD targets [236,237].

Although clinical superiority has not been conclusively demonstrated for prolonged CFT-TAZ infusions, theoretical advantages exist. Pilmis et al. prospectively analyzed 72 *P. aeruginosa*-infected patients (79% ICU, 66.7% respiratory focus), comparing intermittent (<1 h), extended (4 h), and continuous infusions of CFT-TAZ (2/1 g every 8 h). They found that intermittent infusions (<1 h) failed to achieve the 100% fT > 4 × MIC target when MICs were ≥4 mg/L, while continuous infusion reached the target even at MICs ≥ 8 mg/L [238].

Similarly, Montero et al. investigated in vitro the behavior of CFT-TAZ against three XDR-PA strains (MICs: 2, 8, 16 mg/L) under intermittent, extended, and continuous infusions. Continuous infusion provided the greatest reduction in bacterial density, especially in strains with higher MICs [239].

For CAZ-AVI, limited data are available regarding prolonged infusion's impact on *P. aeruginosa* infections. However, Tumbarello et al. found that continuous infusion of CAZ-

AVI reduced mortality in treating *Klebsiella pneumoniae* KPC producers [240]. Continuous infusion of CAZ-AVI also increases the likelihood of achieving pK/pD targets with lower doses in MDR Gram-negative infections [241].

A systematic review suggests the optimal dosing of fosfomycin as an 8 g loading dose followed by 16–24 g of continuous infusion every 24 h [242].

Despite limited evidence, a 2023 consensus document recommends extended or continuous beta-lactam infusions with a loading dose in critically ill patients, particularly for Gram-negative infections, to improve cure rates and reduce mortality. The document also suggests individualized therapeutic drug monitoring (TDM) for beta-lactams, although routine TDM is not universally recommended [243].

7.2. Combination Therapy

Combining antibiotics aims to achieve synergistic effects, improving patient outcomes or reducing the risk of resistance selection. Although evidence is limited, most studies report additive or synergistic effects when combining CFT-TAZ, CAZ-AVI, IMI-REL, or cefiderocol with agents like amikacin, colistin, fosfomycin, meropenem, or aztreonam [244–246].

CFT-TAZ shows synergy with aminoglycosides, even against CFT-TAZ-resistant and GES carbapenemase-producing strains [244,247,248]. An in vitro study using CFT-TAZ and meropenem against XDR-PA (ST 175) strains maintained bacterial suppression over 14 days, whereas monotherapy failed [249].

In in vitro mortality curve studies, a synergistic or additive effect of CAZ-AVI with colistin, aztreonam, amikacin, fosfomycin, and meropenem was observed, even in strains resistant to CAZ-AVI [250,251]. In the study by Mikhail et al., the combination of CAZ-AVI with meropenem demonstrated the greatest reduction in the MICs of CAZ-AVI against 21 MDR-PA isolates [250]. The combination of CAZ-AVI with imipenem or fosfomycin showed similar results against XDR-PA and MDR-PA (non-MBL producers) [178,252]. Against 18 *P. aeruginosa* strains producing GES-type carbapenemases, the combination of CAZ-AVI and meropenem has proven to be an alternative treatment, demonstrating activity against 100% of the strains [253].

The combination of CAZ-AVI and aztreonam showed in vitro efficacy against MBL-producing *P. aeruginosa* strains [251,254]. However, clinical evidence is very limited, and the data published in a systematic review conclude that the efficacy of this combination is greater against Enterobacteriaceae than against *P. aeruginosa* [205].

Synergy has been observed in the combination of CAZ-AVI with aztreonam and amikacin, and there are published cases in which its clinical efficacy against VIM-producing *P. aeruginosa* has been confirmed [255].

Gatti et al. found that continuous fosfomycin combined with extended cefiderocol or continuous CAZ-AVI achieved optimal pK/pD targets and microbiological eradication in five out of six patients with DTR-PA infections [256]. There is evidence to suggest that fosfomycin is more effective when used as part of a combination regimen [257].

A 2021 meta-analysis associated CFT-TAZ combination therapy with reduced all-cause mortality in Gram-negative infections but could not establish a clear link between combination therapy and improved clinical outcomes [258]. Another review comparing CAZ-AVI monotherapy and combination therapy in carbapenem-resistant Enterobacterales and *P. aeruginosa* found no differences in mortality, clinical cure, or resistance development [259].

To sum up, the use of prolonged infusions and/or the combination of synergistic drugs may be helpful in managing DTR-PA infections with low sensitivity to new beta-lactams and high inoculum. However, the available evidence is limited and of low quality.

7.3. Inhaled/Nebulized Therapy

Despite theoretical benefits, such as achieving high pulmonary antibiotic concentrations [260], the clinical advantages of inhaled antibiotic therapies remain unproven, and treatment guidelines do not recommend their use [45,235]. Most studies predate the introduction of newer beta-lactams and included heterogeneous populations with *P. aeruginosa* strains often only susceptible to colistin and aminoglycosides [261].

A 2011 systematic review limited the potential benefits of aerosolized therapy to inhaled colistin or aminoglycosides (always combined with systemic antibiotics) in treating MDR bacteria or poorly responding pneumonia [262], and findings were reiterated in 2017 [263].

Nebulized amikacin combined with systemic therapies in VAP was evaluated in a 2021 meta-analysis, showing improved microbiological eradication but no benefits in mortality, MV duration, or ICU length of stay [264]. The IASIS trial found no clinical benefits despite reduced bacterial loads with inhaled amikacin and fosfomycin [265].

The lack of benefit may stem from formulations not optimized for inhalation, compromising lung tissue penetration, even with appropriate nebulization devices. Furthermore, inhaled/nebulized therapies are not without adverse effects, primarily bronchospasm.

8. Guidelines and Recommendations

IDSA guidelines recommend the treatment of non-urinary tract infections caused by DTR-PA with ceftolozane–tazobactam, ceftazidime–avibactam, or imipenem–relebactam as the first options. They suggest cefiderocol as an alternative, which is the preferred option in cases of MBL production. If DTR-PA is susceptible to any of these antibiotics, monotherapy is recommended [266].

ESCMID guidelines, endorsed by ESICM, do not establish recommendations on the preferred treatment or new antibiotics and recommend using combination therapy in the case of severe CR-PA infections if treatment with aminoglycosides, colistin, or fosfomycin is required [235].

9. Treatment Proposal

When prescribing empirical antimicrobial treatment for an infection that may be caused by a DTR-PA in a critically ill patient, it is important to consider the microbiology of our ICU and the patient's colonization status.

As we have seen, risk factors and scores have low predictive value, so, before the microbiological results are available, it is not possible to determine whether the infection (for example, a VAP) is caused by *P. aeruginosa* or another GNB. Therefore, the resistance mechanisms present in the GNB in our unit must be taken into account. When establishing a threshold of 10%, as recommended by other authors [267], if the prevalence of carbapenemase-producing GNB exceeds 10% in our setting, we should prescribe treatment active against these carbapenemases. If it is below this 10%, our first option would be CFT-TAZ.

Similarly, if a critically ill patient is colonized by an MDR GNB and develops a severe infection, this must be considered, and treatment should be active against the bacteria colonizing the patient.

Figure 2 shows the proposed empirical treatment algorithm.

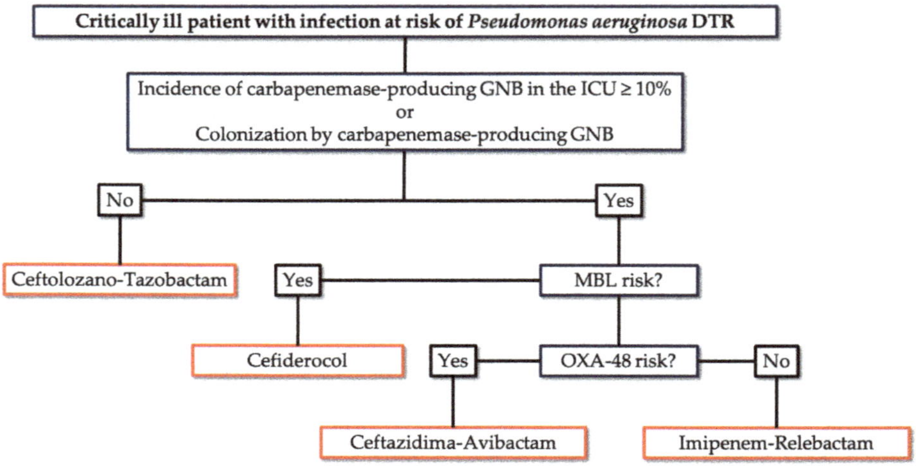

Figure 2. Empirical treatment algorithm for critically ill patients with infection at risk of difficult-to-treat *Peudomonas aeruginosa*.

Once the microbiological results are available, our order of preference, considering efficacy, the impact on antimicrobial flora, and antibiotic stewardship, would be CFT-TAZ, IMI-REL, CAZ-AVI, and cefiderocol (as long as its in vitro sensitivity has been demonstrated and regardless of the selected empirical treatment).

Both empirical and targeted treatments can be given as monotherapy, provided it is possible to treat with one of the first-line antibiotics (CFT-TAZ, IMI-REL, CAZ-AVI, or cefiderocol).

10. Conclusions

Infection by DTR-PA is a challenge in critically ill patients due to its severity or the difficulty in selecting an appropriate antibiotic treatment, both empirically and even when targeted. In this review, we have analyzed the available therapeutic options and propose a therapeutic algorithm to facilitate decision making, which should always be based on local resistance patterns.

Author Contributions: Conceptualization, P.V.-C.; investigation, P.V.-C., S.C.-F., E.C.-F., L.d.R.-C., P.F.-U., V.J.L.-C., J.N.-d.O., A.R.-V., and A.I.T.-V.; writing—original draft preparation, P.V.-C.; writing—review and editing, S.C.-F., E.C.-F., L.d.R.-C., P.F.-U., V.J.L.-C., J.N.-d.O., A.R.-V., and A.I.T.-V. All authors have read and agreed to the published version of the manuscript.

Funding: This research received no external funding.

Institutional Review Board Statement: Not applicable.

Informed Consent Statement: Not applicable.

Data Availability Statement: Not applicable.

Acknowledgments: We also acknowledge the use of the AI tool ChatGPT for language refinement and coherence in the preparation of this manuscript. The intellectual content, writing, analysis, and interpretations remain entirely the work of the authors.

Conflicts of Interest: P.V.-C. has received honoraria for lectures from Pfizer, MSD, Shionogi, and Menarini. The other authors declare no conflicts of interest.

References

1. Díaz Santos, E.; Mora Jiménez, C.; Del Río-Carbajo, L.; Vidal-Cortés, P. Treatment of severe multi-drug resistant *Pseudomonas aeruginosa* infections. *Med. Intensiv. (Engl. Ed.)* **2022**, *46*, 508–520. [CrossRef]
2. Segata, N.; Haake, S.K.; Mannon, P.; Lemon, K.P.; Waldron, L.; Gevers, D.; Huttenhower, C.; Izard, J. Composition of the adult digestive tract bacterial microbiome based on seven mouth surfaces, tonsils, throat and stool samples. *Genome Biol.* **2012**, *13*, R42. [CrossRef]
3. Mensa, J.; Barberán, J.; Soriano, A.; Llinares, P.; Marco, F.; Cantón, R.; Bou, G.; González Del Castillo, J.; Maseda, E.; Azanza, J.R.; et al. Antibiotic selection in the treatment of acute invasive infections by *Pseudomonas aeruginosa*: Guidelines by the Spanish Society of Chemotherapy. *Rev. Esp. Quimioter.* **2018**, *31*, 78–100.
4. WHO. Publishes List of Bacteria for Which New Antibiotics Are Urgently Needed [Internet]. Available online: https://www.who.int/news/item/27-02-2017-who-publishes-list-of-bacteria-for-which-new-antibiotics-are-urgently-needed (accessed on 22 November 2021).
5. World Health Organization. WHO Bacterial Priority Pathogens List, 2024: Bacterial Pathogens of Public Health Importance to Guide Research, Development and Strategies to Prevent and Control Antimicrobial Resistance. [Internet]. 2024. Available online: https://www.who.int/publications/i/item/9789240093461 (accessed on 5 November 2024).
6. Reynolds, D.; Kollef, M. The Epidemiology and Pathogenesis and Treatment of *Pseudomonas aeruginosa* Infections: An Update. *Drugs* **2021**, *81*, 2117–2131. [CrossRef] [PubMed]
7. Weiner-Lastinger, L.M.; Abner, S.; Edwards, J.R.; Kallen, A.J.; Karlsson, M.; Magill, S.S.; Pollock, D.; See, I.; Soe, M.M.; Walters, M.S.; et al. Antimicrobial-resistant pathogens associated with adult healthcare-associated infections: Summary of data reported to the National Healthcare Safety Network, 2015–2017. *Infect. Control Hosp. Epidemiol.* **2020**, *41*, 1–18. [CrossRef] [PubMed]
8. Vincent, J.-L.; Sakr, Y.; Singer, M.; Martin-Loeches, I.; Machado, F.R.; Marshall, J.C.; Finfer, S.; Pelosi, P.; Brazzi, L.; Aditianingsih, D.; et al. Prevalence and Outcomes of Infection Among Patients in Intensive Care Units in 2017. *JAMA* **2020**, *323*, 1478–1487. [CrossRef] [PubMed]
9. ENVIN-HELICS. Available online: https://hws.vhebron.net/envin-helics/ (accessed on 28 May 2024).
10. Bergin, S.P.; Coles, A.; Calvert, S.B.; Farley, J.; Powers, J.H.; Zervos, M.J.; Sims, M.; Kollef, M.H.; Durkin, M.J.; Kabchi, B.A.; et al. PROPHETIC: Prospective Identification of Pneumonia in Hospitalized Patients in the ICU. *Chest* **2020**, *158*, 2370–2380. [CrossRef]
11. Ibn Saied, W.; Mourvillier, B.; Cohen, Y.; Ruckly, S.; Reignier, J.; Marcotte, G.; Siami, S.; Bouadma, L.; Darmon, M.; de Montmollin, E.; et al. A Comparison of the Mortality Risk Associated with Ventilator-Acquired Bacterial Pneumonia and Nonventilator ICU-Acquired Bacterial Pneumonia. *Crit. Care Med.* **2019**, *47*, 345–352. [CrossRef]
12. Sader, H.S.; Castanheira, M.; Arends, S.J.R.; Goossens, H.; Flamm, R.K. Geographical and temporal variation in the frequency and antimicrobial susceptibility of bacteria isolated from patients hospitalized with bacterial pneumonia: Results from 20 years of the SENTRY Antimicrobial Surveillance Program (1997–2016). *J. Antimicrob. Chemother.* **2019**, *74*, 1595–1606. [CrossRef] [PubMed]
13. Moise, P.A.; Gonzalez, M.; Alekseeva, I.; Lopez, D.; Akrich, B.; DeRyke, C.A.; Chen, W.-T.; Pavia, J.; Palermo, B.; Hackel, M.; et al. Collective assessment of antimicrobial susceptibility among the most common Gram-negative respiratory pathogens driving therapy in the ICU. *JAC Antimicrob. Resist.* **2021**, *3*, dlaa129. [CrossRef] [PubMed]
14. Luyt, C.-E.; Sahnoun, T.; Gautier, M.; Vidal, P.; Burrel, S.; Pineton de Chambrun, M.; Chommeloux, J.; Desnos, C.; Arzoine, J.; Nieszkowska, A.; et al. Ventilator-associated pneumonia in patients with SARS-CoV-2-associated acute respiratory distress syndrome requiring ECMO: A retrospective cohort study. *Ann. Intensive Care* **2020**, *10*, 158. [CrossRef]
15. Contou, D.; Claudinon, A.; Pajot, O.; Micaëlo, M.; Longuet Flandre, P.; Dubert, M.; Cally, R.; Logre, E.; Fraissé, M.; Mentec, H.; et al. Bacterial and viral co-infections in patients with severe SARS-CoV-2 pneumonia admitted to a French ICU. *Ann. Intensive Care* **2020**, *10*, 119. [CrossRef]
16. European Centre for Disease Prevention Control. Healthcare-associated infections acquired in intensive care units. In *E.C.D.C. Annual Epidemiological Report for 2020*; ECDC: Stockholm, Sweden, 2024.
17. Mittal, R.; Aggarwal, S.; Sharma, S.; Chhibber, S.; Harjai, K. Urinary tract infections caused by *Pseudomonas aeruginosa*: A minireview. *J. Infect. Public Health* **2009**, *2*, 101–111. [CrossRef] [PubMed]
18. Elgohari, S.; Wilson, J.; Saei, A.; Sheridan, E.A.; Lamagni, T. Impact of national policies on the microbial aetiology of surgical site infections in acute NHS hospitals in England: Analysis of trends between 2000 and 2013 using multi-centre prospective cohort data. *Epidemiol. Infect.* **2017**, *145*, 957–969. [CrossRef]
19. Tabah, A.; Buetti, N.; Staiquly, Q.; Ruckly, S.; Akova, M.; Aslan, A.T.; Leone, M.; Conway Morris, A.; Bassetti, M.; Arvaniti, K.; et al. Epidemiology and outcomes of hospital-acquired bloodstream infections in intensive care unit patients: The EUROBACT-2 international cohort study. *Intensive Care Med.* **2023**, *49*, 178–190. [CrossRef] [PubMed]
20. Giacobbe, D.R.; Battaglini, D.; Ball, L.; Brunetti, I.; Bruzzone, B.; Codda, G.; Crea, F.; De Maria, A.; Dentone, C.; Di Biagio, A.; et al. Bloodstream infections in critically ill patients with COVID-19. *Eur. J. Clin. Investig.* **2020**, *50*, e13319. [CrossRef] [PubMed]

21. Martínez Pérez-Crespo, P.M.; Rojas, Á.; Lanz-García, J.F.; Retamar-Gentil, P.; Reguera-Iglesias, J.M.; Lima-Rodríguez, O.; Del Arco Jiménez, A.; Fernández Suárez, J.; Jover-Saenz, A.; Goikoetxea Aguirre, J.; et al. *Pseudomonas aeruginosa* Community-Onset Bloodstream Infections: Characterization, Diagnostic Predictors, and Predictive Score Development-Results from the PRO-BAC Cohort. *Antibiotics* **2022**, *11*, 707. [CrossRef]
22. Ewig, S.; Ruiz, M.; Mensa, J.; Marcos, M.A.; Martinez, J.A.; Arancibia, F.; Niederman, M.S.; Torres, A. Severe community-acquired pneumonia. Assessment of severity criteria. *Am. J. Respir. Crit. Care Med.* **1998**, *158*, 1102–1108. [CrossRef]
23. Cillóniz, C.; Dominedò, C.; Garcia-Vidal, C.; Torres, A. Community-acquired pneumonia as an emergency condition. *Curr. Opin. Crit. Care* **2018**, *24*, 531–539. [CrossRef] [PubMed]
24. Aurora, A.; Le, T.D.; Akers, K.S.; Blyth, D.M.; Graybill, J.C.; Clemens, M.S.; Chung, K.K.; Rizzo, J.A. Recurrent bacteremia: A 10-year retrospective study in combat-related burn casualties. *Burns* **2019**, *45*, 579–588. [CrossRef] [PubMed]
25. Döring, G.; Hoiby, N.; Consensus Study Group. Early intervention and prevention of lung disease in cystic fibrosis: A European consensus. *J. Cyst. Fibros.* **2004**, *3*, 67–91. [CrossRef] [PubMed]
26. Sanders, D.B.; Fink, A.K. Background and Epidemiology. *Pediatr. Clin. N. Am.* **2016**, *63*, 567–584. [CrossRef] [PubMed]
27. Salsgiver, E.L.; Fink, A.K.; Knapp, E.A.; LiPuma, J.J.; Olivier, K.N.; Marshall, B.C.; Saiman, L. Changing Epidemiology of the Respiratory Bacteriology of Patients with Cystic Fibrosis. *Chest* **2016**, *149*, 390–400. [CrossRef]
28. Crull, M.R.; Somayaji, R.; Ramos, K.J.; Caldwell, E.; Mayer-Hamblett, N.; Aitken, M.L.; Nichols, D.P.; Rowhani-Rahbar, A.; Goss, C.H. Changing Rates of Chronic *Pseudomonas aeruginosa* Infections in Cystic Fibrosis: A Population-Based Cohort Study. *Clin. Infect. Dis.* **2018**, *67*, 1089–1095. [CrossRef] [PubMed]
29. Hatziagorou, E.; Orenti, A.; Drevinek, P.; Kashirskaya, N.; Mei-Zahav, M.; De Boeck, K. Changing epidemiology of the respiratory bacteriology of patients with cystic fibrosis-data from the European cystic fibrosis society patient registry. *J. Cyst. Fibros.* **2020**, *19*, 376–383. [CrossRef] [PubMed]
30. Bilton, D. Update on non-cystic fibrosis bronchiectasis. *Curr. Opin. Pulm. Med.* **2008**, *14*, 595–599. [CrossRef]
31. López-Causapé, C.; Cabot, G.; Del Barrio-Tofiño, E.; Oliver, A. The Versatile Mutational Resistome of *Pseudomonas aeruginosa*. *Front. Microbiol.* **2018**, *9*, 685. [CrossRef] [PubMed]
32. Prestel, C.; Moulton-Meissner, H.; Gable, P.; Stanton, R.A.; Glowicz, J.; Franco, L.; McConnell, M.; Torres, T.; John, D.; Blackwell, G.; et al. Dialysis Water Supply Faucet as Reservoir for Carbapenemase-Producing *Pseudomonas aeruginosa*. *Emerg. Infect. Dis.* **2022**, *28*, 2069–2073. [CrossRef] [PubMed]
33. versen, B.G.; Eriksen, H.-M.; Bø, G.; Hagestad, K.; Jacobsen, T.; Engeset, E.; Lassen, J.; Aavitsland, P. *Pseudomonas aeruginosa* contamination of mouth swabs during production causing a major outbreak. *Ann. Clin. Microbiol. Antimicrob.* **2007**, *6*, 3.
34. Do Rego, H.; Timsit, J.F. Management strategies for severe *Pseudomonas aeruginosa* infections. *Curr. Opin. Infect. Dis.* **2023**, *36*, 585–595. [CrossRef]
35. Bassetti, M.; Vena, A.; Russo, A.; Croxatto, A.; Calandra, T.; Guery, B. Rational approach in the management of *Pseudomonas aeruginosa* infections. *Curr. Opin. Infect. Dis.* **2018**, *31*, 578–586. [CrossRef] [PubMed]
36. Bassetti, M.; Vena, A.; Croxatto, A.; Righi, E.; Guery, B. How to manage *Pseudomonas aeruginosa* infections. *Drugs Context* **2018**, *7*, 212527. [CrossRef] [PubMed]
37. Torrens, G.; van der Schalk, T.E.; Cortes-Lara, S.; Timbermont, L.; Del Barrio-Tofiño, E.; Xavier, B.B.; Zamorano, L.; Lammens, C.; Ali, O.; Ruzin, A.; et al. Susceptibility profiles and resistance genomics of *Pseudomonas aeruginosa* isolates from European ICUs participating in the ASPIRE-ICU trial. *J. Antimicrob. Chemother.* **2022**, *77*, 1862–1872. [CrossRef] [PubMed]
38. O'Donnell, J.N.; Bidell, M.R.; Lodise, T.P. Approach to the Treatment of Patients with Serious Multidrug-Resistant *Pseudomonas aeruginosa* Infections. *Pharmacotherapy* **2020**, *40*, 952–969. [CrossRef] [PubMed]
39. Giovagnorio, F.; De Vito, A.; Madeddu, G.; Parisi, S.G.; Geremia, N. Resistance in *Pseudomonas aeruginosa*: A Narrative Review of Antibiogram Interpretation and Emerging Treatments. *Antibiotics* **2023**, *12*, 1621. [CrossRef]
40. Livermore, D.M. Interplay of impermeability and chromosomal beta-lactamase activity in imipenem-resistant *Pseudomonas aeruginosa*. *Antimicrob. Agents Chemother.* **1992**, *36*, 2046–2048. [CrossRef]
41. Botelho, J.; Grosso, F.; Peixe, L. Antibiotic resistance in *Pseudomonas aeruginosa*—Mechanisms, epidemiology and evolution. *Drug Resist. Updates* **2019**, *44*, 100640. [CrossRef] [PubMed]
42. Pang, Z.; Raudonis, R.; Glick, B.R.; Lin, T.J.; Cheng, Z. Antibiotic resistance in *Pseudomonas aeruginosa*: Mechanisms and alternative therapeutic strategies. *Biotechnol. Adv.* **2019**, *37*, 177–192. [CrossRef] [PubMed]
43. Magiorakos, A.-P.; Srinivasan, A.; Carey, R.B.; Carmeli, Y.; Falagas, M.E.; Giske, C.G.; Harbarth, S.; Hindler, J.F.; Kahlmeter, G.; Olsson-Liljequist, B.; et al. Multidrug-resistant, extensively drug-resistant and pandrug-resistant bacteria: An international expert proposal for interim standard definitions for acquired resistance. *Clin. Microbiol. Infect.* **2012**, *18*, 268–281. [CrossRef] [PubMed]
44. Kadri, S.S.; Adjemian, J.; Lai, Y.L.; Spaulding, A.B.; Ricotta, E.; Prevots, D.R.; Palmore, T.N.; Rhee, C.; Klompas, M.; Dekker, J.P.; et al. Difficult-to-Treat Resistance in Gram-negative Bacteremia at 173 US Hospitals: Retrospective Cohort Analysis of Prevalence, Predictors, and Outcome of Resistance to All First-line Agents. *Clin. Infect. Dis.* **2018**, *67*, 1803–1814. [CrossRef] [PubMed]

45. Tamma, P.D.; Aitken, S.L.; Bonomo, R.A.; Mathers, A.J.; van Duin, D.; Clancy, C.J. Infectious Diseases Society of America 2022 Guidance on the Treatment of Extended-Spectrum β-lactamase Producing Enterobacterales (ESBL-E), Carbapenem-Resistant Enterobacterales (CRE), and *Pseudomonas aeruginosa* with Difficult-to-Treat Resistance (DTR-*P. aeruginosa*). *Clin. Infect. Dis.* **2022**, *75*, 187–212. [PubMed]
46. Kanj, S.S.; Bassetti, M.; Kiratisin, P.; Rodrigues, C.; Villegas, M.V.; Yu, Y.; van Duin, D. Clinical data from studies involving novel antibiotics to treat multidrug-resistant Gram-negative bacterial infections. *Int. J. Antimicrob. Agents* **2022**, *60*, 106633. [CrossRef]
47. Del Barrio-Tofiño, E.; Zamorano, L.; Cortes-Lara, S.; López-Causapé, C.; Sánchez-Diener, I.; Cabot, G.; Bou, G.; Martínez-Martínez, L.; Oliver, A.; GEMARA-SEIMC/REIPI Pseudomonas study Group. Spanish nationwide survey on *Pseudomonas aeruginosa* antimicrobial resistance mechanisms and epidemiology. *J. Antimicrob. Chemother.* **2019**, *74*, 1825–1835. [CrossRef] [PubMed]
48. Rosenthal, V.D.; Bat-Erdene, I.; Gupta, D.; Belkebir, S.; Rajhans, P.; Zand, F.; Myatra, S.N.; Afeef, M.; Tanzi, V.L.; Muralidharan, S.; et al. International Nosocomial Infection Control Consortium (INICC) report, data summary of 45 countries for 2012–2017: Device-associated module. *Am. J. Infect. Control* **2020**, *48*, 423–432. [CrossRef] [PubMed]
49. Sader, H.S.; Carvalhaes, C.G.; Shortridge, D.; Castanheira, M. Comparative activity of newer β-lactam/β-lactamase inhibitor combinations against *Pseudomonas aeruginosa* from patients hospitalized with pneumonia in European medical centers in 2020. *Eur. J. Clin. Microbiol. Infect. Dis.* **2022**, *41*, 319–324. [CrossRef]
50. Fernández-Esgueva, M.; López-Calleja, A.I.; Mulet, X.; Fraile-Ribot, P.A.; Cabot, G.; Huarte, R.; Rezusta, A.; Oliver, A. Characterization of AmpC β-lactamase mutations of extensively drug-resistant *Pseudomonas aeruginosa* isolates that develop resistance to ceftolozane/tazobactam during therapy. *Enferm. Infecc. Microbiol. Clin. (Engl. Ed.)* **2020**, *38*, 474–478. [CrossRef] [PubMed]
51. Arca-Suárez, J.; Vázquez-Ucha, J.C.; Fraile-Ribot, P.A.; Lence, E.; Cabot, G.; Martínez-Guitián, M.; Lasarte-Monterrubio, C.; Rodríguez-Iglesias, M.; Beceiro, A.; González-Bello, C.; et al. Molecular and biochemical insights into the in vivo evolution of AmpC-mediated resistance to ceftolozane/tazobactam during treatment of an MDR *Pseudomonas aeruginosa* infection. *J. Antimicrob. Chemother.* **2020**, *75*, 3209–3217. [CrossRef]
52. Fournier, D.; Carrière, R.; Bour, M.; Grisot, E.; Triponney, P.; Muller, C.; Lemoine, J.; Jeannot, K.; Plésiat, P. Mechanisms of Resistance to Ceftolozane/Tazobactam in *Pseudomonas aeruginosa*: Results of the GERPA Multicenter Study. *Antimicrob. Agents Chemother.* **2021**, *65*, e01117-20. [CrossRef] [PubMed]
53. Ruedas-López, A.; Alonso-García, I.; Lasarte-Monterrubio, C.; Guijarro-Sánchez, P.; Gato, E.; Vázquez-Ucha, J.C.; Vallejo, J.A.; Fraile-Ribot, P.A.; Fernández-Pérez, B.; Velasco, D.; et al. Selection of AmpC β-Lactamase Variants and Metallo-β-Lactamases Leading to Ceftolozane/Tazobactam and Ceftazidime/Avibactam Resistance during Treatment of MDR/XDR *Pseudomonas aeruginosa* Infections. *Antimicrob. Agents Chemother.* **2022**, *66*, e0206721. [CrossRef]
54. Candel, F.J.; Santerre Henriksen, A.; Longshaw, C.; Yamano, Y.; Oliver, A. In vitro activity of the novel siderophore cephalosporin, cefiderocol, in Gram-negative pathogens in Europe by site of infection. *Clin. Microbiol. Infect.* **2022**, *28*, 447.e1–447.e6. [CrossRef] [PubMed]
55. PÉrez-VÁzquez, M.; Sola-Campoy, P.J.; Zurita, Á.M.; Ávila, A.; GÓmez-Bertomeu, F.; SolÍs, S.; LÓpez-Urrutia, L.; GÓnzalez-BarberÁ, E.M.; Cercenado, E.; Bautista, V.; et al. Carbapenemase-producing *Pseudomonas aeruginosa* in Spain: Interregional dissemination of the high-risk clones ST175 and ST244 carrying blaVIM-2, blaVIM-1, blaIMP-8, blaVIM-20 and blaKPC-2. *Int. J. Antimicrob. Agents* **2020**, *56*, 106026. [CrossRef] [PubMed]
56. Simner, P.J.; Beisken, S.; Bergman, Y.; Posch, A.E.; Cosgrove, S.E.; Tamma, P.D. Cefiderocol Activity Against Clinical *Pseudomonas aeruginosa* Isolates Exhibiting Ceftolozane-Tazobactam Resistance. *Open Forum Infect. Dis.* **2021**, *8*, ofab311. [CrossRef]
57. Lee, Y.L.; Ko, W.C.; Hsueh, P.R. In vitro activities of ceftazidime-avibactam, ceftolozane-tazobactam, meropenem-vaborbactam and other comparators against *Pseudomonas aeruginosa* isolates with discrepant resistance to carbapenems: Data from the Antimicrobial Testing Leadership and Surveillance (ATLAS) program, 2012–2021. *Int. J. Antimicrob. Agents.* **2023**, *62*, 106867. [PubMed]
58. Carrillo-Larco, R.M.; Anza-Ramírez, C.; Saal-Zapata, G.; Villarreal-Zegarra, D.; Zafra-Tanaka, J.H.; Ugarte-Gil, C.; Bernabé-Ortiz, A. Type 2 diabetes mellitus and antibiotic-resistant infections: A systematic review and meta-analysis. *J. Epidemiol. Community Health* **2022**, *76*, 75–84. [CrossRef]
59. Lee, Y.L.; Ko, W.C.; Hsueh, P.R. Geographic Patterns of Carbapenem-Resistant *Pseudomonas aeruginosa* in the Asia-Pacific Region: Results from the Antimicrobial Testing Leadership and Surveillance (ATLAS) Program, 2015–2019. *Antimicrob. Agents Chemother.* **2022**, *66*, e0200021. [CrossRef] [PubMed]
60. Weiner, L.M.; Webb, A.K.; Limbago, B.; Dudeck, M.A.; Patel, J.; Kallen, A.J.; Edwards, J.R.; Sievert, D.M. Antimicrobial-Resistant Pathogens Associated with Healthcare-Associated Infections: Summary of Data Reported to the National Healthcare Safety Network at the Centers for Disease Control and Prevention, 2011–2014. *Infect. Control Hosp. Epidemiol.* **2016**, *37*, 1288–1301. [CrossRef] [PubMed]
61. Blomquist, K.C.; Nix, D.E. A Critical Evaluation of Newer β-Lactam Antibiotics for Treatment of *Pseudomonas aeruginosa* Infections. *Ann. Pharmacother.* **2021**, *55*, 1010–1024. [CrossRef]

62. Sastre-Femenia, M.À.; Fernández-Muñoz, A.; Gomis-Font, M.A.; Taltavull, B.; López-Causapé, C.; Arca-Suárez, J.; Martínez-Martínez, L.; Cantón, R.; Larrosa, N.; Oteo-Iglesias, J.; et al. *Pseudomonas aeruginosa* antibiotic susceptibility profiles, genomic epidemiology and resistance mechanisms: A nation-wide five-year time lapse analysis. *Lancet Reg. Health Eur.* **2023**, *34*, 100736. [CrossRef] [PubMed]
63. Cillóniz, C.; Dominedò, C.; Torres, A. Multidrug Resistant Gram-Negative Bacteria in Community-Acquired Pneumonia. *Crit. Care* **2019**, *23*, 79. [CrossRef] [PubMed]
64. Zaragoza, R.; Vidal-Cortés, P.; Aguilar, G.; Borges, M.; Diaz, E.; Ferrer, R.; Maseda, E.; Nieto, M.; Nuvials, F.X.; Ramirez, P.; et al. Update of the treatment of nosocomial pneumonia in the ICU. *Crit. Care* **2020**, *24*, 383. [CrossRef] [PubMed]
65. Kollef, M.H.; Chastre, J.; Fagon, J.-Y.; François, B.; Niederman, M.S.; Rello, J.; Torres, A.; Vincent, J.-L.; Wunderink, R.G.; Go, K.W.; et al. Global prospective epidemiologic and surveillance study of ventilator-associated pneumonia due to *Pseudomonas aeruginosa*. *Crit. Care Med.* **2014**, *42*, 2178–2187. [CrossRef] [PubMed]
66. Ibrahim, D.; Jabbour, J.F.; Kanj, S.S. Current choices of antibiotic treatment for *Pseudomonas aeruginosa* infections. *Curr. Opin. Infect. Dis.* **2020**, *33*, 464–473. [CrossRef]
67. Raman, G.; Avendano, E.E.; Chan, J.; Merchant, S.; Puzniak, L. Risk factors for hospitalized patients with resistant or multidrug-resistant *Pseudomonas aeruginosa* infections: A systematic review and meta-analysis. *Antimicrob. Resist. Infect. Control* **2018**, *7*, 79. [CrossRef] [PubMed]
68. Khadem, T.; Stevens, V.; Holt, K.; Hoffmann, C.; Dumyati, G.; Brown, J. Risk factors for carbapenem-nonsusceptible *Pseudomonas aeruginosa*: Case-control study. *Diagn. Microbiol. Infect. Dis.* **2017**, *89*, 146–150. [CrossRef]
69. Hernández-Jiménez, P.; López-Medrano, F.; Fernández-Ruiz, M.; Silva, J.T.; Corbella, L.; San-Juan, R.; Lizasoain, M.; Díaz-Regañón, J.; Viedma, E.; Aguado, J.M. Risk Factors and Outcomes for Multidrug Resistant *Pseudomonas aeruginosa* Infection in Immunocompromised Patients. *Antibiotics* **2022**, *11*, 1459. [CrossRef] [PubMed]
70. Walters, M.S.; Grass, J.E.; Bulens, S.N.; Hancock, E.B.; Phipps, E.C.; Muleta, D.; Mounsey, J.; Kainer, M.A.; Concannon, C.; Dumyati, G.; et al. Carbapenem-Resistant *Pseudomonas aeruginosa* at US Emerging Infections Program Sites, 2015. *Emerg. Infect. Dis.* **2019**, *25*, 1281–1288. [CrossRef] [PubMed]
71. Wei, X.; Li, L.; Li, M.; Liang, H.; He, Y.; Li, S. Risk Factors and Outcomes of Patients with Carbapenem-Resistant *Pseudomonas aeruginosa* Bloodstream Infection. *Infect. Drug. Resist.* **2023**, *16*, 337–346. [CrossRef]
72. Herrera, S.; Morata, L.; Sempere, A.; Verdejo, M.; Del Rio, A.; Martínez, J.A.; Cuervo, G.; Hernández-Meneses, M.; Chumbita, M.; Pitart, C.; et al. *Pseudomonas aeruginosa* Bloodstream Infection, Resistance, and Mortality: Do Solid Organ Transplant Recipients Do Better or Worse? *Antibiotics* **2023**, *12*, 380. [CrossRef]
73. Palavutitotai, N.; Jitmuang, A.; Tongsai, S.; Kiratisin, P.; Angkasekwinai, N. Epidemiology and risk factors of extensively drug-resistant *Pseudomonas aeruginosa* infections. *PLoS ONE* **2018**, *13*, e0193431. [CrossRef] [PubMed]
74. Fernández-Barat, L.; Ferrer, M.; De Rosa, F.; Gabarrús, A.; Esperatti, M.; Terraneo, S.; Rinaudo, M.; Li Bassi, G.; Torres, A. Intensive care unit-acquired pneumonia due to *Pseudomonas aeruginosa* with and without multidrug resistance. *J. Infect.* **2017**, *74*, 142–152. [CrossRef] [PubMed]
75. Alonso, B.; Fernández-Barat, L.; Di Domenico, E.G.; Marín, M.; Cercenado, E.; Merino, I.; de Pablos, M.; Muñoz, P.; Guembe, M. Characterization of the virulence of *Pseudomonas aeruginosa* strains causing ventilator-associated pneumonia. *BMC Infect. Dis.* **2020**, *20*, 909.
76. Lodise, T.P.; Bonine, N.G.; Ye, J.M.; Folse, H.J.; Gillard, P. Development of a bedside tool to predict the probability of drug-resistant pathogens among hospitalized adult patients with gram-negative infections. *BMC Infect. Dis.* **2019**, *19*, 718. [CrossRef] [PubMed]
77. Ferrer, R.; Soriano, A.; Cantón, R.; Del Pozo, J.L.; García-Vidal, C.; Garnacho-Montero, J.; Larrosa, N.; Rascado, P.; Salavert, M.; Pintado, V.; et al. A systematic literature review and expert consensus on risk factors associated to infection progression in adult patients with respiratory tract or rectal colonisation by carbapenem-resistant Gram-negative bacteria. *Rev. Esp. Quimioter.* **2022**, *35*, 455–467. [CrossRef] [PubMed]
78. Tartof, S.Y.; Kuntz, J.L.; Chen, L.H.; Wei, R.; Puzniak, L.; Tian, Y.; Im, T.M.; Takhar, H.S.; Merchant, S.; Lodise, T. Development and Assessment of Risk Scores for Carbapenem and Extensive β-Lactam Resistance Among Adult Hospitalized Patients with *Pseudomonas aeruginosa* Infection. *JAMA Netw. Open* **2018**, *1*, e183927. [CrossRef]
79. Thaden, J.T.; Park, L.P.; Maskarinec, S.A.; Ruffin, F.; Fowler, V.G.; van Duin, D. Results from a 13-Year Prospective Cohort Study Show Increased Mortality Associated with Bloodstream Infections Caused by *Pseudomonas aeruginosa* Compared to Other Bacteria. *Antimicrob. Agents Chemother.* **2017**, *61*, e02671-16. [CrossRef]
80. Babich, T.; Naucler, P.; Valik, J.K.; Giske, C.G.; Benito, N.; Cardona, R.; Rivera, A.; Pulcini, C.; Fattah, M.A.; Haquin, J.; et al. Risk factors for mortality among patients with *Pseudomonas aeruginosa* bacteraemia: A retrospective multicentre study. *Int. J. Antimicrob. Agents* **2020**, *55*, 105847. [CrossRef]
81. Kern, W.V.; Roth, J.A.; Bertz, H.; Götting, T.; Dettenkofer, M.; Widmer, A.F.; Theilacker, C. Contribution of specific pathogens to bloodstream infection mortality in neutropenic patients with hematologic malignancies: Results from a multicentric surveillance cohort study. *Transpl. Infect. Dis.* **2019**, *21*, e13186. [CrossRef]

82. Prina, E.; Ranzani, O.T.; Polverino, E.; Cillóniz, C.; Ferrer, M.; Fernandez, L.; Puig de la Bellacasa, J.; Menéndez, R.; Mensa, J.; Torres, A. Risk factors associated with potentially antibiotic-resistant pathogens in community-acquired pneumonia. *Ann. Am. Thorac. Soc.* **2015**, *12*, 153–160. [CrossRef] [PubMed]
83. Micek, S.T.; Wunderink, R.G.; Kollef, M.H.; Chen, C.; Rello, J.; Chastre, J.; Antonelli, M.; Welte, T.; Clair, B.; Ostermann, H.; et al. An international multicenter retrospective study of *Pseudomonas aeruginosa* nosocomial pneumonia: Impact of multidrug resistance. *Crit. Care* **2015**, *19*, 219. [CrossRef]
84. Peng, Y.; Bi, J.; Shi, J.; Li, Y.; Ye, X.; Chen, X.; Yao, Z. Multidrug-resistant *Pseudomonas aeruginosa* infections pose growing threat to health care-associated infection control in the hospitals of Southern China: A case-control surveillance study. *Am. J. Infect. Control* **2014**, *42*, 1308–1311. [CrossRef] [PubMed]
85. Lucena, A.; Dalla Costa, L.M.; Nogueira, K.S.; Matos, A.P.; Gales, A.C.; Paganini, M.C.; Castro, M.E.S.; Raboni, S. Nosocomial infections with metallo-beta-lactamase-producing *Pseudomonas aeruginosa*: Molecular epidemiology, risk factors, clinical features and outcomes. *J. Hosp. Infect.* **2014**, *87*, 234–240. [CrossRef] [PubMed]
86. ighi, E.; Peri, A.M.; Harris, P.N.A.; Wailan, A.M.; Liborio, M.; Lane, S.W.; Paterson, D.L. Global prevalence of carbapenem resistance in neutropenic patients and association with mortality and carbapenem use: Systematic review and meta-analysis. *J. Antimicrob. Chemother.* **2017**, *72*, 668–677.
87. Reyes, J.; Komarow, L.; Chen, L.; Ge, L.; Hanson, B.M.; Cober, E.; Herc, E.; Alenazi, T.; Kaye, K.S.; Garcia-Diaz, J.; et al. Global epidemiology and clinical outcomes of carbapenem-resistant *Pseudomonas aeruginosa* and associated carbapenemases (POP): A prospective cohort study. *Lancet Microbe* **2023**, *4*, e159-70. [CrossRef] [PubMed]
88. Tabak, Y.P.; Merchant, S.; Ye, G.; Vankeepuram, L.; Gupta, V.; Kurtz, S.G.; Puzniak, L.A. Incremental clinical and economic burden of suspected respiratory infections due to multi-drug-resistant *Pseudomonas aeruginosa* in the United States. *J. Hosp. Infect.* **2019**, *103*, 134–141. [CrossRef] [PubMed]
89. Tumbarello, M.; De Pascale, G.; Trecarichi, E.M.; Spanu, T.; Antonicelli, F.; Maviglia, R.; Pennisi, M.A.; Bello, G.; Antonelli, M. Clinical outcomes of *Pseudomonas aeruginosa* pneumonia in intensive care unit patients. *Intensive Care Med.* **2013**, *39*, 682–692. [CrossRef] [PubMed]
90. Paulsson, M.; Granrot, A.; Ahl, J.; Tham, J.; Resman, F.; Riesbeck, K.; Månsson, F. Antimicrobial combination treatment including ciprofloxacin decreased the mortality rate of *Pseudomonas aeruginosa* bacteraemia: A retrospective cohort study. *Eur. J. Clin. Microbiol. Infect. Dis.* **2017**, *36*, 1187–1196. [CrossRef] [PubMed]
91. Peña, C.; Cabot, G.; Gómez-Zorrilla, S.; Zamorano, L.; Ocampo-Sosa, A.; Murillas, J.; Almirante, B.; Pomar, V.; Aguilar, M.; Granados, A.; et al. Influence of virulence genotype and resistance profile in the mortality of *Pseudomonas aeruginosa* bloodstream infections. *Clin. Infect. Dis.* **2015**, *60*, 539–548. [CrossRef]
92. Zhang, Y.; Chen, X.-L.; Huang, A.-W.; Liu, S.-L.; Liu, W.-J.; Zhang, N.; Lu, X.-Z. Mortality attributable to carbapenem-resistant *Pseudomonas aeruginosa* bacteremia: A meta-analysis of cohort studies. *Emerg. Microbes Infect.* **2016**, *5*, e27. [CrossRef]
93. Juan, C.; Peña, C.; Oliver, A. Host and Pathogen Biomarkers for Severe *Pseudomonas aeruginosa* Infections. *J. Infect. Dis.* **2017**, *215* (Suppl. S1), S44–S51. [CrossRef] [PubMed]
94. Horcajada, J.P.; Montero, M.; Oliver, A.; Sorlí, L.; Luque, S.; Gómez-Zorrilla, S.; Benito, N.; Grau, S. Epidemiology and Treatment of Multidrug-Resistant and Extensively Drug-Resistant *Pseudomonas aeruginosa* Infections. *Clin. Microbiol. Rev.* **2019**, *32*, e00031-19. [CrossRef] [PubMed]
95. Herrera, S.; Bodro, M.; Soriano, A. Predictors of multidrug resistant *Pseudomonas aeruginosa* involvement in bloodstream infections. *Curr. Opin. Infect. Dis.* **2021**, *34*, 686–692. [CrossRef] [PubMed]
96. Potron, A.; Poirel, L.; Nordmann, P. Emerging broad-spectrum resistance in *Pseudomonas aeruginosa* and *Acinetobacter baumannii*: Mechanisms and epidemiology. *Int. J. Antimicrob. Agents* **2015**, *45*, 568–585. [CrossRef]
97. The European Committee on Antimicrobial Susceptibility Testing. Breakpoint Tables for Interpretation of MICs and Zone Diameters. Version 14.0. 2024. Available online: https://www.eucast.org/clinical_breakpoints (accessed on 20 October 2024).
98. European Committee on Antimicrobial Susceptibility Testing. Amikacin: Rationale for the Clinical Breakpoints. Version 3.1. 2024. Available online: https://www.eucast.org/publications-and-documents/rd (accessed on 20 October 2024).
99. Saravolatz, L.D.; Stein, G.E. Plazomicin: A new aminoglycoside. *Clin. Infect. Dis.* **2020**, *70*, 704–709. [CrossRef] [PubMed]
100. Corona, A.; De Santis, V.; Agarossi, A.; Prete, A.; Cattaneo, D.; Tomasini, G.; Bonetti, G.; Patroni, A.; Latronico, N. Antibiotic Therapy Strategies for Treating Gram-Negative Severe Infections in the Critically Ill: A Narrative Review. *Antibiotics* **2023**, *12*, 1262. [CrossRef] [PubMed]
101. EMA European Medicines Agency. Zemdri: Withdrawn Application. 2020. Available online: https://www.ema.europa.eu/en/medicines/human/withdrawn-applications/zemdri (accessed on 3 November 2023).
102. Sader, H.S.; Mendes, R.E.; Streit, J.M.; Carvalhaes, C.G.; Castanheira, M. Antimicrobial susceptibility of Gram-negative bacteria from intensive care unit and non-intensive care unit patients from United States hospitals (2018–2020). *Diagn. Microbiol. Infect. Dis.* **2022**, *102*, 115557. [CrossRef] [PubMed]

103. Scudeller, L.; Righi, E.; Chiamenti, M.; Bragantini, D.; Menchinelli, G.; Cattaneo, P.; Giske, C.G.; Lodise, T.; Sanguinetti, M.; Piddock, L.J.V.; et al. Systematic review and meta-analysis of in vitro efficacy of antibiotic combination therapy against carbapenem-resistant Gram-negative bacilli. *Int. J. Antimicrob. Agents* **2021**, *57*, 106344. [CrossRef]
104. Brasseur, A.; Hites, M.; Roisin, S.; Cotton, F.; Vincent, J.-L.; De Backer, D.; Jacobs, F.; Taccone, F.S. A high-dose aminoglycoside regimen combined with renal replacement therapy for the treatment of MDR pathogens: A proof-of-concept study. *J. Antimicrob. Chemother.* **2016**, *71*, 1386–1394. [CrossRef] [PubMed]
105. Pogue, J.M.; Kaye, K.S.; Veve, M.P.; Patel, T.S.; Gerlach, A.T.; Davis, S.L.; Puzniak, L.A.; File, T.M.; Olson, S.; Dhar, S.; et al. Ceftolozane/Tazobactam vs Polymyxin or Aminoglycoside-based Regimens for the Treatment of Drug-resistant *Pseudomonas aeruginosa*. *Clin. Infect. Dis.* **2020**, *71*, 304–310. [CrossRef]
106. Díaz-Cañestro, M.; Periañez, L.; Mulet, X.; Martin-Pena, M.L.; Fraile-Ribot, P.A.; Ayestarán, I.; Colomar, A.; Nuñez, A.; Maciá, M.; Novo, A.; et al. Ceftolozane/tazobactam for the treatment of multidrug resistant *Pseudomonas aeruginosa*: Experience from the Balearic Islands. *Eur. J. Clin. Microbiol. Infect. Dis.* **2018**, *37*, 2191–2200. [CrossRef]
107. orgensen, S.C.J.; Trinh, T.D.; Zasowski, E.J.; Lagnf, A.M.; Bhatia, S.; Melvin, S.M.; Steed, M.E.; Simon, S.P.; Estrada, S.J.; Morrisette, T.; et al. Real-World Experience with Ceftazidime-Avibactam for Multidrug-Resistant Gram-Negative Bacterial Infections. *Open Forum Infect. Dis.* **2019**, *6*, ofz522. [CrossRef]
108. Ito, A.; Nishikawa, T.; Matsumoto, S.; Yoshizawa, H.; Sato, T.; Nakamura, R.; Tsuji, M.; Yamano, Y. Siderophore Cephalosporin Cefiderocol Utilizes Ferric Iron Transporter Systems for Antibacterial Activity against *Pseudomonas aeruginosa*. *Antimicrob. Agents Chemother.* **2016**, *60*, 7396–7401. [CrossRef] [PubMed]
109. Andrews, S.C.; Robinson, A.K.; Rodríguez-Quiñones, F. Bacterial iron homeostasis. *FEMS Microbiol. Rev.* **2003**, *27*, 215–237. [CrossRef] [PubMed]
110. Ito-Horiyama, T.; Ishii, Y.; Ito, A.; Sato, T.; Nakamura, R.; Fukuhara, N.; Tsuji, M.; Yamano, Y.; Yamaguchi, K.; Tateda, K. Stability of Novel Siderophore Cephalosporin S-649266 against Clinically Relevant Carbapenemases. *Antimicrob. Agents Chemother.* **2016**, *60*, 4384–4386. [CrossRef] [PubMed]
111. Ito, A.; Kohira, N.; Bouchillon, S.K.; West, J.; Rittenhouse, S.; Sader, H.S.; Rhomberg, P.R.; Jones, R.N.; Yoshizawa, H.; Nakamura, R.; et al. In vitro antimicrobial activity of S-649266, a catechol-substituted siderophore cephalosporin, when tested against non-fermenting Gram-negative bacteria. *J. Antimicrob. Chemother.* **2016**, *71*, 670–677. [CrossRef]
112. Wu, J.Y.; Srinivas, P.; Pogue, J.M. Cefiderocol: A Novel Agent for the Management of Multidrug-Resistant Gram-Negative Organisms. *Infect. Dis. Ther.* **2020**, *9*, 17–40. [CrossRef] [PubMed]
113. Aoki, T.; Yoshizawa, H.; Yamawaki, K.; Yokoo, K.; Sato, J.; Hisakawa, S.; Hasegawa, Y.; Kusano, H.; Sano, M.; Sugimoto, H.; et al. Cefiderocol (S-649266), A new siderophore cephalosporin exhibiting potent activities against *Pseudomonas aeruginosa* and other gram-negative pathogens including multi-drug resistant bacteria: Structure activity relationship. *Eur. J. Med. Chem.* **2018**, *155*, 847–868. [CrossRef]
114. Kohira, N.; West, J.; Ito, A.; Ito-Horiyama, T.; Nakamura, R.; Sato, T.; Rittenhouse, S.; Tsuji, M.; Yamano, Y. In Vitro Antimicrobial Activity of a Siderophore Cephalosporin, S-649266, against Enterobacteriaceae Clinical Isolates, Including Carbapenem-Resistant Strains. *Antimicrob. Agents Chemother.* **2016**, *60*, 729–734. [CrossRef]
115. Longshaw, C.; Manissero, D.; Tsuji, M.; Echols, R.; Yamano, Y. In vitro activity of the siderophore cephalosporin, cefiderocol, against molecularly characterized, carbapenem-non-susceptible Gram-negative bacteria from Europe. *JAC Antimicrob. Resist.* **2020**, *2*, dlaa060. [CrossRef]
116. Gill, C.M.; Santini, D.; Nicolau, D.P.; ERACE-PA Global Study Group. In vitro activity of cefiderocol against a global collection of carbapenem-resistant *Pseudomonas aeruginosa* with a high level of carbapenemase diversity. *J. Antimicrob. Chemother.* **2024**, *79*, 412–416. [CrossRef] [PubMed]
117. Karlowsky, J.A.; Hackel, M.A.; Takemura, M.; Yamano, Y.; Echols, R.; Sahm, D.F. In Vitro Susceptibility of Gram-Negative Pathogens to Cefiderocol in Five Consecutive Annual Multinational SIDERO-WT Surveillance Studies, 2014 to 2019. *Antimicrob. Agents Chemother.* **2022**, *66*, e0199021. [CrossRef]
118. Takemura, M.; Wise, M.G.; Hackel, M.A.; Sahm, D.F.; Yamano, Y. In vitro activity of cefiderocol against MBL-producing Gram-negative bacteria collected in North America and Europe in five consecutive annual multinational SIDERO-WT surveillance studies (2014–2019). *J. Antimicrob. Chemother.* **2023**, *78*, 2019–2027. [CrossRef] [PubMed]
119. Shortridge, D.; Streit, J.M.; Mendes, R.; Castanheira, M. In Vitro Activity of Cefiderocol against U.S. and European Gram-Negative Clinical Isolates Collected in 2020 as Part of the SENTRY Antimicrobial Surveillance Program. *Microbiol. Spectr.* **2022**, *10*, e0271221. [CrossRef] [PubMed]
120. Portsmouth, S.; van Veenhuyzen, D.; Echols, R.; Machida, M.; Ferreira, J.C.A.; Ariyasu, M.; Tenke, P.; Nagata, T.D. Cefiderocol versus imipenem-cilastatin for the treatment of complicated urinary tract infections caused by Gram-negative uropathogens: A phase 2, randomised, double-blind, non-inferiority trial. *Lancet Infect. Dis.* **2018**, *18*, 1319–1328. [CrossRef] [PubMed]

121. Wunderink, R.G.; Matsunaga, Y.; Ariyasu, M.; Clevenbergh, P.; Echols, R.; Kaye, K.S.; Kollef, M.; Menon, A.; Pogue, J.M.; Shorr, A.F.; et al. Cefiderocol versus high-dose, extended-infusion meropenem for the treatment of Gram-negative nosocomial pneumonia (APEKS-NP): A randomised, double-blind, phase 3, non-inferiority trial. *Lancet Infect. Dis.* **2021**, *21*, 213–225. [CrossRef] [PubMed]
122. Bassetti, M.; Echols, R.; Matsunaga, Y.; Ariyasu, M.; Doi, Y.; Ferrer, R.; Lodise, T.P.; Naas, T.; Niki, Y.; Paterson, D.L.; et al. Efficacy and safety of cefiderocol or best available therapy for the treatment of serious infections caused by carbapenem-resistant Gram-negative bacteria (CREDIBLE-CR): A randomised, open-label, multicentre, pathogen-focused, descriptive, phase 3 trial. *Lancet Infect. Dis.* **2021**, *21*, 226–240. [CrossRef]
123. Satlin, M.J.; Simner, P.J.; Slover, C.M.; Yamano, Y.; Nagata, T.D.; Portsmouth, S. Cefiderocol Treatment for Patients with Multidrug- and Carbapenem-Resistant *Pseudomonas aeruginosa* Infections in the Compassionate Use Program. *Antimicrob. Agents Chemother.* **2023**, *67*, e0019423. [CrossRef] [PubMed]
124. Risco-Risco, C.; Henriquez-Camacho, C.; Herrera-Rueda, M.; Barberán, J.; Andaluz-Ojeda, D. Cefiderocol Versus Best Available Therapy in the Treatment of Critically Ill Patients with Severe Infections Due to Resistant Gram-Negative Bacteria: A Systematic Review and Meta-Analysis. *Antibiotics* **2024**, *13*, 1048. [CrossRef] [PubMed]
125. Tuon, F.F.; Rocha, J.L.; Formigoni-Pinto, M.R. Pharmacological aspects and spectrum of action of ceftazidime-avibactam: A systematic review. *Infection* **2018**, *46*, 165–181. [CrossRef] [PubMed]
126. Bassetti, M.; Vena, A.; Battaglini, D.; Pelosi, P.; Giacobbe, D.R. The role of new antimicrobials for Gram-negative infections in daily clinical practice. *Curr. Opin. Infect. Dis.* **2020**, *33*, 495–500. [CrossRef]
127. de Jonge, B.L.M.; Karlowsky, J.A.; Kazmierczak, K.M.; Biedenbach, D.J.; Sahm, D.F.; Nichols, W.W. In Vitro Susceptibility to Ceftazidime-Avibactam of Carbapenem-Nonsusceptible Enterobacteriaceae Isolates Collected during the INFORM Global Surveillance Study (2012 to 2014). *Antimicrob. Agents Chemother.* **2016**, *60*, 3163–3169. [CrossRef]
128. Karlowsky, J.A.; Biedenbach, D.J.; Kazmierczak, K.M.; Stone, G.G.; Sahm, D.F. Activity of Ceftazidime-Avibactam against Extended-Spectrum- and AmpC β-Lactamase-Producing Enterobacteriaceae Collected in the INFORM Global Surveillance Study from 2012 to 2014. *Antimicrob. Agents Chemother.* **2016**, *60*, 2849–2857. [CrossRef] [PubMed]
129. Sader, H.S.; Castanheira, M.; Duncan, L.R.; Mendes, R.E. Antimicrobial activities of ceftazidime/avibactam, ceftolozane/tazobactam, imipenem/relebactam, meropenem/vaborbactam, and comparators against *Pseudomonas aeruginosa* from patients with skin and soft tissue infections. *Int. J. Infect. Dis.* **2021**, *113*, 279–281. [CrossRef]
130. Wagenlehner, F.M.; Sobel, J.D.; Newell, P.; Armstrong, J.; Huang, X.; Stone, G.G.; Yates, K.; Gasink, L.B. Ceftazidime-avibactam Versus Doripenem for the Treatment of Complicated Urinary Tract Infections, Including Acute Pyelonephritis: RECAPTURE, a Phase 3 Randomized Trial Program. *Clin. Infect. Dis.* **2016**, *63*, 754–762. [CrossRef]
131. Torres, A.; Zhong, N.; Pachl, J.; Timsit, J.-F.; Kollef, M.; Chen, Z.; Song, J.; Taylor, D.; Laud, P.J.; Stone, G.G.; et al. Ceftazidime-avibactam versus meropenem in nosocomial pneumonia, including ventilator-associated pneumonia (REPROVE): A randomised, double-blind, phase 3 non-inferiority trial. *Lancet Infect. Dis.* **2018**, *18*, 285–295. [CrossRef] [PubMed]
132. Carmeli, Y.; Armstrong, J.; Laud, P.J.; Newell, P.; Stone, G.; Wardman, A.; Gasink, L.B. Ceftazidime-avibactam or best available therapy in patients with ceftazidime-resistant Enterobacteriaceae and *Pseudomonas aeruginosa* complicated urinary tract infections or complicated intra-abdominal infections (REPRISE): A randomised, pathogen-directed, phase 3 study. *Lancet Infect. Dis.* **2016**, *16*, 661–673. [PubMed]
133. Qin, X.; Tran, B.G.; Kim, M.J.; Wang, L.; Nguyen, D.A.; Chen, Q.; Song, J.; Laud, P.J.; Stone, G.G.; Chow, J.W. A randomised, double-blind, phase 3 study comparing the efficacy and safety of ceftazidime/avibactam plus metronidazole versus meropenem for complicated intra-abdominal infections in hospitalised adults in Asia. *Int. J. Antimicrob. Agents* **2017**, *49*, 579–588. [CrossRef] [PubMed]
134. Mazuski, J.E.; Gasink, L.B.; Armstrong, J.; Broadhurst, H.; Stone, G.G.; Rank, D.; Llorens, L.; Newell, P.; Pachl, J. Efficacy and Safety of Ceftazidime-Avibactam Plus Metronidazole Versus Meropenem in the Treatment of Complicated Intra-abdominal Infection: Results From a Randomized, Controlled, Double-Blind, Phase 3 Program. *Clin. Infect. Dis.* **2016**, *62*, 1380–1389. [CrossRef] [PubMed]
135. Stone, G.G.; Newell, P.; Gasink, L.B.; Broadhurst, H.; Wardman, A.; Yates, K.; Chen, Z.; Song, J.; Chow, J.W. Clinical activity of ceftazidime/avibactam against MDR Enterobacteriaceae and *Pseudomonas aeruginosa*: Pooled data from the ceftazidime/avibactam Phase III clinical trial programme. *J. Antimicrob. Chemother.* **2018**, *73*, 2519–2523. [CrossRef]
136. Torres, A.; Wible, M.; Tawadrous, M.; Irani, P.; Stone, G.G.; Quintana, A.; Debabov, D.; Burroughs, M.; Bradford, P.A.; Kollef, M. Efficacy and safety of ceftazidime/avibactam in patients with infections caused by β-lactamase-producing Gram-negative pathogens: A pooled analysis from the Phase 3 clinical trial programme. *J. Antimicrob. Chemother.* **2023**, *78*, 2672–2682. [CrossRef] [PubMed]
137. Corbella, L.; Boán, J.; San-Juan, R.; Fernández-Ruiz, M.; Carretero, O.; Lora, D.; Hernández-Jiménez, P.; Ruiz-Ruigómez, M.; Rodríguez-Goncer, I.; Silva, J.T.; et al. Effectiveness of ceftazidime-avibactam for the treatment of infections due to *Pseudomonas aeruginosa*. *Int. J. Antimicrob. Agents* **2022**, *59*, 106517. [CrossRef]

138. Xu, C.; Zeng, F.; Huang, Y.; Xu, Q.; Yang, Y.; Gong, W.; Shi, C.; Zhang, Y. Clinical efficacy of ceftazidime/avibactam combination therapy for severe hospital-acquired pulmonary infections caused by carbapenem-resistant and difficult-to-treat *Pseudomonas aeruginosa*. *Int. J. Antimicrob. Agents* **2024**, *63*, 107021. [CrossRef] [PubMed]
139. Almangour, T.A.; Ghonem, L.; Alassiri, D.; Aljurbua, A.; Al Musawa, M.; Alharbi, A.; Almohaizeie, A.; Almuhisen, S.; Alghaith, J.; Damfu, N.; et al. Ceftolozane-Tazobactam Versus Ceftazidime-Avibactam for the Treatment of Infections Caused by Multidrug-Resistant *Pseudomonas aeruginosa*: A Multicenter Cohort Study. *Antimicrob. Agents Chemother.* **2023**, *67*, e0040523. [CrossRef] [PubMed]
140. Zhanel, G.G.; Chung, P.; Adam, H.; Zelenitsky, S.; Denisuik, A.; Schweizer, F.; Lagacé-Wiens, P.R.S.; Rubinstein, E.; Gin, A.S.; Walkty, A.; et al. Ceftolozane/tazobactam: A novel cephalosporin/β-lactamase inhibitor combination with activity against multidrug-resistant gram-negative bacilli. *Drugs* **2014**, *74*, 31–51. [CrossRef] [PubMed]
141. Rodríguez, A.; Moreno, G.; Bodi, M.; Martín-Loeches, I. Antibiotics in development for multiresistant gram-negative bacilli. *Med. Intensiv. (Engl. Ed.)* **2022**, *46*, 630–640. [CrossRef]
142. Shortridge, D.; Pfaller, M.A.; Streit, J.M.; Flamm, R.K. Antimicrobial activity of ceftolozane/tazobactam tested against contemporary (2015–2017) *Pseudomonas aeruginosa* isolates from a global surveillance programme. *J. Glob. Antimicrob. Resist.* **2020**, *21*, 60–64. [CrossRef]
143. Wagenlehner, F.M.; Umeh, O.; Steenbergen, J.; Yuan, G.; Darouiche, R.O. Ceftolozane-tazobactam compared with levofloxacin in the treatment of complicated urinary-tract infections, including pyelonephritis: A randomised, double-blind, phase 3 trial (ASPECT-cUTI). *Lancet* **2015**, *385*, 1949–1956. [CrossRef]
144. Solomkin, J.; Hershberger, E.; Miller, B.; Popejoy, M.; Friedland, I.; Steenbergen, J.; Yoon, M.; Collins, S.; Yuan, G.; Barie, P.S.; et al. Ceftolozane/Tazobactam Plus Metronidazole for Complicated Intra-abdominal Infections in an Era of Multidrug Resistance: Results from a Randomized, Double-Blind, Phase 3 Trial (ASPECT-cIAI). *Clin. Infect. Dis.* **2015**, *60*, 1462–1471. [CrossRef]
145. Kollef, M.H.; Nováček, M.; Kivistik, Ü.; Réa-Neto, Á.; Shime, N.; Martin-Loeches, I.; Timsit, J.-F.; Wunderink, R.G.; Bruno, C.J.; Huntington, J.A.; et al. Ceftolozane-tazobactam versus meropenem for treatment of nosocomial pneumonia (ASPECT-NP): A randomised, controlled, double-blind, phase 3, non-inferiority trial. *Lancet Infect. Dis.* **2019**, *19*, 1299–1311. [CrossRef]
146. Timsit, J.-F.; Huntington, J.A.; Wunderink, R.G.; Shime, N.; Kollef, M.H.; Kivistik, Ü.; Nováček, M.; Réa-Neto, Á.; Martin-Loeches, I.; Yu, B.; et al. Ceftolozane/tazobactam versus meropenem in patients with ventilated hospital-acquired bacterial pneumonia: Subset analysis of the ASPECT-NP randomized, controlled phase 3 trial. *Crit. Care* **2021**, *25*, 290. [CrossRef]
147. Balandin, B.; Ballesteros, D.; Ruiz De Luna, R.; López-Vergara, L.; Pintado, V.; Sancho-González, M.; Soriano-Cuesta, C.; Pérez-Pedrero, M.J.; Asensio-Martín, M.J.; Fernández-Simón, I.; et al. Multicenter study of ceftolozane/tazobactam for treatment of *Pseudomonas aeruginosa* infections in critically ill patients. *Int. J. Antimicrob. Agents* **2021**, *57*, 106270. [CrossRef] [PubMed]
148. Almangour, T.A.; Aljabri, A.; Al Musawa, M.; Almohaizeie, A.; Almuhisen, S.; Damfu, N.; Alfozan, A.; Alraddadi, B.M.; Alattas, M.; Qutub, M.; et al. Ceftolozane-tazobactam vs. colistin for the treatment of infections due to multidrug-resistant *Pseudomonas aeruginosa*: A multicentre cohort study. *J. Glob. Antimicrob. Resist.* **2022**, *28*, 288–294. [CrossRef] [PubMed]
149. Gallagher, J.C.; Satlin, M.J.; Elabor, A.; Saraiya, N.; McCreary, E.K.; Molnar, E.; El-Beyrouty, C.; Jones, B.M.; Dixit, D.; Heil, E.L.; et al. Ceftolozane-Tazobactam for the Treatment of Multidrug-Resistant *Pseudomonas aeruginosa* Infections: A Multicenter Study. *Open Forum Infect. Dis.* **2018**, *5*, ofy280. [CrossRef]
150. Haidar, G.; Philips, N.J.; Shields, R.K.; Snyder, D.; Cheng, S.; Potoski, B.A.; Doi, Y.; Hao, B.; Press, E.G.; Cooper, V.S.; et al. Ceftolozane-Tazobactam for the Treatment of Multidrug-Resistant *Pseudomonas aeruginosa* Infections: Clinical Effectiveness and Evolution of Resistance. *Clin. Infect. Dis.* **2017**, *65*, 110–120. [CrossRef]
151. Munita, J.M.; Aitken, S.L.; Miller, W.R.; Perez, F.; Rosa, R.; Shimose, L.A.; Lichtenberger, P.N.; Abbo, L.M.; Jain, R.; Nigo, M.; et al. Multicenter Evaluation of Ceftolozane/Tazobactam for Serious Infections Caused by Carbapenem-Resistant *Pseudomonas aeruginosa*. *Clin. Infect. Dis.* **2017**, *65*, 158–161. [CrossRef]
152. Bassetti, M.; Castaldo, N.; Cattelan, A.; Mussini, C.; Righi, E.; Tascini, C.; Menichetti, F.; Mastroianni, C.M.; Tumbarello, M.; Grossi, P.; et al. Ceftolozane/tazobactam for the treatment of serious *Pseudomonas aeruginosa* infections: A multicentre nationwide clinical experience. *Int. J. Antimicrob. Agents* **2019**, *53*, 408–415. [CrossRef]
153. Falagas, M.E.; Kasiakou, S.K. Colistin: The revival of polymyxins for the management of multidrug-resistant gram-negative bacterial infections. *Clin. Infect. Dis.* **2005**, *40*, 1333–1341. [CrossRef] [PubMed]
154. Dijkmans, A.C.; Wilms, E.B.; Kamerling, I.M.C.; Birkhoff, W.; Ortiz-Zacarías, N.V.; van Nieuwkoop, C.; Verbrugh, H.A.; Touw, D.J. Colistin: Revival of an Old Polymyxin Antibiotic. *Ther. Drug Monit.* **2015**, *37*, 419–427. [CrossRef]
155. Son, S.J.; Huang, R.; Squire, C.J.; Leung, I.K.H. MCR-1: A promising target for structure-based design of inhibitors to tackle polymyxin resistance. *Drug Discov. Today* **2019**, *24*, 206–216. [CrossRef] [PubMed]
156. Zavascki, A.P.; Nation, R.L. Nephrotoxicity of Polymyxins: Is There Any Difference between Colistimethate and Polymyxin B? *Antimicrob. Agents Chemother.* **2017**, *61*, e02319-16. [CrossRef] [PubMed]
157. Falagas, M.E.; Kasiakou, S.K.; Tsiodras, S.; Michalopoulos, A. The use of intravenous and aerosolized polymyxins for the treatment of infections in critically ill patients: A review of the recent literature. *Clin. Med. Res.* **2006**, *4*, 138–146. [CrossRef]

158. Martis, N.; Leroy, S.; Blanc, V. Colistin in multi-drug resistant *Pseudomonas aeruginosa* blood-stream infections: A narrative review for the clinician. *J. Infect.* **2014**, *69*, 1–12. [CrossRef]
159. Haagensen, J.A.J.; Klausen, M.; Ernst, R.K.; Miller, S.I.; Folkesson, A.; Tolker-Nielsen, T.; Molin, S. Differentiation and distribution of colistin- and sodium dodecyl sulfate-tolerant cells in *Pseudomonas aeruginosa* biofilms. *J. Bacteriol.* **2007**, *189*, 28–37. [CrossRef]
160. Pamp, S.J.; Gjermansen, M.; Johansen, H.K.; Tolker-Nielsen, T. Tolerance to the antimicrobial peptide colistin in *Pseudomonas aeruginosa* biofilms is linked to metabolically active cells, and depends on the pmr and mexAB-oprM genes. *Mol. Microbiol.* **2008**, *68*, 223–240. [CrossRef]
161. Delgado-Valverde, M.; Portillo-Calderón, I.; Alcalde-Rico, M.; Conejo, M.C.; Hidalgo, C.; Del Toro Esperón, C.; Pascual, Á. Activity of imipenem/relebactam and comparators against KPC-producing Klebsiella pneumoniae and imipenem-resistant *Pseudomonas aeruginosa*. *Eur. J. Clin. Microbiol. Infect. Dis.* **2024**, *43*, 445–457. [CrossRef] [PubMed]
162. Carvalhaes, C.G.; Shortridge, D.; Sader, H.S.; Castanheira, M. Activity of Meropenem-Vaborbactam against Bacterial Isolates Causing Pneumonia in Patients in U.S. Hospitals during 2014 to 2018. *Antimicrob. Agents Chemother.* **2020**, *64*, e02177-19. [CrossRef] [PubMed]
163. Zhang, H.; Zhang, Q. Clinical efficacy and safety of colistin treatment in patients with pulmonary infection caused by *Pseudomonas aeruginosa* or *Acinetobacter baumannii*: A meta-analysis. *Arch. Med. Sci.* **2015**, *11*, 34–42. [CrossRef] [PubMed]
164. Cisneros, J.M.; Rosso-Fernández, C.M.; Roca-Oporto, C.; De Pascale, G.; Jiménez-Jorge, S.; Fernández-Hinojosa, E.; Matthaiou, D.K.; Ramírez, P.; Díaz-Miguel, R.O.; Estella, A.; et al. Colistin versus meropenem in the empirical treatment of ventilator-associated pneumonia (Magic Bullet study): An investigator-driven, open-label, randomized, noninferiority controlled trial. *Crit. Care* **2019**, *23*, 383. [CrossRef] [PubMed]
165. Kaye, K.S.; Marchaim, D.; Thamlikitkul, V.; Carmeli, Y.; Chiu, C.-H.; Daikos, G.; Dhar, S.; Durante-Mangoni, E.; Gikas, A.; Kotanidou, A.; et al. Colistin Monotherapy versus Combination Therapy for Carbapenem-Resistant Organisms. *NEJM Evid.* **2023**, *2*, EVIDoa2200131. [CrossRef] [PubMed]
166. Dickstein, Y.; Lellouche, J.; Schwartz, D.; Nutman, A.; Rakovitsky, N.; Dishon Benattar, Y.; Altunin, S.; Bernardo, M.; Iossa, D.; Durante-Mangoni, E.; et al. Colistin Resistance Development Following Colistin-Meropenem Combination Therapy Versus Colistin Monotherapy in Patients with Infections Caused by Carbapenem-Resistant Organisms. *Clin. Infect. Dis.* **2020**, *71*, 2599–2607. [CrossRef] [PubMed]
167. Paul, M.; Daikos, G.L.; Durante-Mangoni, E.; Yahav, D.; Carmeli, Y.; Benattar, Y.D.; Skiada, A.; Andini, R.; Eliakim-Raz, N.; Nutman, A.; et al. Colistin alone versus colistin plus meropenem for treatment of severe infections caused by carbapenem-resistant Gram-negative bacteria: An open-label, randomised controlled trial. *Lancet Infect. Dis.* **2018**, *18*, 391–400. [CrossRef]
168. Tsuji, B.T.; Pogue, J.M.; Zavascki, A.P.; Paul, M.; Daikos, G.L.; Forrest, A.; Giacobbe, D.R.; Viscoli, C.; Giamarellou, H.; Karaiskos, I.; et al. International Consensus Guidelines for the Optimal Use of the Polymyxins: Endorsed by the American College of Clinical Pharmacy (ACCP), European Society of Clinical Microbiology and Infectious Diseases (ESCMID), Infectious Diseases Society of America (IDSA), International Society for Anti-infective Pharmacology (ISAP), Society of Critical Care Medicine (SCCM), and Society of Infectious Diseases Pharmacists (SIDP). *Pharmacotherapy* **2019**, *39*, 10–39.
169. Motsch, J.; Murta de Oliveira, C.; Stus, V.; Köksal, I.; Lyulko, O.; Boucher, H.W.; Kaye, K.S.; File, T.M.; Brown, M.L.; Khan, I.; et al. RESTORE-IMI 1: A Multicenter, Randomized, Double-blind Trial Comparing Efficacy and Safety of Imipenem/Relebactam vs Colistin Plus Imipenem in Patients with Imipenem-nonsusceptible Bacterial Infections. *Clin. Infect. Dis.* **2020**, *70*, 1799–1808. [CrossRef]
170. Falagas, M.E.; Rafailidis, P.I.; Ioannidou, E.; Alexiou, V.G.; Matthaiou, D.K.; Karageorgopoulos, D.E.; Kapaskelis, A.; Nikita, D.; Michalopoulos, A. Colistin therapy for microbiologically documented multidrug-resistant Gram-negative bacterial infections: A retrospective cohort study of 258 patients. *Int. J. Antimicrob. Agents* **2010**, *35*, 194–199. [CrossRef] [PubMed]
171. Wu, Y.; Jiang, S.; Li, D.; Wu, Y.; Li, Q.; Wang, X.; Liu, B.; Bao, H.; Wu, D.; Hu, X. Clinical Efficacy and Safety of Colistin Sulfate in the Treatment of Carbapenem-Resistant Organism Infections in Patients with Hematological Diseases. *Infect. Dis. Ther.* **2024**, *13*, 141–154. [CrossRef] [PubMed]
172. Karaiskos, I.; Lagou, S.; Pontikis, K.; Rapti, V.; Poulakou, G. The "Old" and the "New" Antibiotics for MDR Gram-Negative Pathogens: For Whom, When, and How. *Front. Public Health* **2019**, *7*, 151. [CrossRef] [PubMed]
173. Pontikis, K.; Karaiskos, I.; Bastani, S.; Dimopoulos, G.; Kalogirou, M.; Katsiari, M.; Oikonomou, A.; Poulakou, G.; Roilides, E.; Giamarellou, H.; et al. Outcomes of critically ill intensive care unit patients treated with fosfomycin for infections due to pandrug-resistant and extensively drug-resistant carbapenemase-producing Gram-negative bacteria. *Int. J. Antimicrob. Agents* **2014**, *43*, 52–59. [CrossRef]
174. Karageorgopoulos, D.E.; Wang, R.; Yu, X.H.; Falagas, M.E. Fosfomycin: Evaluation of the published evidence on the emergence of antimicrobial resistance in Gram-negative pathogens. *J. Antimicrob. Chemother.* **2012**, *67*, 255–268. [CrossRef] [PubMed]
175. Flamm, R.K.; Rhomberg, P.R.; Watters, A.A.; Sweeney, K.; Ellis-Grosse, E.J.; Shortridge, D. Activity of fosfomycin when tested against US contemporary bacterial isolates. *Diagn. Microbiol. Infect. Dis.* **2019**, *93*, 143–146. [CrossRef] [PubMed]

176. Díez-Aguilar, M.; Morosini, M.I.; Del Campo, R.; García-Castillo, M.; Zamora, J.; Cantón, R. In Vitro Activity of Fosfomycin against a Collection of Clinical *Pseudomonas aeruginosa* Isolates from 16 Spanish Hospitals: Establishing the Validity of Standard Broth Microdilution as Susceptibility Testing Method. *Antimicrob. Agents Chemother.* **2013**, *57*, 5701–5703. [CrossRef]
177. Falagas, M.E.; Kastoris, A.C.; Karageorgopoulos, D.E.; Rafailidis, P.I. Fosfomycin for the treatment of infections caused by multidrug-resistant non-fermenting Gram-negative bacilli: A systematic review of microbiological, animal and clinical studies. *Int. J. Antimicrob. Agents* **2009**, *34*, 111–120. [CrossRef]
178. Papp-Wallace, K.M.; Zeiser, E.T.; Becka, S.A.; Park, S.; Wilson, B.M.; Winkler, M.L.; D'Souza, R.; Singh, I.; Sutton, G.; Fouts, D.E.; et al. Ceftazidime-Avibactam in Combination with Fosfomycin: A Novel Therapeutic Strategy Against Multidrug-Resistant *Pseudomonas aeruginosa*. *J. Infect. Dis.* **2019**, *220*, 666–676. [CrossRef] [PubMed]
179. Albiero, J.; Mazucheli, J.; Barros, J.P.D.R.; Szczerepa, M.M.D.A.; Nishiyama, S.A.B.; Carrara-Marroni, F.E.; Sy, S.; Fidler, M.; Sy, S.K.B.; Tognim, M.C.B. Pharmacodynamic Attainment of the Synergism of Meropenem and Fosfomycin Combination against *Pseudomonas aeruginosa* Producing Metallo-β-Lactamase. *Antimicrob. Agents Chemother.* **2019**, *63*, e00126-19. [CrossRef] [PubMed]
180. Apisarnthanarak, A.; Mundy, L.M. Carbapenem-resistant *Pseudomonas aeruginosa* pneumonia with intermediate minimum inhibitory concentrations to doripenem: Combination therapy with high-dose, 4-h infusion of doripenem plus fosfomycin versus intravenous colistin plus fosfomycin. *Int. J. Antimicrob. Agents* **2012**, *39*, 271–272. [CrossRef] [PubMed]
181. Frattari, A.; Savini, V.; Polilli, E.; Cibelli, D.; Talamazzi, S.; Bosco, D.; Consorte, A.; Fazii, P.; Parruti, G. Ceftolozane-tazobactam and Fosfomycin for rescue treatment of otogenous meningitis caused by XDR *Pseudomonas aeruginosa*: Case report and review of the literature. *IDCases* **2018**, *14*, e00451. [CrossRef] [PubMed]
182. Zhanel, G.G.; Lawrence, C.K.; Adam, H.; Schweizer, F.; Zelenitsky, S.; Zhanel, M.; Lagacé-Wiens, P.R.S.; Walkty, A.; Denisuik, A.; Golden, A.; et al. Imipenem-Relebactam and Meropenem-Vaborbactam: Two Novel Carbapenem-β-Lactamase Inhibitor Combinations. *Drugs* **2018**, *78*, 65–98. [CrossRef] [PubMed]
183. Young, K.; Painter, R.E.; Raghoobar, S.L.; Hairston, N.N.; Racine, F.; Wisniewski, D.; Balibar, C.J.; Villafania, A.; Zhang, R.; Sahm, D.F.; et al. In vitro studies evaluating the activity of imipenem in combination with relebactam against *Pseudomonas aeruginosa*. *BMC Microbiol.* **2019**, *19*, 150. [CrossRef] [PubMed]
184. Mansour, H.; Ouweini, A.E.L.; Chahine, E.B.; Karaoui, L.R. Imipenem/cilastatin/relebactam: A new carbapenem β-lactamase inhibitor combination. *Am. J. Health Syst. Pharm.* **2021**, *78*, 674–683. [CrossRef]
185. Lob, S.H.; Karlowsky, J.A.; Young, K.; Motyl, M.R.; Hawser, S.; Kothari, N.D.; Sahm, D.F. In vitro activity of imipenem-relebactam against resistant phenotypes of Enterobacteriaceae and *Pseudomonas aeruginosa* isolated from intraabdominal and urinary tract infection samples—SMART Surveillance Europe 2015–2017. *J. Med. Microbiol.* **2020**, *69*, 207–217. [CrossRef]
186. Hernández-García, M.; García-Castillo, M.; Melo-Cristino, J.; Pinto, M.F.; Gonçalves, E.; Alves, V.; Vieira, A.R.; Ramalheira, E.; Sancho, L.; Diogo, J.; et al. In vitro activity of imipenem/relebactam against *Pseudomonas aeruginosa* isolates recovered from ICU patients in Spain and Portugal (SUPERIOR and STEP studies). *J. Antimicrob. Chemother.* **2022**, *77*, 3163–3172. [CrossRef] [PubMed]
187. Lasarte-Monterrubio, C.; Fraile-Ribot, P.A.; Vázquez-Ucha, J.C.; Cabot, G.; Guijarro-Sánchez, P.; Alonso-García, I.; Rumbo-Feal, S.; Galán-Sánchez, F.; Beceiro, A.; Arca-Suárez, J.; et al. Activity of cefiderocol, imipenem/relebactam, cefepime/taniborbactam and cefepime/zidebactam against ceftolozane/tazobactam- and ceftazidime/avibactam-resistant *Pseudomonas aeruginosa*. *J. Antimicrob. Chemother.* **2022**, *77*, 2809–2815. [CrossRef] [PubMed]
188. Peñuelas, M.; García-Salguero, C.; Iñigo, M.; Viñuela-Prieto, J.M.; Candel, F.J.; Del Pozo, J.L.; Culebras, E. In vitro activity of imipenem/relebactam against Gram-negative clinical isolates in two Spanish tertiary hospitals. *Rev. Esp. Quimioter.* **2021**, *34*, 668–671. [CrossRef] [PubMed]
189. Mushtaq, S.; Meunier, D.; Vickers, A.; Woodford, N.; Livermore, D.M. Activity of imipenem/relebactam against *Pseudomonas aeruginosa* producing ESBLs and carbapenemases. *J. Antimicrob. Chemother.* **2021**, *76*, 434–442. [CrossRef]
190. Bail, L.; Ito, C.A.S.; Arend, L.N.V.S.; Nogueira, K.d.S.; Tuon, F.F. Activity of imipenem-relebactam and ceftolozane-tazobactam against carbapenem-resistant *Pseudomonas aeruginosa* and KPC-producing Enterobacterales. *Diagn. Microbiol. Infect. Dis.* **2021**, *102*, 115568. [CrossRef] [PubMed]
191. Fraile-Ribot, P.A.; Zamorano, L.; Orellana, R.; Del Barrio-Tofiño, E.; Sánchez-Diener, I.; Cortes-Lara, S.; López-Causapé, C.; Cabot, G.; Bou, G.; Martínez-Martínez, L.; et al. Activity of Imipenem-Relebactam against a Large Collection of *Pseudomonas aeruginosa* Clinical Isolates and Isogenic β-Lactam-Resistant Mutants. *Antimicrob. Agents Chemother.* **2020**, *64*, e02165-19. [CrossRef]
192. Titov, I.; Wunderink, R.G.; Roquilly, A.; Rodríguez Gonzalez, D.; David-Wang, A.; Boucher, H.W.; Kaye, K.S.; Losada, M.C.; Du, J.; Tipping, R.; et al. A Randomized, Double-blind, Multicenter Trial Comparing Efficacy and Safety of Imipenem/Cilastatin/Relebactam Versus Piperacillin/Tazobactam in Adults with Hospital-acquired or Ventilator-associated Bacterial Pneumonia (RESTORE-IMI 2 Study). *Clin. Infect. Dis.* **2020**, *73*, e4539–e4548. [CrossRef] [PubMed]
193. Leanza, C.; Mascellino, M.T.; Volpicelli, L.; Covino, S.; Falletta, A.; Cancelli, F.; Franchi, C.; Carnevalini, M.; Mastroianni, C.M.; Oliva, A. Real-world use of imipenem/cilastatin/relebactam for the treatment of KPC-producing Klebsiella pneumoniae complex and difficult-to-treat resistance (DTR) *Pseudomonas aeruginosa* infections: A single-center preliminary experience. *Front. Microbiol.* **2024**, *15*, 1432296. [CrossRef]

194. Patel, T.S.; Pogue, J.M.; Mills, J.P.; Kaye, K.S. Meropenem-vaborbactam: A new weapon in the war against infections due to resistant Gram-negative bacteria. *Future Microbiol.* **2018**, *13*, 971–983. [CrossRef] [PubMed]
195. Bhowmick, T.; Weinstein, M.P. Microbiology of Meropenem-Vaborbactam: A Novel Carbapenem Beta-Lactamase Inhibitor Combination for Carbapenem-Resistant Enterobacterales Infections. *Infect. Dis. Ther.* **2020**, *9*, 757–767. [CrossRef]
196. Castanheira, M.; Doyle, T.B.; Hubler, C.M.; DeVries, S.; Shortridge, D. Vaborbactam increases meropenem susceptibility in *Pseudomonas aeruginosa* clinical isolates displaying MexXY and AmpC upregulation. *mSphere* **2023**, *8*, e0016223. [CrossRef] [PubMed]
197. Shortridge, D.; Carvalhaes, C.; Deshpande, L.; Castanheira, M. Activity of meropenem/vaborbactam and comparators against Gram-negative isolates from Eastern and Western European patients hospitalized with pneumonia including ventilator-associated pneumonia (2014–19). *J. Antimicrob. Chemother.* **2021**, *76*, 2600–2605. [CrossRef] [PubMed]
198. Kaye, K.S.; Bhowmick, T.; Metallidis, S.; Bleasdale, S.C.; Sagan, O.S.; Stus, V.; Vazquez, J.; Zaitsev, V.; Bidair, M.; Chorvat, E.; et al. Effect of Meropenem-Vaborbactam vs Piperacillin-Tazobactam on Clinical Cure or Improvement and Microbial Eradication in Complicated Urinary Tract Infection: The TANGO I Randomized Clinical Trial. *JAMA* **2018**, *319*, 788–799. [CrossRef] [PubMed]
199. Wunderink, R.G.; Giamarellos-Bourboulis, E.J.; Rahav, G.; Mathers, A.J.; Bassetti, M.; Vazquez, J.; Cornely, O.A.; Solomkin, J.; Bhowmick, T.; Bishara, J.; et al. Effect and Safety of Meropenem-Vaborbactam versus Best-Available Therapy in Patients with Carbapenem-Resistant Enterobacteriaceae Infections: The TANGO II Randomized Clinical Trial. *Infect. Dis. Ther.* **2018**, *7*, 439–455. [CrossRef]
200. Alosaimy, S.; Lagnf, A.M.; Morrisette, T.; Scipione, M.R.; Zhao, J.J.; Jorgensen, S.C.J.; Mynatt, R.; Carlson, T.J.; Jo, J.; Garey, K.W.; et al. Real-world, Multicenter Experience with Meropenem-Vaborbactam for Gram-Negative Bacterial Infections Including Carbapenem-Resistant Enterobacterales and *Pseudomonas aeruginosa*. *Open Forum Infect. Dis.* **2021**, *8*, ofab371. [CrossRef] [PubMed]
201. Sader, H.S.; Mendes, R.E.; Kimbrough, J.H.; Hubler, C.M.; Castanheira, M. Activity of Aztreonam/Avibactam and Recently Approved β-Lactamase Inhibitor Combinations against Enterobacterales and *Pseudomonas aeruginosa* from Intensive Care Unit and Non-Intensive Care Unit Patients. *Antibiotics* **2024**, *13*, 564. [CrossRef]
202. Sangiorgio, G.; Calvo, M.; Stefani, S. Aztreonam and avibactam combination therapy for metallo-β-lactamase-producing gram-negative bacteria: A comprehensive review. *Clin. Microbiol. Infect.* 2024; *in press*. [CrossRef]
203. Kang, Y.; Xie, L.; Yang, J.; Cui, J. Optimal treatment of ceftazidime-avibactam and aztreonam-avibactam against bloodstream infections or lower respiratory tract infections caused by extensively drug-resistant or pan drug-resistant (XDR/PDR) *Pseudomonas aeruginosa*. *Front. Cell Infect. Microbiol.* **2023**, *13*, 1023948. [CrossRef] [PubMed]
204. Carmeli, Y.; Cisneros, J.M.; Paul, M.; Daikos, G.L.; Wang, M.; Torre-Cisneros, J.; Singer, G.; Titov, I.; Gumenchuk, I.; Zhao, Y.; et al. Aztreonam-avibactam versus meropenem for the treatment of serious infections caused by Gram-negative bacteria (REVISIT): A descriptive, multinational, open-label, phase 3, randomised trial. *Lancet Infect. Dis.* **2024**, *25*, 218–230. [CrossRef] [PubMed]
205. Mauri, C.; Maraolo, A.E.; Di Bella, S.; Luzzaro, F.; Principe, L. The Revival of Aztreonam in Combination with Avibactam against Metallo-β-Lactamase-Producing Gram-Negatives: A Systematic Review of In Vitro Studies and Clinical Cases. *Antibiotics* **2021**, *10*, 1012. [CrossRef]
206. Kaye, K.S.; Belley, A.; Barth, P.; Lahlou, O.; Knechtle, P.; Motta, P.; Velicitat, P. Effect of Cefepime/Enmetazobactam vs Piperacillin/Tazobactam on Clinical Cure and Microbiological Eradication in Patients with Complicated Urinary Tract Infection or Acute Pyelonephritis: A Randomized Clinical Trial. *JAMA* **2022**, *328*, 1304–1314. [CrossRef]
207. Morrissey, I.; Magnet, S.; Hawser, S.; Shapiro, S.; Knechtle, P. In Vitro Activity of Cefepime-Enmetazobactam against Gram-Negative Isolates Collected from U.S. and European Hospitals during 2014–2015. *Antimicrob. Agents Chemother.* **2019**, *63*, e00514-19. [CrossRef]
208. Bonnin, R.A.; Jeannot, K.; Santerre Henriksen, A.; Quevedo, J.; Dortet, L. In vitro activity of cefepime-enmetazobactam on carbapenem-resistant gram negatives. *Clin. Microbiol. Infect.* **2024**, *31*, 240–249. [CrossRef] [PubMed]
209. Gerges, B.; Rosenblatt, J.; Truong, Y.-L.; Jiang, Y.; Shelburne, S.A.; Chaftari, A.-M.; Hachem, R.; Raad, I. In vitro activity of cefepime/taniborbactam and comparator agents against Gram-negative bacterial bloodstream pathogens recovered from patients with cancer. *JAC Antimicrob. Resist.* **2024**, *6*, dlae060. [CrossRef] [PubMed]
210. Karlowsky, J.A.; Wise, M.G.; Hackel, M.A.; Six, D.A.; Uehara, T.; Daigle, D.M.; Pevear, D.C.; Moeck, G.; Sahm, D. Cefepime-taniborbactam activity against antimicrobial-resistant clinical isolates of Enterobacterales and *Pseudomonas aeruginosa*: GEARS global surveillance programme 2018–22. *J. Antimicrob. Chemother.* **2024**, *79*, 3116–3131. [CrossRef] [PubMed]
211. Hernández-García, M.; García-Castillo, M.; Ruiz-Garbajosa, P.; Bou, G.; Siller-Ruiz, M.; Pitart, C.; Gracia-Ahufinger, I.; Mulet, X.; Pascual, Á.; Tormo, N.; et al. In Vitro Activity of Cefepime-Taniborbactam against Carbapenemase-Producing Enterobacterales and *Pseudomonas aeruginosa* Isolates Recovered in Spain. *Antimicrob. Agents Chemother.* **2022**, *66*, e0216121. [CrossRef]

212. Hernández-García, M.; García-Castillo, M.; Nieto-Torres, M.; Bou, G.; Ocampo-Sosa, A.; Pitart, C.; Gracia-Ahufinger, I.; Mulet, X.; Pascual, Á.; Tormo, N.; et al. Deciphering mechanisms affecting cefepime-taniborbactam in vitro activity in carbapenemase-producing Enterobacterales and carbapenem-resistant *Pseudomonas* spp. isolates recovered during a surveillance study in Spain. *Eur. J. Clin. Microbiol. Infect. Dis.* **2024**, *43*, 279–296. [CrossRef] [PubMed]
213. Wagenlehner, F.M.; Gasink, L.B.; McGovern, P.C.; Moeck, G.; McLeroth, P.; Dorr, M.; Dane, A.; Henkel, T. Cefepime-Taniborbactam in Complicated Urinary Tract Infection. *N. Engl. J. Med.* **2024**, *390*, 611–622. [CrossRef] [PubMed]
214. Moeck, G.; Gasink, L.B.; Mendes, R.E.; Woosley, L.N.; Dorr, M.; Chen, H.; Wagenlehner, F.M.; Henkel, T.; McGovern, P.C. Patient outcomes by baseline pathogen resistance phenotype and genotype in CERTAIN-1, a Phase 3 study of cefepime-taniborbactam versus meropenem in adults with complicated urinary tract infection. *Antimicrob. Agents Chemother.* **2024**, *68*, e0023624. [CrossRef] [PubMed]
215. Khan, Z.; Iregui, A.; Landman, D.; Quale, J. Activity of cefepime/zidebactam (WCK 5222) against Enterobacteriaceae, *Pseudomonas aeruginosa* and *Acinetobacter baumannii* endemic to New York City medical centres. *J. Antimicrob. Chemother.* **2019**, *74*, 2938–2942. [CrossRef] [PubMed]
216. Mullane, E.M.; Avery, L.M.; Nicolau, D.P. Comparative Evaluation of the In Vitro Activities of WCK 5222 (Cefepime-Zidebactam) and Combination Antibiotic Therapies against Carbapenem-Resistant *Pseudomonas aeruginosa*. *Antimicrob. Agents Chemother.* **2020**, *64*, e01669-19. [CrossRef] [PubMed]
217. Mushtaq, S.; Garello, P.; Vickers, A.; Woodford, N.; Livermore, D.M. Activity of cefepime/zidebactam (WCK 5222) against "problem" antibiotic-resistant Gram-negative bacteria sent to a national reference laboratory. *J. Antimicrob. Chemother.* **2021**, *76*, 1511–1522. [CrossRef]
218. Dubey, D.; Roy, M.; Shah, T.H.; Bano, N.; Kulshrestha, V.; Mitra, S.; Sangwan, P.; Dubey, M.; Imran, A.; Jain, B.; et al. Compassionate use of a novel β-lactam enhancer-based investigational antibiotic cefepime/zidebactam (WCK 5222) for the treatment of extensively-drug-resistant NDM-expressing *Pseudomonas aeruginosa* infection in an intra-abdominal infection-induced sepsis patient: A case report. *Ann. Clin. Microbiol. Antimicrob.* **2023**, *22*, 55.
219. Tirlangi, P.K.; Wanve, B.S.; Dubbudu, R.R.; Yadav, B.S.; Kumar, L.S.; Gupta, A.; Sree, R.A.; Challa, H.P.R.; Reddy, P.N. Successful Use of Cefepime-Zidebactam (WCK 5222) as a Salvage Therapy for the Treatment of Disseminated Extensively Drug-Resistant New Delhi Metallo-β-Lactamase-Producing *Pseudomonas aeruginosa* Infection in an Adult Patient with Acute T-Cell Leukemia. *Antimicrob. Agents Chemother.* **2023**, *67*, e0050023. [CrossRef] [PubMed]
220. Soman, R.; Sirsat, R.; Sunavala, A.; Punatar, N.; Mehta, J.; Rodrigues, C.; Veeraraghavan, B. Successful treatment of sino-pulmonary infection & skull base osteomyelitis caused by New Delhi metallo-β-lactamase-producing *Pseudomonas aeruginosa* in a renal transplant recipient by using an investigational antibiotic cefepime/zidebactam (WCK 5222). *Eur. J. Clin. Microbiol. Infect. Dis.* 2024; *ahead of print*. [CrossRef]
221. Asempa, T.E.; Motos, A.; Abdelraouf, K.; Bissantz, C.; Zampaloni, C.; Nicolau, D.P. Meropenem-nacubactam activity against AmpC-overproducing and KPC-expressing *Pseudomonas aeruginosa* in a neutropenic murine lung infection model. *Int. J. Antimicrob. Agents* **2020**, *55*, 105838. [CrossRef]
222. Monogue, M.L.; Giovagnoli, S.; Bissantz, C.; Zampaloni, C.; Nicolau, D.P. In Vivo Efficacy of Meropenem with a Novel Non-β-Lactam-β-Lactamase Inhibitor, Nacubactam, against Gram-Negative Organisms Exhibiting Various Resistance Mechanisms in a Murine Complicated Urinary Tract Infection Model. *Antimicrob. Agents Chemother.* **2018**, *62*, e02596-17. [CrossRef]
223. Tamma, P.D.; Beisken, S.; Bergman, Y.; Posch, A.E.; Avdic, E.; Sharara, S.L.; Cosgrove, S.E.; Simner, P.J. Modifiable Risk Factors for the Emergence of Ceftolozane-tazobactam Resistance. *Clin. Infect. Dis.* **2021**, *73*, e4599–e4606. [CrossRef] [PubMed]
224. Gatti, M.; Cojutti, P.G.; Pascale, R.; Tonetti, T.; Laici, C.; Dell'Olio, A.; Siniscalchi, A.; Giannella, M.; Viale, P.; Pea, F. Assessment of a PK/PD Target of Continuous Infusion Beta-Lactams Useful for Preventing Microbiological Failure and/or Resistance Development in Critically Ill Patients Affected by Documented Gram-Negative Infections. *Antibiotics* **2021**, *10*, 1311. [CrossRef] [PubMed]
225. Felton, T.W.; Goodwin, J.; O'Connor, L.; Sharp, A.; Gregson, L.; Livermore, J.; Howard, S.J.; Neely, M.N.; Hope, W.W. Impact of Bolus dosing versus continuous infusion of Piperacillin and Tazobactam on the development of antimicrobial resistance in *Pseudomonas aeruginosa*. *Antimicrob. Agents Chemother.* **2013**, *57*, 5811–5819. [CrossRef] [PubMed]
226. Tam, V.H.; Chang, K.-T.; Zhou, J.; Ledesma, K.R.; Phe, K.; Gao, S.; Van Bambeke, F.; Sánchez-Díaz, A.M.; Zamorano, L.; Oliver, A.; et al. Determining β-lactam exposure threshold to suppress resistance development in Gram-negative bacteria. *J. Antimicrob. Chemother.* **2017**, *72*, 1421–1428. [CrossRef] [PubMed]
227. Abdul-Aziz, M.H.; Lipman, J.; Akova, M.; Bassetti, M.; De Waele, J.J.; Dimopoulos, G.; Dulhunty, J.; Kaukonen, K.-M.; Koulenti, D.; Martin, C.; et al. Is prolonged infusion of piperacillin/tazobactam and meropenem in critically ill patients associated with improved pharmacokinetic/pharmacodynamic and patient outcomes? An observation from the Defining Antibiotic Levels in Intensive care unit patients (DALI) cohort. *J. Antimicrob. Chemother.* **2016**, *71*, 196–207.

228. Vardakas, K.Z.; Voulgaris, G.L.; Maliaros, A.; Samonis, G.; Falagas, M.E. Prolonged versus short-term intravenous infusion of antipseudomonal β-lactams for patients with sepsis: A systematic review and meta-analysis of randomised trials. *Lancet Infect. Dis.* **2018**, *18*, 108–120. [CrossRef]
229. Kondo, Y.; Ota, K.; Imura, H.; Hara, N.; Shime, N. Prolonged versus intermittent β-lactam antibiotics intravenous infusion strategy in sepsis or septic shock patients: A systematic review with meta-analysis and trial sequential analysis of randomized trials. *J. Intensive Care* **2020**, *8*, 77. [CrossRef] [PubMed]
230. Tamma, P.D.; Putcha, N.; Suh, Y.D.; Van Arendonk, K.J.; Rinke, M.L. Does prolonged β-lactam infusions improve clinical outcomes compared to intermittent infusions? A meta-analysis and systematic review of randomized, controlled trials. *BMC Infect. Dis.* **2011**, *11*, 181. [CrossRef] [PubMed]
231. Monti, G.; Bradić, N.; Marzaroli, M.; Konkayev, A.; Fominskiy, E.; Kotani, Y.; Likhvantsev, V.V.; Momesso, E.; Nogtev, P.; Lobreglio, R.; et al. Continuous vs Intermittent Meropenem Administration in Critically Ill Patients with Sepsis: The MERCY Randomized Clinical Trial. *JAMA* **2023**, *330*, 141. [CrossRef] [PubMed]
232. Bilal, M.; Zoller, M.; Fuhr, U.; Jaehde, U.; Ullah, S.; Liebchen, U.; Büsker, S.; Zander, J.; Babouee Flury, B.; Taubert, M. Cefepime Population Pharmacokinetics, Antibacterial Target Attainment, and Estimated Probability of Neurotoxicity in Critically Ill Patients. *Antimicrob. Agents Chemother.* **2023**, *67*, e0030923. [CrossRef]
233. Tamma, P.D.; Aitken, S.L.; Bonomo, R.A.; Mathers, A.J.; van Duin, D.; Clancy, C.J. Infectious Diseases Society of America 2023 Guidance on the Treatment of Antimicrobial Resistant Gram-Negative Infections. *Clin. Infect. Dis.* **2023**, ciad428. [CrossRef]
234. Pintado, V.; Ruiz-Garbajosa, P.; Aguilera-Alonso, D.; Baquero-Artigao, F.; Bou, G.; Cantón, R.; Grau, S.; Gutiérrez-Gutiérrez, B.; Larrosa, N.; Machuca, I.; et al. Executive summary of the consensus document of the Spanish Society of Infectious Diseases and Clinical Microbiology (SEIMC) on the diagnosis and antimicrobial treatment of infections due to carbapenem-resistant Gram-negative bacteria. *Enferm. Infecc. Microbiol. Clin. (Engl. Ed.)* **2023**, *41*, 360–370. [CrossRef]
235. Paul, M.; Carrara, E.; Retamar, P.; Tängdén, T.; Bitterman, R.; Bonomo, R.A.; de Waele, J.; Daikos, G.L.; Akova, M.; Harbarth, S.; et al. European Society of Clinical Microbiology and Infectious Diseases (ESCMID) guidelines for the treatment of infections caused by multidrug-resistant Gram-negative bacilli (endorsed by European society of intensive care medicine). *Clin. Microbiol. Infect.* **2022**, *28*, 521–547. [CrossRef]
236. Gatti, M.; Pea, F. Continuous versus intermittent infusion of antibiotics in Gram-negative multidrug-resistant infections. *Curr. Opin. Infect. Dis.* **2021**, *34*, 737–747. [CrossRef]
237. Gatti, M.; Pea, F. Jumping into the future: Overcoming pharmacokinetic/pharmacodynamic hurdles to optimize the treatment of severe difficult to treat-Gram-negative infections with novel beta-lactams. *Expert Rev. Anti. Infect. Ther.* **2023**, *21*, 149–166. [CrossRef]
238. Pilmis, B.; Petitjean, G.; Lesprit, P.; Lafaurie, M.; El Helali, N.; Le Monnier, A. Continuous infusion of ceftolozane/tazobactam is associated with a higher probability of target attainment in patients infected with *Pseudomonas aeruginosa*. *Eur. J. Clin. Microbiol. Infect. Dis.* **2019**, *38*, 1457–1461. [CrossRef] [PubMed]
239. Montero, M.M.; Domene-Ochoa, S.; López-Causapé, C.; López-Montesinos, I.; Luque, S.; Sorlí, L.; Campillo, N.; Padilla, E.; Prim, N.; Ferrer Alapont, L.; et al. Comparison of Ceftolozane/Tazobactam Infusion Regimens in a Hollow-Fiber Infection Model against Extensively Drug-Resistant *Pseudomonas aeruginosa* Isolates. *Microbiol. Spectr.* **2022**, *10*, e0089222. [CrossRef] [PubMed]
240. Tumbarello, M.; Raffaelli, F.; Giannella, M.; Mantengoli, E.; Mularoni, A.; Venditti, M.; De Rosa, F.G.; Sarmati, L.; Bassetti, M.; Brindicci, G.; et al. Ceftazidime-Avibactam Use for Klebsiella pneumoniae Carbapenemase-Producing K. pneumoniae Infections: A Retrospective Observational Multicenter Study. *Clin. Infect. Dis.* **2021**, *73*, 1664–1676. [CrossRef]
241. Fresan, D.; Luque, S.; Benítez-Cano, A.; Sorlí, L.; Milagro Montero, M.; De-Antonio, M.; Prim, N.; Vega, V.; Horcajada, J.P.; Grau, S. Pharmacokinetics/pharmacodynamics and therapeutic drug monitoring of ceftazidime/avibactam administered by continuous infusion in patients with MDR Gram-negative bacterial infections. *J. Antimicrob. Chemother.* **2023**, *78*, 678–683. [CrossRef]
242. Antonello, R.M.; Di Bella, S.; Maraolo, A.E.; Luzzati, R. Fosfomycin in continuous or prolonged infusion for systemic bacterial infections: A systematic review of its dosing regimen proposal from in vitro, in vivo and clinical studies. *Eur. J. Clin. Microbiol. Infect. Dis.* **2021**, *40*, 1117–1126. [CrossRef]
243. Hong, L.T.; Downes, K.J.; FakhriRavari, A.; Abdul-Mutakabbir, J.C.; Kuti, J.L.; Jorgensen, S.; Young, D.C.; Alshaer, M.H.; Bassetti, M.; Bonomo, R.A.; et al. International consensus recommendations for the use of prolonged-infusion beta-lactam antibiotics: Endorsed by the American College of Clinical Pharmacy, British Society for Antimicrobial Chemotherapy, Cystic Fibrosis Foundation, European Society of Clinical Microbiology and Infectious Diseases, Infectious Diseases Society of America, Society of Critical Care Medicine, and Society of Infectious Diseases Pharmacists. *Pharmacotherapy* **2023**, *43*, 740–777.
244. Rico Caballero, V.; Almarzoky Abuhussain, S.; Kuti, J.L.; Nicolau, D.P. Efficacy of Human-Simulated Exposures of Ceftolozane-Tazobactam Alone and in Combination with Amikacin or Colistin against Multidrug-Resistant *Pseudomonas aeruginosa* in an In Vitro Pharmacodynamic Model. *Antimicrob. Agents Chemother.* **2018**, *62*, e02384-17. [CrossRef]

245. Montero, M.; Domene Ochoa, S.; López-Causapé, C.; VanScoy, B.; Luque, S.; Sorlí, L.; Campillo, N.; Angulo-Brunet, A.; Padilla, E.; Prim, N.; et al. Efficacy of Ceftolozane-Tazobactam in Combination with Colistin against Extensively Drug-Resistant *Pseudomonas aeruginosa*, Including High-Risk Clones, in an In Vitro Pharmacodynamic Model. *Antimicrob. Agents Chemother.* **2020**, *64*, e02542-19. [CrossRef] [PubMed]
246. Jacqueline, C.; Howland, K.; Chesnel, L. In vitro activity of ceftolozane/tazobactam in combination with other classes of antibacterial agents. *J. Glob. Antimicrob. Resist.* **2017**, *10*, 326–329. [CrossRef]
247. Nasomsong, W.; Nulsopapon, P.; Changpradub, D.; Pungcharoenkijkul, S.; Hanyanunt, P.; Chatreewattanakul, T.; Santimaleeworagun, W. Optimizing Doses of Ceftolozane/Tazobactam as Monotherapy or in Combination with Amikacin to Treat Carbapenem-Resistant *Pseudomonas aeruginosa*. *Antibiotics* **2022**, *11*, 517. [CrossRef]
248. Galani, I.; Papoutsaki, V.; Karantani, I.; Karaiskos, I.; Galani, L.; Adamou, P.; Deliolanis, I.; Kodonaki, A.; Papadogeorgaki, E.; Markopoulou, M.; et al. In vitro activity of ceftolozane/tazobactam alone and in combination with amikacin against MDR/XDR *Pseudomonas aeruginosa* isolates from Greece. *J. Antimicrob. Chemother.* **2020**, *75*, 2164–2172. [CrossRef]
249. Montero, M.; VanScoy, B.D.; López-Causapé, C.; Conde, H.; Adams, J.; Segura, C.; Zamorano, L.; Oliver, A.; Horcajada, J.P.; Ambrose, P.G. Evaluation of Ceftolozane-Tazobactam in Combination with Meropenem against *Pseudomonas aeruginosa* Sequence Type 175 in a Hollow-Fiber Infection Model. *Antimicrob. Agents Chemother.* **2018**, *62*, e00026-18. [CrossRef]
250. Mikhail, S.; Singh, N.B.; Kebriaei, R.; Rice, S.A.; Stamper, K.C.; Castanheira, M.; Rybak, M.J. Evaluation of the Synergy of Ceftazidime-Avibactam in Combination with Meropenem, Amikacin, Aztreonam, Colistin, or Fosfomycin against Well-Characterized Multidrug-Resistant Klebsiella pneumoniae and *Pseudomonas aeruginosa*. *Antimicrob. Agents Chemother.* **2019**, *63*, e00779-19. [CrossRef]
251. Montero, M.M.; Domene Ochoa, S.; López-Causapé, C.; Luque, S.; Sorlí, L.; Campillo, N.; López Montesinos, I.; Padilla, E.; Prim, N.; Angulo-Brunet, A. Time-Kill Evaluation of Antibiotic Combinations Containing Ceftazidime-Avibactam against Extensively Drug-Resistant *Pseudomonas aeruginosa* and Their Potential Role against Ceftazidime-Avibactam-Resistant Isolates. *Microbiol. Spectr.* **2021**, *9*, e00585-21. [CrossRef]
252. Zhang, Y.; Zhao, J.; Han, J.; Fan, Y.; Xiong, Z.; Zou, X.; Li, B.; Liu, X.; Li, Z.; Lu, B.; et al. Synergistic Activity of Imipenem in Combination with Ceftazidime/Avibactam or Avibactam against Non-MBL-Producing Extensively Drug-Resistant *Pseudomonas aeruginosa*. *Microbiol. Spectr.* **2022**, *10*, e02740-21. [CrossRef]
253. Abouelhassan, Y.; Gill, C.M.; Nicolau, D.P. Assessing the in vivo efficacy of rational antibiotics and combinations against difficult-to-treat *Pseudomonas aeruginosa* producing GES β-lactamases. *J. Antimicrob. Chemother.* **2023**, *78*, 1843–1847. [CrossRef]
254. Lee, M.; Abbey, T.; Biagi, M.; Wenzler, E. Activity of aztreonam in combination with ceftazidime-avibactam against serine- and metallo-β-lactamase-producing *Pseudomonas aeruginosa*. *Diagn. Microbiol. Infect. Dis.* **2021**, *99*, 115227. [CrossRef]
255. Mularoni, A.; Mezzatesta, M.L.; Pilato, M.; Medaglia, A.A.; Cervo, A.; Bongiorno, D.; Aprile, A.; Luca, A.; Stefani, S.; Grossi, P. Combination of aztreonam, ceftazidime–avibactam and amikacin in the treatment of VIM-1 *Pseudomonas aeruginosa* ST235 osteomyelitis. *Int. J. Infect. Dis.* **2021**, *108*, 510–512. [CrossRef]
256. Gatti, M.; Giannella, M.; Rinaldi, M.; Gaibani, P.; Viale, P.; Pea, F. Pharmacokinetic/Pharmacodynamic Analysis of Continuous-Infusion Fosfomycin in Combination with Extended-Infusion Cefiderocol or Continuous-Infusion Ceftazidime-Avibactam in a Case Series of Difficult-to-Treat Resistant *Pseudomonas aeruginosa* Bloodstream Infections and/or Hospital-Acquired Pneumonia. *Antibiotics* **2022**, *11*, 1739. [CrossRef]
257. Asuphon, O.; Montakantikul, P.; Houngsaitong, J.; Kiratisin, P.; Sonthisombat, P. Optimizing intravenous fosfomycin dosing in combination with carbapenems for treatment of *Pseudomonas aeruginosa* infections in critically ill patients based on pharmacokinetic/pharmacodynamic (PK/PD) simulation. *Int. J. Infect. Dis.* **2016**, *50*, 23–29. [CrossRef]
258. Fiore, M.; Corrente, A.; Pace, M.C.; Alfieri, A.; Simeon, V.; Ippolito, M.; Giarratano, A.; Cortegiani, A. Ceftolozane-Tazobactam Combination Therapy Compared to Ceftolozane-Tazobactam Monotherapy for the Treatment of Severe Infections: A Systematic Review and Meta-Analysis. *Antibiotics* **2021**, *10*, 79. [CrossRef]
259. Aslan, A.T.; Ezure, Y.; Horcajada, J.P.; Harris, P.N.A.; Paterson, D.L. In vitro, in vivo and clinical studies comparing the efficacy of ceftazidime-avibactam monotherapy with ceftazidime-avibactam-containing combination regimens against carbapenem-resistant Enterobacterales and multidrug-resistant *Pseudomonas aeruginosa* isolates or infections: A scoping review. *Front. Med.* **2023**, *10*, 1249030.
260. Candel, F.J.; Salavert, M.; Estella, A.; Ferrer, M.; Ferrer, R.; Gamazo, J.J.; García-Vidal, C.; del Castillo, J.G.; González-Ramallo, V.J.; Gordo, F.; et al. Ten Issues to Update in Nosocomial or Hospital-Acquired Pneumonia: An Expert Review. *J. Clin. Med.* **2023**, *12*, 6526. [CrossRef]
261. Lu, Q.; Luo, R.; Bodin, L.; Yang, J.; Zahr, N.; Aubry, A.; Golmard, J.-L.; Rouby, J.-J. Efficacy of High-dose Nebulized Colistin in Ventilator-associated Pneumonia Caused by Multidrug-resistant *Pseudomonas aeruginosa* and *Acinetobacter baumannii*. *Anesthesiology* **2012**, *117*, 1335–1347. [CrossRef]
262. Wood, G.C. Aerosolized antibiotics for treating hospital-acquired and ventilator-associated pneumonia. *Expert Rev. Anti. Infect. Ther.* **2011**, *9*, 993–1000. [CrossRef]

263. Wood, G.C.; Swanson, J.M. An Update on Aerosolized Antibiotics for Treating Hospital-Acquired and Ventilator-Associated Pneumonia in Adults. *Ann. Pharmacother.* **2017**, *51*, 1112–1121. [CrossRef]
264. Qin, J.P.; Huang, H.B.; Zhou, H.; Zhu, Y.; Xu, Y.; Du, B. Amikacin nebulization for the adjunctive therapy of gram-negative pneumonia in mechanically ventilated patients: A systematic review and meta-analysis of randomized controlled trials. *Sci. Rep.* **2021**, *11*, 6969. [CrossRef]
265. Kollef, M.H.; Ricard, J.-D.; Roux, D.; Francois, B.; Ischaki, E.; Rozgonyi, Z.; Boulain, T.; Ivanyi, Z.; János, G.; Garot, D.; et al. A Randomized Trial of the Amikacin Fosfomycin Inhalation System for the Adjunctive Therapy of Gram-Negative Ventilator-Associated Pneumonia: IASIS Trial. *Chest* **2017**, *151*, 1239–1246. [CrossRef]
266. Tamma, P.D.; Heil, E.L.; Justo, J.A.; Mathers, A.J.; Satlin, M.J.; Bonomo, R.A. Infectious Diseases Society of America 2024 Guidance on the Treatment of Antimicrobial-Resistant Gram-Negative Infections. *Clin. Infect. Dis.* **2024**, ciae403. [CrossRef]
267. Torres, A.; Niederman, M.S.; Chastre, J.; Ewig, S.; Fernandez-Vandellos, P.; Hanberger, H.; Kollef, M.; Li Bassi, G.; Luna, C.M.; Martin-Loeches, I.; et al. International ERS/ESICM/ESCMID/ALAT guidelines for the management of hospital-acquired pneumonia and ventilator-associated pneumonia: Guidelines for the management of hospital-acquired pneumonia (HAP)/ventilator-associated pneumonia (VAP) of the European Respiratory Society (ERS), European Society of Intensive Care Medicine (ESICM), European Society of Clinical Microbiology and Infectious Diseases (ESCMID) and Asociación Latinoamericana del Tórax (ALAT). *Eur. Respir. J.* **2017**, *50*, 1700582.

antibiotics

Article

Optimizing Antibiotic Therapy for *Stenotrophomonas maltophilia* Infections in Critically Ill Patients: A Pharmacokinetic/Pharmacodynamic Approach

Helena Barrasa [1,2,*], Miguel Angel Morán [2,3], Leire Fernández-Ciriza [4], Arantxa Isla [2,5], María Ángeles Solinís [2,5], Andrés Canut-Blasco [2,6] and Alicia Rodríguez-Gascón [2,5,*]

1 Intensive Care Unit, Araba University Hospital, Osakidetza Basque Health Service, 01009 Vitoria-Gasteiz, Spain
2 Bioaraba Health Research Institute, 01009 Vitoria-Gasteiz, Spain; miguelangel.moranrodriguez@osakidetza.eus (M.A.M.); arantxa.isla@ehu.eus (A.I.); marian.solinis@ehu.eus (M.Á.S.); andres.canutblasco@osakidetza.eus (A.C.-B.)
3 Infectious Disease Division, Araba University Hospital, Osakidetza Basque Health Service, 01009 Vitoria-Gasteiz, Spain
4 Microbiology Laboratory, Biomedical Diagnostic Service, Hospital San Pedro, 26006 Logroño, Spain; lfciriza@riojasalud.es
5 Pharmacokinetic, Nanotechnology and Gene Therapy Group (PharmaNanoGene), Faculty of Pharmacy, Lascaray Research Centre, University of the Basque Country UPV/EHU, 01006 Vitoria-Gasteiz, Spain
6 Microbiology Service, Araba University Hospital, Osakidetza Basque Health Service, 01009 Vitoria-Gasteiz, Spain
* Correspondence: helena.barrasagonzalez@osakidetza.eus (H.B.); alicia.rodriguez@ehu.eus (A.R.-G.); Tel.: +34-945-007000 (ext. 4737) (H.B.); +34-945-013094 (A.R.-G.)

Abstract: *Stenotrophomonas maltophilia* is an opportunistic, multidrug-resistant non-fermentative Gram-negative bacillus, posing a significant challenge in clinical treatment due to its numerous intrinsic and acquired resistance mechanisms. This study aimed to evaluate the adequacy of antibiotics used for the treatment of *S. maltophilia* infections in critically ill patients using a pharmacokinetic/pharmacodynamic (PK/PD) approach. The antibiotics studied included cotrimoxazole, levofloxacin, minocycline, tigecycline, cefiderocol, and the new combination aztreonam/avibactam, which is not yet approved. By Monte Carlo simulations, the probability of target attainment (PTA), the PK/PD breakpoints, and the cumulative fraction of response (CFR) were estimated. PK parameters and MIC distributions were sourced from the literature, the European Committee on Antimicrobial Susceptibility Testing (EUCAST), and the SENTRY Antimicrobial Surveillance Program collection. Cefiderocol 2 g q8h, minocycline 200 mg q12h, tigecycline 100 mg q12h, and aztreonam/avibactam 1500/500 mg q6h were the best options to treat empirically infections due to *S. maltophilia*. Cotrimoxazole provided a higher probability of treatment success for the U.S. isolates than for European isolates. For all antibiotics, discrepancies between the PK/PD breakpoints and the clinical breakpoints defined by EUCAST (or the ECOFF) and CLSI were detected.

Keywords: *Stenotrophomonas maltophilia*; PK/PD; cotrimoxazole; levofloxacin; minocycline; tigecycline; aztreonam/avibactam; cefiderocol

1. Introduction

Stenotrophomonas maltophilia is an opportunistic, multidrug-resistant non-fermentative Gram-negative bacilli that causes a variety of clinical syndromes including hospital-acquired pneumonia (HAP) or ventilator-associated pneumonia (VAP) as well as bloodstream infections (BSIs), particularly in debilitated or immunocompromised patients, with high mortality rates [1]. *S. maltophilia* ranks among the most frequent pathogens isolated from hospitalized pneumonia patients in Europe, and it is the primary Gram-negative pathogen resistant to carbapenems isolated from BSIs in the USA [2]. *S. maltophilia* is commonly found in cystic fibrosis (CF) airways which can cause colonization and chronic infection in patients with CF [3].

According to the latest guidelines of The Infectious Diseases Society of America (IDSA) [4,5] for mild infections, the recommended treatment includes cotrimoxazole and minocycline either as monotherapy, or alternatively, tigecycline, levofloxacin, or cefiderocol as monotherapy. It is strongly advised to refrain from using ceftazidime due to its probable ineffectiveness, and improvement is not expected when combined with avibactam without aztreonam. For moderate to severe infections, at least three distinct approaches are suggested: (1) combination therapy comprising cotrimoxazole plus minocycline; (2) initial treatment with cotrimoxazole alone, with the subsequent addition of minocycline (preferred), tigecycline, levofloxacin, or cefiderocol if clinical improvement is delayed with cotrimoxazole alone; and (3) cefiderocol or ceftazidime/avibactam in conjunction with aztreonam, particularly when intolerance toward or ineffectiveness of other agents are anticipated.

S. maltophilia is intrinsically resistant to many classes of antibiotics, including aminoglycosides, quinolones, and beta-lactams, through the production of aminoglycoside-modifying enzymes (AMEs), Qnr-like resistance determinants (Sm*qnr* genes), and two inducible beta-lactamases, L1 and L2 [6,7]. L1 metallo-beta-lactamase hydrolyse penicillins, cephalosporins, and carbapenems, but not aztreonam, and are not inhibited by any beta-lactamase inhibitor (BLI). L2 is a class A cephalosporinase susceptible to inhibition by clavulanic acid and avibactam. The overexpression of efflux pumps also contributes to resistance to tetracyclines, quinolones, cotrimoxazole (trimethoprim/sulfamethoxazole), tigecycline, and polymyxins. *S. maltophilia* also acquire genes horizontally that confer resistance to cotrimoxazole (*sul* and *dfrA*) and beta-lactams (*bla*) [4,8].

Although the Clinical and Laboratory Standards Institute (CLSI) has established susceptibility interpretative criteria for ticarcillin/clavulanate, ceftazidime, cefiderocol, minocycline, levofloxacin, cotrimoxazole, and chloramphenicol [9], the European Committee on Antimicrobial Susceptibility Testing (EUCAST) has only established interpretative criteria for cotrimoxazole [10]. The scarcity of available antimicrobial agents with clinical breakpoints recognized, the poor correlation data between MICs and clinical outcomes, and the lack of updated pharmacokinetic/pharmacodynamic studies make it difficult to treat *S. maltophilia* infections, especially in immunocompromised and critically ill patients when the first-line antimicrobial, cotrimoxazole, is contraindicated.

The aim of our study was to evaluate the adequacy of commonly prescribed antibiotics for the treatment of *S. maltophilia* infections in critically ill patients, including cotrimoxazole (trimethoprim/sulfamethoxazole), levofloxacin, minocycline, tigecycline, and cefiderocol, using a pharmacokinetic/pharmacodynamic (PK/PD) approach. The new combination, aztreonam/avibactam, which is not yet approved, was also studied. Our goal was to provide clinicians with additional insights to enhance antibiotic therapy and to combat antimicrobial resistance.

2. Results

Figure 1 shows the probability of target attainment (PTA, or the probability that the specific value of the PK/PD index reaches the values associated with the efficacy at a certain MIC value) of all the antimicrobials included in the study and the MIC distribution of *S. maltophilia* against these antibiotics. For the aztreonam/avibactam combination, since the PTA for avibactam ($\%fT_{>2.5\ mg/L} > 50\%$) is 100%, the joint PTA corresponds to the PTA for aztreonam ($\%fT_{>MIC} \geq 60\%$). MIC distributions of *S. maltophilia* for cotrimoxazole (trimethoprim/sulfamethoxazole), levofloxacin, minocycline, tigecycline, cefiderocol, and aztreonam/avibactam are available from European isolates (reported by EUCAST [11]); for trimethoprim/sulfamethoxazole, minocycline, and levofloxacin, MIC values from U.S. isolates were also available [7].

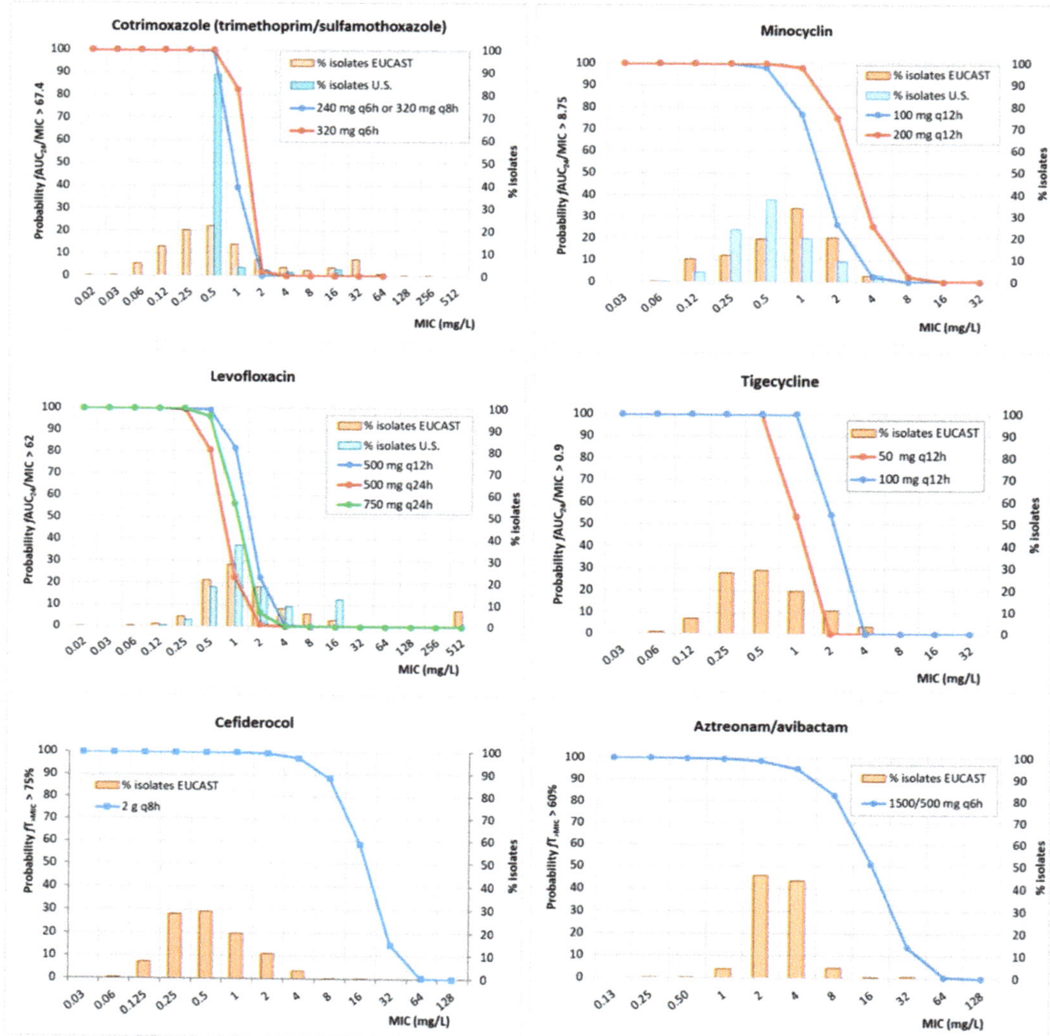

Figure 1. Probability of target attainment (PTA) and MIC distribution of *S. maltophilia* against cotrimoxazole, levofloxacin, minocycline, tigecycline, cefiderocol, and aztreonam/avibactam. For aztreonam/avibactam, PTA corresponds to the joint PTA (target of aztreonam and target for avibactam achieved simultaneously). For cotrimoxazole, the PTA refers to trimethoprim.

The most relevant differences in the susceptibility profile depending on the geographical area (Europe vs. U.S.) were observed for trimethoprim/sulfamethoxazole; while the MIC_{90} of the U.S. isolates is 1 mg/L, European isolates present an MIC_{90} of 16 mg/L. By comparing the PTA values and the MIC distributions, the best options to treat infections due to *S. maltophilia* in Europe are cefiderocol, aztreonam/avibactam, a higher dose of tigecycline, and a higher dose of minocycline. In the U.S., trimethoprim/sulfamethoxazole is also a good option. The MIC distributions of U.S. isolates against tigecycline, cefiderocol, and aztreonam/avibactam were not available, and therefore, we could not compare the PTA with the susceptibility profile of U.S. isolates.

The PK/PD breakpoint, that is, the highest MIC value at which there is a high probability of target attainment (≥97.5%), can be estimated by representing the values of the PK/PD index ($fAUC_{24}$/MIC or %$fT_{>MIC}$) against the MIC values. The PK/PD breakpoint can be read directly from the intersection of the horizontal line at the PK/PD target and the lower limit of the 95% confidence interval (2.5% percentile). Figure 2 features the relationship between the values of the $fAUC_{24}$/MIC and the MIC for cotrimoxazole (trimethoprim component). With the three dose levels analyzed, the PK/PD breakpoint was 0.5 mg/L.

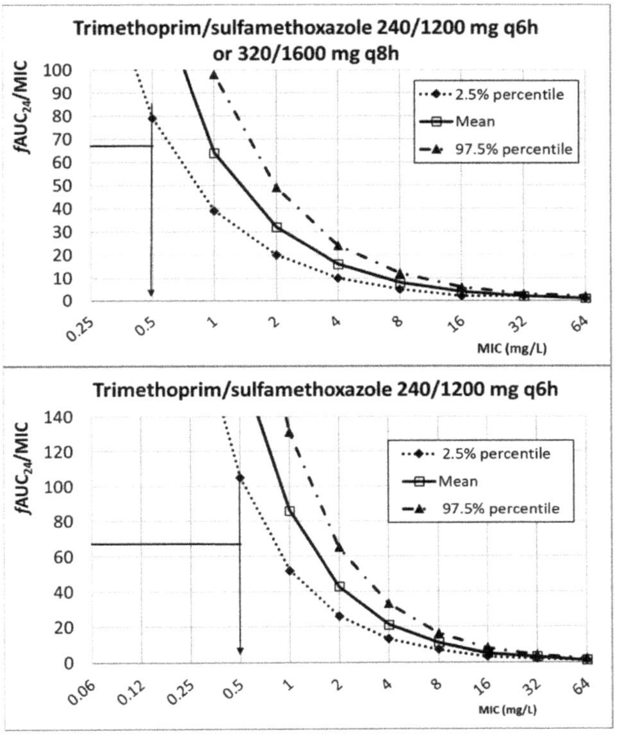

Figure 2. Relationship between $fAUC_{24}$/MIC and MIC for different dosing regimens of cotrimoxazole (trimethoprim component). PK/PD target (horizontal line): 67.4.

Figure 3 shows the relationship between the PK/PD index of levofloxacin ($fAUC_{24}$/MIC) and the MIC. According to these results, and considering the target ($fAUC_{24}$/MIC ≥ 62), the PK/PD breakpoint is 0.5 mg/L for 500 mg q12h and 0.25 mg/L for 500 mg q24h and 750 mg q24h.

In Figure 4, the relationship between the PK/PD index of minocycline ($fAUC_{24}$/MIC) and the MIC is featured. Considering the target ($fAUC_{24}$/MIC ≥ 8.75), the PK/PD breakpoint is 0.5 mg/L and 1 mg/L for 100 mg q12h and 200 mg q12h, respectively.

Figure 5 shows the relationship between the PK/PD index of tigecycline ($fAUC_{24}$/MIC), and the MIC is featured. Considering the target ($fAUC_{24}$/MIC ≥ 0.9), the PK/PD breakpoint is 0.5 mg/L and 1 mg/L for 50 mg q12h and 100 mg q12h, respectively.

The relationship between the PK/PD index of cefiderocol (%$fT_{>MIC}$) and the MIC is featured in Figure 6. Considering the target (%$fT_{>MIC}$ ≥ 75%), the PK/PD breakpoint for the dosing regimen of 2 g q8h is 4 mg/L.

Figure 7 presents the relationship between the PK/PD index of aztreonam ($\%fT_{>MIC}$) and the MIC. Considering the target ($\%fT_{>MIC} \geq 60\%$ for aztreonam), the PK/PD breakpoint for the dosing regimen of 1500 mg q6h is 2 mg/L.

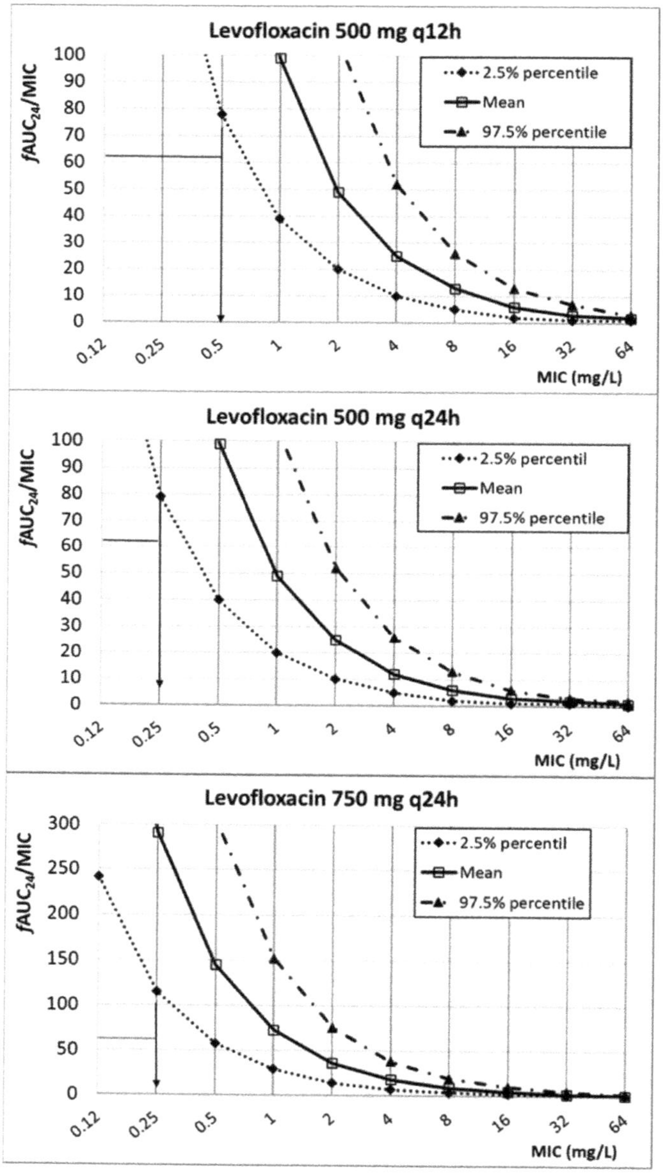

Figure 3. Relationship between $fAUC_{24}$/MIC and MIC for different dosing regimens of levofloxacin. PK/PD target (horizontal line): 62.

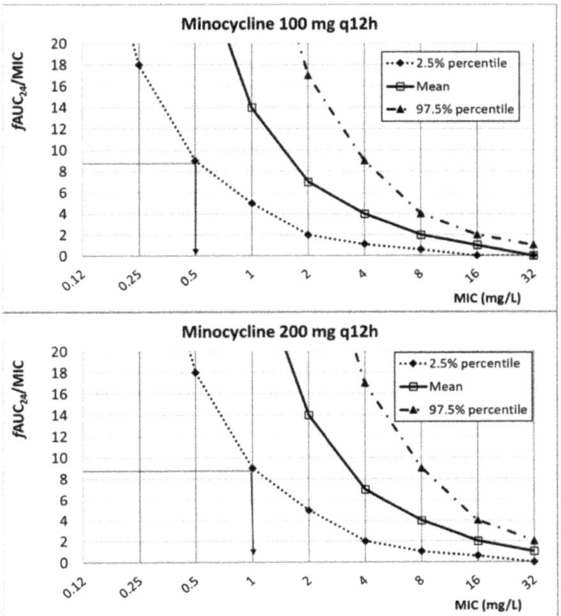

Figure 4. Relationship between $fAUC_{24}/MIC$ and MIC for different dosing regimens of minocycline. PK/PD target (horizontal line): 8.75.

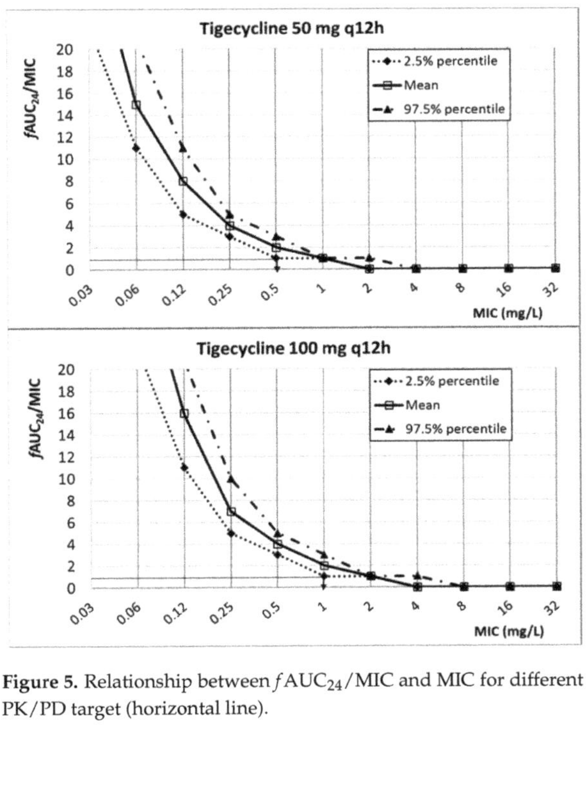

Figure 5. Relationship between $fAUC_{24}/MIC$ and MIC for different dosing regimens of tigecycline. PK/PD target (horizontal line).

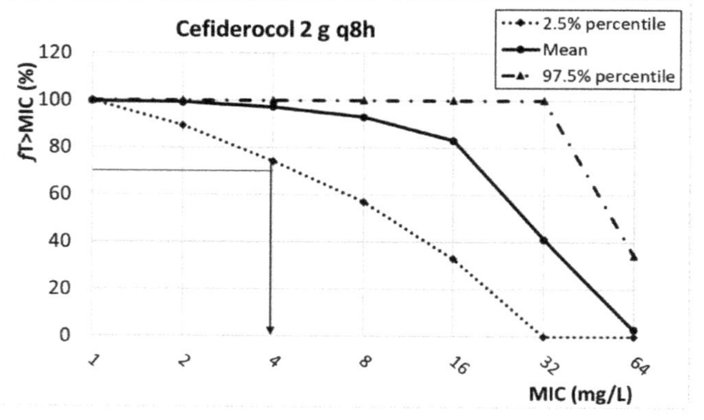

Figure 6. Relationship between $fAUC_{24}/MIC$ and MIC for cefiderocol. PK/PD target (horizontal line): 75%.

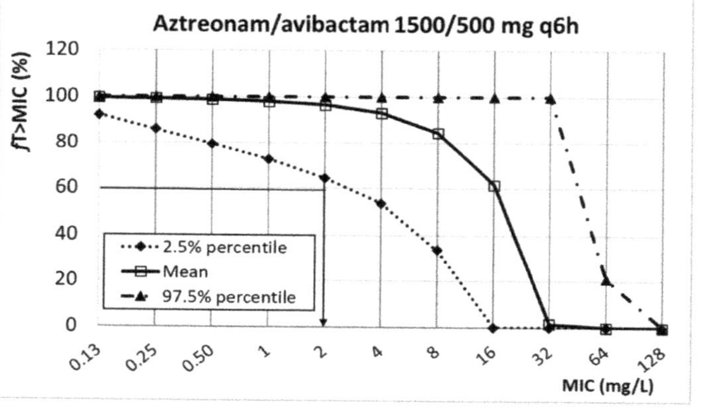

Figure 7. Relationship between $\%fT_{>MIC}$ and MIC for aztreonam/avibactam. PK/PD target (horizontal line): 60%.

Table 1 summarizes the PK/PD breakpoints calculated and the breakpoints published by CLSI [9] and EUCAST [10,11].

By Monte Carlo simulations, we also estimated the cumulative fraction of response (CFR), defined as the expected population PTA for a specific drug dose and a specific population of microorganisms. The CFR is considered the expected probability of success of a dosing regimen against bacteria when a specific value of MIC is not available, and thus, the population distribution of MICs is used. Table 2 shows the CFR values for all antimicrobials included in the study calculated from the corresponding MIC distribution of *S. maltophilia* isolates.

Considering the EUCAST MIC distribution, cotrimoxazole did not provide CFR values >90% at any of the dose levels analyzed. However, for the U.S. isolates, CFR $\geq$ 90% was obtained with all of the doses. For levofloxacin, regardless of the dose level and the precedence of the isolates, CFR was always <60%. Regarding minocycline, only the high dose provided CFR > 90%, regardless of the precedence of the isolates. Tigecycline only provided CFR > 90% at the high dose (100 mg q12h) for the EUCAST isolates. With cefiderocol and aztreonam/avibactam, CFR was 99% and 95%, respectively.

Table 1. Comparison of the pharmacokinetic/pharmacodynamic (PK/PD), European Committee on Antimicrobial Susceptibility Testing (EUCAST), and Clinical and Laboratory Standards Institute (CLSI) breakpoints (mg/L) for *S. maltophilia*.

Antibiotic	PK/PD Breakpoint	Clinical Breakpoint		ECOFFs [a]
		CLSI	EUCAST	
Cotrimoxazole (trimethoprim/sulfamethoxazole)				
240/1200 mg q6h	0.5	≤2 [b]	≤4 [b,c]	2
320/1600 mg q8h	0.5			
320/1600 mg q6h	0.5			
Levofloxacin				
500 mg q24h	0.25	≤2	n.d.	4
500 mg q12h	0.5			
750 mg q24h	0.25			
Minocycline				
100 mg q12h	0.5	≤4	n.d.	1
200 mg q12h	1			
Tigecycline				
50 mg q12h	0.5	n.d.	n.d.	4
100 mg q12h	1			
Cefiderocol				
2 g q8h	4	≤1	n.d.	0.125
Aztreonam/avibactam				
1500/500 mg q6h	2	n.d.	n.d.	8 [d]

[a]: Epidemiological cut-off values according to EUCAST; [b]: trimethoprim component; [c]: susceptible, increased exposure: [d]: tentative ECOFF (TECOFF). n.d.: not defined.

Table 2. CFR values of all antimicrobials included in the study for EUCAST and U.S. isolates.

Antibiotic	CFR (%)	
	EUCAST Isolates	U.S.Isolates
Cotrimoxazole (trimethoprim/sulfamethoxazole)		
240/1200 mg q6h	66	90
320/1600 mg q8h	66	90
320/1600 mg q6h	73	91
Levofloxacin		
500 mg q24h	30	28
500 mg q12h	55	57
750 mg q24h	44	44
Minocycline		
100 mg q12h	74	84
200 mg q12h	92	94
Tigecycline		
50 mg q12h	76	*
100 mg q12h	91	*
Cefiderocol		
2 g q8h	99	*
Aztreonam/avibactam		
1500/500 mg q6h	95	*

*: no MIC distribution was available, and therefore, CFR was not estimated.

3. Discussion

Currently, the management of *S. maltophilia* infections remains a challenge due, among other factors, to (1) the significant number of intrinsic and acquired resistance mechanisms it presents, (2) the occasional difficulty in distinguishing colonization from a true infection, (3) the common polymicrobial presentation (specially in immunocompromised patients), (4) the absence of a standard of care to assess the effectiveness of therapeutic alternatives, and (5) the challenge in determining the sensitivity profile [4]. In this regard, adequate therapy is essential for survival. In a recent meta-analysis, patients with bacteremia treated with inappropriate antimicrobial therapy had higher mortality [12]. Apart from the selection of the most appropriate antibiotic, the success of therapy depends on optimizing the dosing regimen. The integration of pharmacokinetic/pharmacodynamic (PKPD) analysis and Monte Carlo simulation (MCS) has made them important tools for optimizing antimicrobial therapy. They enable the selection of the optimal antibiotic and dosing regimen taking into account the microorganism and the patient, increasing the chance of therapy success and reducing side effects and the emergence of resistant strains [13–15].

In this work, we have identified minocycline 200 mg q12h, tigecycline 100 mg q12h, cefiderocol 2 g q8h, and aztreonam/avibactam 1500/500 mg q6h as the best options to treat infections due to *S. maltophilia* considering the susceptibility of European isolates. For U.S. strains, cotrimoxazole at any dose level and minocycline 200 mg q12h are also good options; the lack of availability of U.S. isolate susceptibility profiles to tigecycline, cefiderocol, and aztreonam/avibactam prevented us from demonstrating the usefulness of these antibiotics. To the knowledge of the authors, this is a more complete study that evaluates, through PK/PD and Monte Carlo simulations, if the antimicrobials used for the treatment of infections due to *S. maltophilia* are adequate considering the susceptibility profile of this microorganism.

The highest MIC value at which a high probability of target attainment (PTA $\geq$ 90%) is obtained can be used to estimate PK/PD breakpoints; however, a much more restrictive PK/PD breakpoint can be obtained from a graphical representation of the PK/PD index as a function of the MIC (EUCAST approach) [16]. PK/PD breakpoints may be especially useful when no clinical breakpoint nor epidemiological cut-off values (ECOFFs) are defined, as is the case of *S. maltophilia*. Contrary to clinical breakpoints, different PK/PD breakpoints can be obtained with different dosages of the same drug, since they are dose regimen-dependent and species-independent [17]. Regarding cotrimoxazole, we detected discrepancies between the PK/PD breakpoint (0.5 mg/L) and the clinical breakpoint defined by EUCAST (susceptible, increased exposure up to 4 mg/L) and CLSI (susceptible up to 2 mg/L) (Table 1). According to the PK/PD breakpoint, cotrimoxazole should not be recommended to treat an infection due to isolates with MICs higher than 0.5 mg/L since drug exposure is insufficient. These results agree with Lasko et al. [18], who demonstrated that cotrimoxazole in monotherapy even at a high dose displays limited activity against cotrimoxazole-susceptible *S. maltophilia* strains. In fact, several authors have pointed out the necessity of redefining the breakpoints of cotrimoxazole for *S. maltophilia* [8,19,20]. Apart from cotrimoxazole, we detected discrepancies between the breakpoints for the rest of the antibiotics. Only with tigecycline and cefiderocol, the PK/PD breakpoints were higher than the ECOFF and the clinical breakpoint by CLSI, respectively; that is, antibiotic exposure is sufficient to treat infections due to isolates with MIC values considered resistant. The PK/PD breakpoints of tigecycline obtained in our study are in agreement with a systematic review, which pointed out that for an MIC < 0.5 mg/L, standard dosing of 50 mg q12h with a loading dose of 100 mg can be used, but if the MIC is $\geq$0.5–1 mg/L, a loading dose of 200 mg and 100 mg q12h is recommended [21]. Discrepancies in the PK/PD and clinical breakpoints have been already detected for other antibiotics [7,22]. In a previous study, the breakpoints of minocycline against *Acinetobacter baumanii* have been questioned since a modern PK/PD evaluation was not carried out for tetracyclines [23].

For empirical therapy, the susceptibility profile of the microorganism responsible for the infection in a certain geographical area is crucial. In this regard, a great difference in the susceptibility of *S. maltophilia* to cotrimoxazole between Europe and the U.S. exists, and therefore, the dose level needed may be different. According to our study, while in the U.S., a high level of treatment success is achieved with any of the three dose regimens studied (CFR $\geq$ 90%), in Europe, even with the highest dose evaluated, the probability of treatment success is much lower (CFR < 75%). In spite of our results, and despite the fact that a recent meta-analysis has shown that the resistance rate of *S. maltophilia* has increased in recent years [24], cotrimoxazole remains the first choice for treatment, with the dosing recommendation ranging from 10 to 15 mg/kg/day of trimethoprim q8h and a maximum daily dose of trimethoprim of 960 mg [1,8].

According to IDSA guidelines [4], minocycline and tigecycline are considered for the treatment of *S. maltophilia* infections. Although minocycline is preferred over tigecycline due to more favorable in vitro data, defined CLSI breakpoints, the availability of an oral formulation, and improved tolerability, our PK/PD study has revealed that both antibiotics at the highest dose (200 mg q12h of minocycline and 100 mg q12h of tigecycline) provide a high probability of treatment success (CFR > 90%) regardless of the geographical area, Europe or the U.S. It is noteworthy that tetracycline derivatives exhibit rapid tissue distribution after administration, leading to low concentrations in urine and serum [25]. Consequently, these derivatives are not advised as treatments of urinary tract infections (UTIs) due to *S. maltophilia* and are only recommended in combination therapy for the management of *S. maltophilia* bloodstream infections [4].

The role of quinolones in the treatment of *S. maltophilia* infections is controversial. While they may serve as an alternative in mild infections, their use in moderate to severe infections is only advised in combination therapy, with monotherapy de-escalation not recommended. This recommendation is based on suboptimal results in in vitro studies [26], low susceptibility in surveillance studies [27], the well-known resistance mechanisms (Sm*qnr* genes), the increasing development of resistance during treatment [24], adverse effects [28], and the lack of high-quality clinical studies supporting their use [29]. Our study has confirmed that levofloxacin is not a good alternative for the empirical treatment of infections due to *S. maltophilia*, neither in Europe nor in the U.S., at least in monotherapy. Only if the MIC is known and up to 0.5 mg/L, levofloxacin at a dose of 500 mg q12h could be an option; if the MIC is $\leq$0.25 mg/L, 500 mg or 750 mg q24 could also be useful. A previous PK/PD study also suggested than levofloxacin monotherapy may not achieve appropriate PK/PD target attainment for *S. maltophilia* infections [30]. Additionally, in a neutropenic murine tight infection model, levofloxacin 750 mg q24h provided probabilities of target attainment for a $1 - \log_{10}$ CFU (colony-forming unit) reduction of 95.8%, 72.2%, and 26% at MICs of 0.5, 1, and 2 mg/L, respectively [31]. As with cotrimoxazole, it has been suggested that the CLSI breakpoint of levofloxacin (2 mg/L) should be redefined. In spite of the less favorable results obtained with levofloxacin, its usefulness for the treatment of *S. maltophilia* infections is controversial due to the lack of robust evidence supporting the superiority of one therapy over others. In this regard, in a recent meta-analysis, significant differences in the mortality of patients with *S. maltophilia* bacteremia among trimethoprim/sulfamethoxazole, fluoroquinolones, and minocycline were not found [12].

In a previous study, cefiderocol and aztreonam/avibactam have been identified as two of the most promising options of treatment for extensively drug-resistant (XDR) *S. maltophilia* infections with resistance to the preferred first-line antimicrobials [21]. Our results are in line with this statement. The susceptibility profile of *S. maltophilia* to cefiderocol, a new, recently approved catechol-conjugated cephalosporin, is very favorable, with global susceptibility higher than 95% [8,32]. Our PK/PD study has confirmed its usefulness for the treatment of infections due to *S. maltophilia* isolates with MICs up to 4 mg/L, and also for empirical treatment, with a probability of success around 100%. These results are in agreement with a recent meta-analysis, which has shown that cefiderocol and minocycline can be considered the preferred treatment alternatives for *S. maltophilia* infections due to low resistance rates, although regional differences in resistance rates to other antibiotics should be considered [33]. Although cefiderocol has shown clinical and microbiological success in some studies [34,35], further research to confirm its efficacy and safety in the real world, that is, in everyday use, is needed.

The combination of aztreonam/avibactam, currently in phase III clinical trials but not yet approved, has shown a global susceptibility rate against *S. maltophilia* of around 98%, including isolates not susceptible to cotrimoxazole [36]. This new beta-lactam/beta-lactam inhibitor combination is an alternative to the use of aztreonam plus ceftazidime/avibactam, which has demonstrated treatment success in complex pancreatic focus [37], bacteremia [38], and pneumonia [39] caused by *S. maltophilia*. While ceftazidime is a substrate of L1 beta-lactamase, it cannot hydrolyze aztreonam, and although L2 hydrolyzes aztreonam, it is inhibited by avibactam. In this way, aztreonam successfully reaches the penicillin-binding proteins (PBPs) of *S. maltophilia*, likely PBP3 [8]. The efficacy and safety of aztreonam/avibactam is being studied, with positive results reported in the interim analysis of two phase III clinical trials [40–42]. PK/PD analysis, at the approved doses for the aztreonam/avibactam combination (1.5/0.5 g q6h), has shown an optimal coverage for infections due to isolates with MICs up to 2 mg/L, and when used empirically, a high probability of treatment success is expected (CFR of 95%). These results confirm that aztreonam/avibactam may represent a valuable alternative for the treatment of *S. maltophilia* infections, addressing a major unmet medical need.

Our study presents several limitations. First, we have evaluated the usefulness of the antimicrobials by PK/PD considering its administration as monotherapy, although clinical guides recommend combination therapy in some situations, mainly to treat moderate to severe infections. Nevertheless, in spite of the fact that in vitro PK/PD studies have revealed that monotherapy is hardly bactericidal against *S. maltophilia* even with susceptible strains, combination therapy does not seem to significantly increase the antibacterial activity [20]. In a systematic review about novel therapies for the treatment of *S. maltophilia* infections, Gibb et al. advise against the routine use of antimicrobial combinations for pneumonia, catheter-associated bacteremia, urinary tract infection, or bacteremia [21]. In the case of abdominal perforation with an undrained abscess, two active agents may be used, and in the case of endocarditis, although there is not enough evidence, combination therapy has been used historically; therefore, dose recommendations based in our results may be not applicable in abdominal perforation and endocarditis. A recent systematic review and meta-analysis to compare the effects of monotherapy and combination therapy on the mortality of patients with *S. maltophilia* infections [43] concluded that combination therapy may have a role in the treatment of severe or complex cases of *S. maltophilia*; however, monotherapy resulted in having more favorable outcomes in terms of mortality in patients with hospital-acquired *S. maltophilia* pneumonia. Due to the low number of studies involved in the meta-analysis (only four), the authors suggest a longitudinal study to further explore this association. The second limitation is that we have the PK/PD analysis to critically ill patients, and the results may not be representative of other patient populations. In spite of these limitations, PK/PD analysis and Monte Carlo simulations are very useful tools to estimate susceptibility breakpoints, mainly when clinical breakpoints are not defined, and to predict the success of antimicrobial agents when used empirically considering the susceptibility profile in a certain geographical area.

4. Materials and Methods

This simulation study was based on literature data only, and therefore, no ethics approval was required.

4.1. Pharmacokinetic Parameters, PK/PD Targets, and Susceptibility Data

The PK parameters of trimethoprim, levofloxacin, minocycline, tigecycline, cefiderocol, aztreonam, and avibactam in critically ill patients, as well as the PK/PD targets (PD endpoints), were obtained from the literature. The PK parameters and the PK/PD targets are presented in Table 3.

Table 3. Pharmacokinetic parameters and PK/PD targets of the antimicrobial agents used for Monte Carlo simulations. Data are expressed as mean ± standard deviation.

Antibiotic	Dosing Regimen	CL (L/h)	Fu	V (L)	PK/PD Target	References
Cotrimoxazole (trimethoprim/ sulfamethoxazole) [a]	240/1200 mg q6h 320/1600 mg q6h 320/1600 mg q8h	1.88 ± 0.44 [b]	0.5 ± 0.017		fAUC$_{24}$/MIC ≥ 67.4	[18,44,45]
Levofloxacin	500 mg q12h 500 mgq24h 750 mgq24h	8.66 ± 3.85	0.71		fAUC$_{24}$/MIC ≥ 62	[30,46,47]
Minocycline	100 mg q12h 200 mgq12h	4.70 ± 2.14	0.28		fAUC$_{24}$/MIC ≥ 8.75	[30,48]
Tigecycline	50 mg q12h 100 mg q12h	22.10 ± 3.82	0.2		fAUC$_{24}$/MIC ≥ 0.9	[30,49]
Cefiderocol	2 g q8h, 3 h infusion	4.04 ± 1.52	0.44 ± 0.04	V1: 7.78 ± 4.43 V2: 5.77 ± 1.94 V3: 0.798	%fT$_{>MIC}$ > 75%	[50,51]
Aztreonam/ avibactam	1500/500 mg q6h 3 h infusion	9.60 ± 5.00 11.09 ± 6.78	0.72 0.92	27.20 ± 20.80 50.81 ± 14.32	%fT$_{>MIC}$ > 60% %fT$_{>2.5\ mg/L}$ > 50%	[52–54]

[a]: pharmacokinetic parameters and PK/PD index refer to trimethoprim. [b]: mL/min/Kg (70 Kg body weight was considered). CL: total body clearance; Fu: unbound fraction; fAUC$_{24}$: area under the unbound concentration–time curve over a period of 24 h; %fT$_{>MIC}$: percentage of time of the dosing interval in which the unbound serum antibiotic concentration remains above the minimum inhibitory concentration (MIC); V: distribution volume.

The PK/PD target of cotrimoxazole (fAUC$_{24}$/MIC ≥ 67.4) refers to the trimethoprim component; however, it was estimated in an in vitro model with trimethoprim and sulfamethoxazole in combination and not separately, and therefore, the activity of the two components is considered [18].

The MIC distributions of trimethoprim/sulfamethoxazole (13 distributions, 2511 observations), levofloxacin (10 distributions, 1979 observations), minocycline (8 distributions, 432 observations), tigecycline (5 distributions, 289 observations), cefiderocol (5 distributions, 338 observations), and aztreonam/avibactam (4 distributions and 805 observations) against *S. maltophilia* were obtained from EUCAST [11]. Additionally, the MIC profile of cotrimoxazole, levofloxacin, and minocycline was also obtained from the study by Pfaller et al. [7], who included 1522 *S. maltophilia* isolates from the SENTRY Antimicrobial Surveillance Program collection, representing 35 U.S. medical centers from 2014 to 2021.

4.2. Pharmacokinetic/Pharmacodynamic Analysis and Monte Carlo Simulation

A 10,000-subject Monte Carlo simulation was conducted for each antibiotic using Oracle® Crystal Ball Fusion Edition v.11.1.2.3.500 (Oracle USA Inc., Redwood City, CA, USA). The PK/PD index and the magnitude or value of the PK/PD index associated with the success of therapy for every antibiotic are listed in Table 3, as well the dosing regimens studied. For trimethoprim, levofloxacin, minocycline, and tigecycline, fAUC$_{24}$/MIC is the PK/PD index that best predicts efficacy, and it was estimated by non-compartmental analysis using the following equation [22]:

$$fAUC_{24}/MIC = D \times Fu/CL$$

where D is the daily dose, Fu is the unbound fraction, and CL is the total clearance.

For cefiderocol and aztreonam, the proportion of time that the unbound serum concentration remains above the MIC in a steady state (%fT$_{>MIC}$) is the PK/PD index related to efficacy, and it was calculated considering a one-compartmental pharmacokinetic model with the following equations [22]:

$$t_1 = \frac{MIC - fC_{min,ss}}{fC_{max,ss} - fC_{min,ss}} \cdot t_{inf}$$

$$t_2 = \left(\frac{fC_{max,ss}}{MIC}\right) \cdot \frac{V_{ss}}{CL_t}$$

$$f\%T_{>MIC} = [(t_2 + t_{inf}) - t_1] \cdot \frac{100}{\tau}$$

where $fC_{min,ss}$ and $fC_{max,ss}$ are the minimum and the maximum serum concentration of the unbound drug (mg/L) in the steady state, respectively, t_{inf} is the infusion length, and t_1 and t_2 are the times at which the antibiotic concentration reaches the MIC during the infusion phase and in the elimination phase, respectively.

In the case of avibactam, the proportion of the dosing interval for which the free drug concentration is >2.5 mg/mL was calculated.

For simulations, a log-normal distribution was assumed for pharmacokinetic parameters, according to statistical criteria. The unbound fraction was included as a fixed value if interindividual variability was not available [55].

For each MIC value, the simulation resulted in a probability distribution, accounting for the variability in the pharmacokinetic parameters. The mean value and the 95% confidence interval (represented as percentiles) of either $\%fT_{>MIC}$ or $fAUC_{24}/MIC$ were then extracted. The highest MIC values at which the PK/PD index reaches the value related to treatment success, that is, the PK/PD breakpoints, were estimated from the lower limit of the 95% CI (2.5% percentile), as EUCAST has established [16].

We estimated the PTA or probability that a PK/PD index reaches the target value, that is, the value associated with efficacy [56]. PTA $\geq$ 90% was associated with a high probability of treatment success, but if 80% $\leq$ PTA < 90%, only a moderate probability of treatment success was considered [22].

The cumulative fraction of response, or CFR, that is, the probability of success of an empirical treatment, was estimated from the PTA at every MIC level and the MIC distribution of the bacterial population. For CFR calculation, the following equation was used [56]:

$$CFR(\%) = \sum_{i=1}^{n} PTA_i \cdot F_i$$

where PTA_i is the PTA at each MIC value (i), and F_i is the percentage of the microorganisms in the population with this MIC value. As with PTA, for CFR $\geq$ 90%, we considered a high probability of treatment success, but it was only moderate if 80% $\leq$ CFR < 90% [22].

Joint PTA, defined as the simultaneous attainment of PTA, was calculated for aztreonam/avibactam [57]. We first determined if the PTA of avibactam was achieved, and if the threshold was met, we then estimated the joint PTA as the PTA calculated for aztreonam.

5. Conclusions

From a PK/PD perspective, the best options to treat empirically *S. maltophilia* infections are cefiderocol, aztreonam/avibactam, and minocycline and tigecycline at the highest doses. While for European isolates, cotrimoxazole provided a low probability of treatment success, this antimicrobial agent may be useful considering the susceptibility of U.S. isolates. For all antibiotics, discrepancies between the PK/PD breakpoints and the clinical breakpoints defined by EUCAST (or the ECOFF) and CLSI were detected. With cotrimoxazole, levofloxacin, minocycline, and aztreonam/avibactam, isolates were considered susceptible based on CLSI and EUCAST breakpoints, and the PK/PD analysis predicted insufficient exposure. Only with tigecycline and cefiderocol were the PK/PD breakpoints higher than the ECOFF and the clinical breakpoint by CLSI, respectively; that is, antibiotic exposure is sufficient to treat infections due to isolates considered resistant.

Author Contributions: Conceptualization, H.B., A.C.-B. and A.R.-G.; formal analysis, L.F.-C., A.I. and A.R.-G.; funding acquisition, M.Á.S. and A.R.-G.; methodology, L.F.-C., A.I., M.Á.S., A.C.-B. and A.R.-G.; software, L.F.-C., A.I. and A.R.-G.; validation, H.B., M.A.M. and M.Á.S.; writing—

original draft, H.B., M.A.M., A.C.-B. and A.R.-G.; writing—review and editing, H.B., M.A.M., L.F.-C., A.I., M.Á.S., A.C.-B. and A.R.-G. All authors have read and agreed to the published version of the manuscript.

Funding: This research was funded by the Basque Government (IT1587-22).

Institutional Review Board Statement: Not applicable.

Informed Consent Statement: Not applicable.

Data Availability Statement: All data are contained within the paper.

Conflicts of Interest: The authors declare no conflicts of interest.

References

1. Chang, Y.T.; Lin, C.Y.; Chen, Y.H.; Hsueh, P.R. Update on infections caused by *Stenotrophomonas maltophilia* with particular attention to resistance mechanisms and therapeutic options. *Front. Microbiol.* **2015**, *6*, 893. [CrossRef] [PubMed]
2. Mojica, M.F.; Humphries, R.; Lipuma, J.J.; Mathers, A.J.; Rao, G.G.; Shelburne, S.A.; Fouts, D.E.; Van Duin, D.; Bonomo, R.A. Clinical challenges treating *Stenotrophomonas maltophilia* infections: An update. *JAC Antimicrob. Resist.* **2022**, *4*, dlac040. [CrossRef] [PubMed]
3. Terlizzi, V.; Tomaselli, M.; Giacomini, G.; Dalpiaz, I.; Chiappini, E. *Stenotrophomonas maltophilia* in people with Cystic Fibrosis: A systematic review of prevalence, risk factors and management. *Eur. J. Clin. Microbiol. Infect. Dis.* **2023**, *42*, 1285–1296. [CrossRef] [PubMed]
4. Tamma, P.D.; Aitken, S.L.; Bonomo, R.A.; Mathers, A.J.; van Duin, D.; Clancy, C.J. Infectious Diseases Society of America 2023 Guidance on the Treatment of Antimicrobial Resistant Gram-Negative Infections. *Clin Infect Dis.* **2023**, ciad428. [CrossRef] [PubMed]
5. Tamma, P.D.; Aitken, S.L.; Bonomo, R.A.; Mathers, A.J.; van Duin, D.; Clancy, C.J. Infectious Diseases Society of America Guidance on the Treatment of AmpC β-Lactamase-Producing Enterobacterales, Carbapenem-Resistant *Acinetobacter baumannii*, and *Stenotrophomonas maltophilia* Infections. *Clin. Infect. Dis.* **2022**, *74*, 2089–2114. [CrossRef] [PubMed]
6. Gales, A.C.; Seifert, H.; Gur, D.; Castanheira, M.; Jones, R.N.; Sader, H.S. Antimicrobial Susceptibility of *Acinetobacter calcoaceticus-Acinetobacter baumannii* Complex and *Stenotrophomonas maltophilia* Clinical Isolates: Results From the SENTRY Antimicrobial Surveillance Program (1997–2016). *Open Forum Infect. Dis.* **2019**, *6* (Suppl. S1), S34–S46. [CrossRef] [PubMed]
7. Pfaller, M.A.; Shortridge, D.; Carvalhaes, C.G.; Castanheira, M. Trends in the susceptibility of U.S. *Acinetobacter baumannii-calcoaceticus* species complex and *Stenotrophomonas maltophilia* isolates to minocycline, 2014–2021. *Microbiol. Spectr.* **2023**, *11*, e0198123. [CrossRef] [PubMed]
8. Mojica, M.F.; Bonomo, R.A.; van Duin, D. Treatment approaches for severe *Stenotrophomonas maltophilia* infections. *Curr. Opin. Infect. Dis.* **2023**, *36*, 572–584. [CrossRef] [PubMed]
9. Clinical and Laboratory Standards Institute (CLSI). *Perfomance Standards for Antimicrobial Susceptibility Testing*, 33rd ed.; CLSI supplement M100; Clinical and Laboratory Standards Institute: Malvern, PA, USA, 2023.
10. EUCAST The European Committee on Antimicrobial Susceptibility Testing. Breakpoint Tables for Interpretation of MICs and Zone Diameters. Version 14.0. 2024. Available online: https://www.eucast.org (accessed on 23 April 2024).
11. EUCAST. The European Committee on Antimicrobial Susceptibility Testing. MIC and Zone Diameter Distributions and ECOFFs. Available online: https://www.eucast.org/mic_and_zone_distributions_and_ecoffs (accessed on 23 April 2024).
12. Huang, C.; Lin, L.; Kuo, S. Risk factors for mortality in *Stenotrophomonas maltophilia* bacteremia—A meta-analysis. *Infect. Dis.* **2024**, *56*, 335–347. [CrossRef]
13. Rodríguez-Gascón, A.; Aguirre-Quiñonero, A.; Aspiazu, M.A.S.; Canut-Blasco, A. Pharmacokinetic/Pharmacodynamic Analysis of Tedizolid Phosphate Compared to Linezolid for the Treatment of Infections Caused by Gram-Positive Bacteria. *Antibiotics* **2021**, *10*, 755. [CrossRef]
14. Valero, A.; Isla, A.; Rodríguez-Gascón, A.; Calvo, B.; Canut, A.; Solinís, M.Á. Pharmacokinetic/pharmacodynamic analysis as a tool for surveillance of the activity of antimicrobials against *Pseudomonas aeruginosa* strains isolated in critically ill patients. *Enfermedades Infecc. Microbiol. Clin.* **2019**, *37*, 380–386. [CrossRef] [PubMed]
15. Rodríguez-Gascón, A.; Solinís, M.Á.; Isla, A. The Role of PK/PD Analysis in the Development and Evaluation of Antimicrobials. *Pharmaceutics* **2021**, *13*, 833. [CrossRef] [PubMed]
16. Mouton, J.W.; Brown, D.F.; Apfalter, P.; Cantón, R.; Giske, C.G.; Ivanova, M.; MacGowan, A.P.; Rodloff, A.; Soussy, C.J.; Steinbakk, M.; et al. The role of pharmacokinetics/pharmacodynamics in setting clinical MIC breakpoints: The EUCAST approach. *Clin. Microbiol. Infect.* **2012**, *18*, E37–E45. [CrossRef] [PubMed]
17. Asín-Prieto, E.; Rodríguez-Gascón, A.; Isla, A. Applications of the pharmacokinetic/pharmacodynamic (PK/PD) analysis of antimicrobial agents. *J. Infect. Chemother.* **2015**, *21*, 319–329. [CrossRef] [PubMed]
18. Lasko, M.J.; Tabor-Rennie, J.L.; Nicolau, D.P.; Kuti, J.L. Trimethoprim/sulfamethoxazole pharmacodynamics against *Stenotrophomonas maltophilia* in the in vitro chemostat model. *J. Antimicrob. Chemother.* **2022**, *77*, 3187–3193. [CrossRef] [PubMed]

19. Lasko, M.J.; Gethers, M.L.; Tabor-Rennie, J.L.; Nicolau, D.P.; Kuti, J.L. In Vitro Time-Kill Studies of Trimethoprim/Sulfamethoxazole against *Stenotrophomonas maltophilia* versus Escherichia coli Using Cation-Adjusted Mueller-Hinton Broth and ISO-Sensitest Broth. *Antimicrob. Agents Chemother.* **2022**, *66*, e0216721. [CrossRef] [PubMed]
20. Kullar, R.; Wenzler, E.; Alexander, J.; Goldstein, E.J.C. Overcoming *Stenotrophomonas maltophilia* Resistance for a More Rational Therapeutic Approach. *Open Forum Infect. Dis.* **2022**, *9*, ofac095. [CrossRef] [PubMed]
21. Gibb, J.; Wong, D.W. Antimicrobial Treatment Strategies for *Stenotrophomonas maltophilia*: A Focus on Novel Therapies. *Antibiotics* **2021**, *10*, 1226. [CrossRef] [PubMed]
22. Asín, E.; Isla, A.; Canut, A.; Rodríguez Gascón, A. Comparison of antimicrobial pharmacokinetic/pharmacodynamic breakpoints with EUCAST and CLSI clinical breakpoints for Gram-positive bacteria. *Int. J. Antimicrob. Agents* **2012**, *40*, 313–322. [CrossRef]
23. Tsakris, A.; Koumaki, V.; Dokoumetzidis, A. Minocycline susceptibility breakpoints for *Acinetobacter baumannii*: Do we need to re-evaluate them? *J. Antimicrob. Chemother.* **2019**, *74*, 295–297. [CrossRef]
24. Banar, M.; Sattari-Maraji, A.; Bayatinejad, G.; Ebrahimi, E.; Jabalameli, L.; Beigverdi, R.; Emaneini, M.; Jabalameli, F. Global prevalence and antibiotic resistance in clinical isolates of *Stenotrophomonas maltophilia*: A systematic review and meta-analysis. *Front. Med.* **2023**, *10*, 1163439. [CrossRef] [PubMed]
25. Agwuh, K.N.; MacGowan, A. Pharmacokinetics and pharmacodynamics of the tetracyclines including glycylcyclines. *J. Antimicrob. Chemother.* **2006**, *58*, 256–265. [CrossRef] [PubMed]
26. Wei, C.; Ni, W.; Cai, X.; Zhao, J.; Cui, J. Evaluation of Trimethoprim/Sulfamethoxazole (SXT), Minocycline, Tigecycline, Moxifloxacin, and Ceftazidime Alone and in Combinations for SXT-Susceptible and SXT-Resistant *Stenotrophomonas maltophilia* by In Vitro Time-Kill Experiments. *PLoS ONE* **2016**, *11*, e0152132. [CrossRef] [PubMed]
27. Farrell, D.J.; Sader, H.S.; Jones, R.N. Antimicrobial susceptibilities of a worldwide collection of *Stenotrophomonas maltophilia* isolates tested against tigecycline and agents commonly used for *S. maltophilia* infections. *Antimicrob. Agents Chemother.* **2010**, *54*, 2735–2737. [CrossRef] [PubMed]
28. Tamma, P.D.; Avdic, E.; Li, D.X.; Dzintars, K.; Cosgrove, S.E. Association of Adverse Events With Antibiotic Use in Hospitalized Patients. *JAMA Intern. Med.* **2017**, *177*, 1308–1315. [CrossRef] [PubMed]
29. Ko, J.H.; Kang, C.I.; Cornejo-Juárez, P.; Yeh, K.M.; Wang, C.H.; Cho, S.Y.; Gözel, M.G.; Kim, S.H.; Hsueh, P.R.; Sekiya, N.; et al. Fluoroquinolones versus trimethoprim-sulfamethoxazole for the treatment of *Stenotrophomonas maltophilia* infections: A systematic review and meta-analysis. *Clin. Microbiol. Infect.* **2019**, *25*, 546–554. [CrossRef] [PubMed]
30. Wei, C.; Ni, W.; Cai, X.; Cui, J. A Monte Carlo pharmacokinetic/pharmacodynamic simulation to evaluate the efficacy of minocycline, tigecycline, moxifloxacin, and levofloxacin in the treatment of hospital-acquired pneumonia caused by *Stenotrophomonas maltophilia*. *Infect. Dis.* **2015**, *47*, 846–851. [CrossRef] [PubMed]
31. Fratoni, A.J.; Nicolau, D.P.; Kuti, J.L. Levofloxacin pharmacodynamics against *Stenotrophomonas maltophilia* in a neutropenic murine thigh infection model: Implications for susceptibility breakpoint revision. *J. Antimicrob. Chemother.* **2021**, *77*, 164–168. [CrossRef] [PubMed]
32. Nakamura, R.; Oota, M.; Matsumoto, S.; Sato, T.; Yamano, Y. In Vitro Activity and In Vivo Efficacy of Cefiderocol against *Stenotrophomonas maltophilia*. *Antimicrob. Agents Chemother.* **2021**, *65*, e01436-20. [CrossRef]
33. Bostanghadiri, N.; Sholeh, M.; Navidifar, T.; Dadgar-Zankbar, L.; Elahi, Z.; van Belkum, A.; Darban-Sarokhalil, D. Global mapping of antibiotic resistance rates among clinical isolates of *Stenotrophomonas maltophilia*: A systematic review and meta-analysis. *Ann. Clin. Microbiol. Antimicrob.* **2024**, *23*, 26. [CrossRef]
34. Fratoni, A.J.; Kuti, J.L.; Nicolau, D.P. Optimised cefiderocol exposures in a successfully treated critically ill patient with polymicrobial *Stenotrophomonas maltophilia* bacteraemia and pneumonia receiving continuous venovenous haemodiafiltration. *Int. J. Antimicrob. Agents* **2021**, *58*, 106395. [CrossRef] [PubMed]
35. Hsu, A.J.; Simner, P.J.; Bergman, Y.; Mathers, A.J.; Tamma, P.D. Successful Treatment of Persistent *Stenotrophomonas maltophilia* Bacteremia With Cefiderocol in an Infant. *Open Forum Infect. Dis.* **2023**, *10*, ofad174. [CrossRef] [PubMed]
36. Sader, H.S.; Duncan, L.R.; Arends, S.J.R.; Carvalhaes, C.G.; Castanheira, M. Antimicrobial Activity of Aztreonam-Avibactam and Comparator Agents When Tested against a Large Collection of Contemporary *Stenotrophomonas maltophilia* Isolates from Medical Centers Worldwide. *Antimicrob. Agents Chemother.* **2020**, *64*, e01433-20. [CrossRef] [PubMed]
37. De Almeida Torres, N.; Morales Junior, R.; Bueno Lopes, L.F.; Zeigler, R.; Everson Uip, D. Synergistic combination of aztreonam and ceftazidime/avibactam against resistant *Stenotrophomonas maltophilia* on pancreatitis. *J. Infect. Dev. Ctries.* **2023**, *17*, 881–885. [CrossRef]
38. Diarra, A.; Pascal, L.; Carpentier, B.; Baclet, N.; Cabaret, P.; Georgel, A.F.; Dubreuil, L.; Weyrich, P. Successful use of avibactam and aztreonam combination for a multiresistant *Stenotrophomonas maltophilia* bloodstream infection in a patient with idiopathic medullary aplasia. *Infect. Dis. Now* **2021**, *51*, 637–638. [CrossRef] [PubMed]
39. Cowart, M.C.; Ferguson, C.L. Optimization of Aztreonam in Combination With Ceftazidime/Avibactam in a Cystic Fibrosis Patient With Chronic *Stenotrophomonas maltophilia* Pneumonia Using Therapeutic Drug Monitoring: A Case Study. *Ther. Drug Monit.* **2021**, *43*, 146–149. [CrossRef] [PubMed]
40. ClinicalTrials.gov [Internet]; Bethesda (MD): National Library of Medicine (US). Efficacy, Safety, and Tolerability of ATM-AVI in the Treatment of Serious Infection Due to MBL-Producing Gram-Negative Bacteria. Identifier NCT03580044; 2018. Available online: https://clinicaltrials.gov/study/NCT03580044?term=NCT03580044&rank=1 (accessed on 23 April 2024).

41. ClinicalTrials.gov [Internet]; Bethesda (MD): National Library of Medicine (US). A Study to Determine the Efficacy, Safety and Tolerability of Aztreonam-Avibactam (ATM-AVI) ± Metronidazole (MTZ) Versus Meropenem (MER) ± Colistin (COL) for the Treatment of Serious Infections Due to Gram Negative Bacteria. (REVISIT). Identifier NCT03329092; 2017. Available online: https://clinicaltrials.gov/study/NCT03329092?term=NCT03329092&rank=1 (accessed on 23 April 2024).
42. Mauri, C.; Maraolo, A.E.; Di Bella, S.; Luzzaro, F.; Principe, L. The Revival of Aztreonam in Combination with Avibactam against Metallo-β-Lactamase-Producing Gram-Negatives: A Systematic Review of In Vitro Studies and Clinical Cases. *Antibiotics* **2021**, *10*, 1012. [CrossRef] [PubMed]
43. Prawang, A.; Chanjamlong, N.; Rungwara, W.; Santimaleeworagun, W.; Paiboonvong, T.; Manapattanasatein, T.; Pitirattanaworranat, P.; Kitseree, P.; Kanchanasurakit, S. Combination Therapy versus Monotherapy in the Treatment of *Stenotrophomonas maltophilia* Infections: A Systematic Review and Meta-Analysis. *Antibiotics* **2022**, *11*, 1788. [CrossRef]
44. Cheng, A.C.; McBryde, E.S.; Wuthiekanun, V.; Chierakul, W.; Amornchai, P.; Day, N.P.; White, N.J.; Peacock, S.J. Dosing regimens of cotrimoxazole (trimethoprim-sulfamethoxazole) for melioidosis. *Antimicrob. Agents Chemother.* **2009**, *53*, 4193–4199. [CrossRef]
45. Chin, T.W.; Vandenbroucke, A.; Fong, I.W. Pharmacokinetics of trimethoprim-sulfamethoxazole in critically ill and non-critically ill AIDS patients. *Antimicrob. Agents Chemother.* **1995**, *39*, 28–33. [CrossRef]
46. Roberts, J.A.; Cotta, M.O.; Cojutti, P.; Lugano, M.; Della Rocca, G.; Pea, F. Does Critical Illness Change Levofloxacin Pharmacokinetics? *Antimicrob. Agents Chemother.* **2015**, *60*, 1459–1463. [CrossRef] [PubMed]
47. Fish, D.N.; Chow, A.T. The clinical pharmacokinetics of levofloxacin. *Clin. Pharmacokinet.* **1997**, *32*, 101–119. [CrossRef] [PubMed]
48. Lodise, T.P.; Van Wart, S.; Sund, Z.M.; Bressler, A.M.; Khan, A.; Makley, A.T.; Hamad, Y.; Salata, R.A.; Silveira, F.P.; Sims, M.D.; et al. Pharmacokinetic and Pharmacodynamic Profiling of Minocycline for Injection following a Single Infusion in Critically Ill Adults in a Phase IV Open-Label Multicenter Study (ACUMIN). *Antimicrob. Agents Chemother.* **2021**, *65*, e01809-20. [CrossRef]
49. Borsuk-De Moor, A.; Rypulak, E.; Potręć, B.; Piwowarczyk, P.; Borys, M.; Sysiak, J.; Onichimowski, D.; Raszewski, G.; Czuczwar, M.; Wiczling, P. Population Pharmacokinetics of High-Dose Tigecycline in Patients with Sepsis or Septic Shock. *Antimicrob. Agents Chemother.* **2018**, *62*, e02273-17. [CrossRef] [PubMed]
50. Kawaguchi, N.; Katsube, T.; Echols, R.; Wajima, T. Population Pharmacokinetic and Pharmacokinetic/Pharmacodynamic Analyses of Cefiderocol, a Parenteral Siderophore Cephalosporin, in Patients with Pneumonia, Bloodstream Infection/Sepsis, or Complicated Urinary Tract Infection. *Antimicrob. Agents Chemother.* **2021**, *65*, e01437-20. [CrossRef] [PubMed]
51. Bilal, M.; El Tabei, L.; Büsker, S.; Krauss, C.; Fuhr, U.; Taubert, M. Clinical Pharmacokinetics and Pharmacodynamics of Cefiderocol. *Clin. Pharmacokinet.* **2021**, *60*, 1495–1508. [CrossRef]
52. Valero, A.; Rodríguez-Gascón, A.; Isla, A.; Barrasa, H.; Del Barrio-Tofiño, E.; Oliver, A.; Canut, A.; Solinís, M.Á. Pseudomonas aeruginosa Susceptibility in Spain: Antimicrobial Activity and Resistance Suppression Evaluation by PK/PD Analysis. *Pharmaceutics* **2021**, *13*, 1899. [CrossRef] [PubMed]
53. Principe, L.; Lupia, T.; Andriani, L.; Campanile, F.; Carcione, D.; Corcione, S.; De Rosa, F.G.; Luzzati, R.; Stroffolini, G.; Steyde, M.; et al. Microbiological, Clinical, and PK/PD Features of the New Anti-Gram-Negative Antibiotics: β-Lactam/β-Lactamase Inhibitors in Combination and Cefiderocol-An All-Inclusive Guide for Clinicians. *Pharmaceuticals* **2022**, *15*, 463. [CrossRef]
54. Nichols, W.W.; Newell, P.; Critchley, I.A.; Riccobene, T.; Das, S. Avibactam Pharmacokinetic/Pharmacodynamic Targets. *Antimicrob. Agents Chemother.* **2018**, *62*, e02446-17. [CrossRef]
55. Owens, R.C., Jr.; Bhavnani, S.M.; Ambrose, P.G. Assessment of pharmacokinetic-pharmacodynamic target attainment of gemifloxacin against *Streptococcus pneumoniae*. *Diagn. Microbiol. Infect. Dis.* **2005**, *51*, 45–49. [CrossRef]
56. Mouton, J.W.; Dudley, M.N.; Cars, O.; Derendorf, H.; Drusano, G.L. Standardization of pharmacokinetic/pharmacodynamic (PK/PD) terminology for anti-infective drugs: An update. *J. Antimicrob. Chemother.* **2005**, *55*, 601–607. [CrossRef] [PubMed]
57. Stein, G.E.; Smith, C.L.; Scharmen, A.; Kidd, J.M.; Cooper, C.; Kuti, J.; Mitra, S.; Nicolau, D.P.; Havlichek, D.H. Pharmacokinetic and Pharmacodynamic Analysis of Ceftazidime/Avibactam in Critically Ill Patients. *Surg. Infect.* **2019**, *20*, 55–61. [CrossRef] [PubMed]

antibiotics

MDPI

Review

Stenotrophomonas maltophilia: The Landscape in Critically Ill Patients and Optimising Management Approaches

Nieves Carbonell [1,*], María Rosa Oltra [2] and María Ángeles Clari [3]

1 Medical Intensive Care Unit, Clinic University Hospital, INCLIVA Biomedical Research Institute, 46010 Valencia, Spain
2 Infectious Disease Unit, Internal Medicine Department, Clinic University Hospital, INCLIVA Biomedical Research Institute, 46010 Valencia, Spain; mrosaoltra@gmail.com
3 Microbiology Service, Clinic University Hospital, INCLIVA Biomedical Research Institute, 46010 Valencia, Spain; maclapons@hotmail.com
* Correspondence: edurnecarbonell@gmail.com

Abstract: The aim of this review is to synthesise the key aspects of the epidemiology, current microbiological diagnostic challenges, antibiotic resistance rates, optimal antimicrobial management, and most effective prevention strategies for *Stenotrophomonas maltophilia* (SM) in the intensive care unit (ICU) population. In recent years, resistance surveillance data indicate that SM accounts for less than 3% of all healthcare-associated infection strains, a percentage that doubles in the case of ventilator-associated pneumonia (VAP). Interestingly, SM ranks as the third most isolated non-glucose fermenter Gram-negative bacilli (NFGNB). Although this NFGNB genus has usually been considered a bystander and colonising strain, recently published data warn about its potential role as a causative pathogen of severe infections, particularly pneumonia and bloodstream infections (BSI), not only for the classical immunocompromised susceptible host patients but also for critically ill ones even without overt immunosuppression. Indeed, it has been associated with crude 28-day mortality as high as 54.8%, despite initial response following targeted therapy. Additionally, alongside its intrinsic resistance to a wide range of common antimicrobials, various worldwide and local surveillance studies raise concerns about an increase in ICU settings regarding resistance to first-line drugs such as cotrimoxazole or tigecycline. This scenario alerts ICU physicians to the need to reconsider the best stewardship approach when SM is isolated in obtained samples from critically ill patients. Despite the coverage of this multidrug-resistant bacterium (MDRB) provided by some traditional and a non-negligible number of current pipeline antimicrobials, an ecological and cost-effective strategy is needed in the present era.

Keywords: ICU; critically ill; sepsis; antimicrobial; multidrug-resistant bacteria; sepsis; antimicrobial stewardship; *Stenotrophomonas maltophilia*

1. Introduction

The genus *Stenotrophomonas* comprises at least eight species, of which *Stenotrophomonas maltophilia* (SM) is the most predominant and the only one known to cause human disease [1]. SM is an environmental non-glucose fermenter Gram-negative bacillus (NFGNB) isolated from aqueous-associated sources both inside and outside the hospital setting [2]. It is ubiquitous and often encountered as a coloniser of plants and medical devices owing to its site adhesion and biofilm formation abilities [3]. Not typically found in the common gut flora, it can colonise the oral cavity and the respiratory tract epithelial cells of cystic fibrosis (CF) and hospitalised patients, causing chronic infection of the airways in this population that contributes to inflammation, lung damage, and premature mortality.

Interestingly, although understudied, SM ranks as the third most isolated unusual NFGNB (after *Pseudomonas aeruginosa* and *Acinetobacter baumannii*) in various reports [4,5].

Most SM isolates are hospital-acquired, with a median delay of 8–14 days of hospital stay, but community-acquired isolates have also been described [4,6].

To date, distinguishing between SM colonisation and true infection represents a significant challenge, especially when more than one pathogen is isolated. This yet unresolved issue needs to be elucidated because although other host and severity clinical factors enable physicians to tailor management decision-making, finding a balance between antimicrobial overuse and the risk of worse prognosis due to absent or delayed treatment remains complicated [7]. SM infection rates have been confirmed to range from 13 to 60% according to definitions for surveillance of healthcare-associated infection established by the National Healthcare Safety Network managed by the Centers for Disease Control and Prevention (CDC/NHSN) [8,9]. Moreover, in a prospective multicentre cohort (33% ICU patients), Fihman V et al. observed that SM caused infection more often than colonisation [RR 1.74 (95% CI 1.15–2.63), p = 0.01] [4]. In a previous review of 13 cohort studies, a considerable mortality rate (up to 37.5%) was attributed to SM infection. These authors warned clinicians against underestimating its clinical significance, even redefining the term "SM colonisation" [10].

As an unusual NFGNB, SM has often been considered less pathogenic than many other nosocomial organisms. However, this is without considering immunocompromised patients or those with chronic respiratory diseases such as CF, who represent a debilitated population at high risk of suffering from severe and mainly nosocomial infections from this opportunistic pathogen [4,11].

Furthermore, SM infections are notable in the ICU population. All patients admitted to ICU are at high risk of infection by MDRB, even without a known immunosuppressed status, and when infected, need timely appropriate treatment due to an increased risk for mortality. In an earlier, classic study in 1995, Laing FPY et al. found that ICU patients were more frequently infected than those in non-ICU settings [12]. Although ICU-acquired colonisation and/or infection related to SM was considered uncommon among immunocompetent ICU patients (two patients per 1000 ICU days) [6], it was nonetheless recognised as a potentially worrisome emerging ICU pathogen; indeed, an ICU-acquired infection related to SM was independently associated with ICU mortality in this study. A recently published study confirms this ominous SM infection prognosis. It has been associated with crude 28-day mortality as high as 54.8% despite initial response after targeted therapy, especially if respiratory-focused [13].

Several studies have investigated the risk factors for SM infection in ICU patients, some of which are related to illness severity and underlying comorbidities such as APACHE-II score > 20, older age, and chronic obstructive pulmonary disease (COPD). Other risk factors that are concerned with invasive procedures at ICU admission include indwelling intravascular catheter devices, mechanical ventilation, tracheotomy, and tracheal intubation. Finally, SM isolation within 30 days, hospitalisation within the last three months, and prolonged antibiotic treatment (specially carbapenems [CP], but also β-lactamase inhibitors, antipseudomonal cephalosporins and aminoglycosides) have been associated with SM infections; COPD and CP use have been demonstrated as independently predictive factors [4,6,7,11,14–16].

Defining the clinical risk factors for SM infection is, therefore, a challenge, but one that would be highly beneficial for adequate antimicrobial treatment in the current MDRB era. Initial CP regimens covering extended-spectrum beta-lactamase-producing *Enterobacteriaceae* (ESBL-PE) bacteria causing community and healthcare infections could lead to inappropriate SM treatment due to its intrinsic CP-resistant profile. Indeed, an association between inappropriate initial antimicrobial treatment and mortality has previously been reported in SM-infected, either critically ill or non-critical cases [4,6,10].

This current situation is a challenge for doctors, who need to raise the index of suspicion. Moreover, knowledge about local epidemiology is essential to become familiar with antibiotic resistance rates and accordingly plan an optimal antimicrobial stewardship strategy. Finally, updated infection control measures such as those included in the Spanish

"Zero Resistance" program [17] should accompany these bundles to improve the prognosis of SM infections in ICU patients.

This review aims to highlight key issues over the last twenty years to help provide clinical guidance for when SM is isolated in critically ill patients.

2. Relevant Sections

2.1. Commensal vs. Pathogenic Status of SM: Relevant Aspects

2.1.1. Why Should We Consider Highlighting the Importance of Colonisation by SM?

While microbial culture isolation of a putative pathogen in the laboratory is often associated with infectious syndromes such as BSIs and other sterile body site infections, the correlation is not well defined for NFGNB when the cultured specimen is from body sites with a high colonisation/contamination potential, especially when more than one pathogen is isolated [7].

In contrast, colonisation by an MDRB has been associated with a significantly higher frequency of subsequent infection with the same MDRB and increased mortality in the ICU population. A meta-analysis including a total of 13 studies (with 15,045 ICU patients) found the risk for subsequent ESBL-PE infection to be almost 50-fold higher in colonised than non-colonised patients. These authors concluded that ESBL-PE colonisation of the digestive tract could be a useful marker to predict ESBL-PE infection [18]. In a single-centre retrospective observational study including 3463 surveillance cultures from 250 haematological patients (11 from ICU), Torres I and colleagues documented MDRB colonisation in 33.7% of admissions, most frequently by NFGNB (55.7%). Colonisation by any MDRB was independently associated with an increased risk of MDRB-BSI (HR, 3.70; 95% CI, 1.38–9.90; $p = 0.009$) [19].

SM is rarely present in the oropharynx microbiome of healthy patients but can often be recovered from the oropharynx of hospitalised and CF patients. In the specific case of SM, infection was predicted (96% sensitivity and 93% specificity) by a relative abundance of 36% of oral *Stenotrophomonas*, as assessed via 16SrRNA gene quantification in a cohort of 90 acute myeloid leukaemia (AML) patients receiving remission induction chemotherapy [14]. An SM infection incidence of 9% was reported in this immunosuppressed non-ICU population. In a previous similar study, which analysed SM colonisation during allogeneic hematopoietic stem cell transplantation, the authors observed that SM colonised patients had a worse prognosis, with a poorer overall survival from 6 to 60 months due to higher non-relapsed mortality after allo-transplant (6 months: 15% vs. 4.8% and 60 months: 40.1% vs. 16.2%, $p = 0.003$) [20]. SM colonised in the oral pharynx tends to form bacterial biofilms in the lining of indwelling catheters, increasing the risk of pulmonary SM infection. The results obtained from immunosuppressed non-ICU patients are quite different from those described with *Enterobacterales*, non-SM NFGNB, and *Enterococcus* spp., which usually involve the importance of negative predictive value for suspected infection, frequently BSI caused by gastrointestinal translocation due to rectal colonisation [18,19].

Several classic prospective case-control studies in the ICU population contain significant findings and suggestions focused on the patient risk profile and outcomes of SM infection. Regarding the former, four studies stand out. First, research performed by the Grupo Andaluz para el Estudio de Enfermedades Infecciosas (GAEI) in six tertiary hospitals (with one-third of patients in ICU) revealed a pooled incidence of SM colonisation or infection of 5.7 cases per 10,000 admissions. About half were considered infected, with pneumonia as the most frequent type of infection in ICU patients (two-thirds VAP). The results of qualitative and quantitative analysis of variables independently associated with an increased risk of acquiring SM pointed to SM as a potential cause of nosocomial infections in patients who had previously received a prolonged course of a carbapenem, ceftazidime, or quinolone, particularly if they were under mechanical ventilation [9]. Second, a more recently published meta-analysis including 2320 ICU patients, of which 306 (13%) were SM-infected, showed a particular risk profile with highly suspected SM origin in ICU-acquired pneumonia, specifically including the above-mentioned criteria. These authors drew attention to a subset of critically ill patients with underlying comorbidities (COPD, malignancy, and high APACHE-II score) who had undergone invasive procedures related to artificial airways and were on broad-spectrum antibiotics due to a combination of host and medical factors [15]. Third, during the pandemic period, a systematic Japanese review of COVID-19-associated SM infection (most patients requiring ICU admission) reported these patients as having similar risk factors as in the above-mentioned studies of patients without COVID-19 [21]. Finally, revisiting the risk factors for the second most common SM infection, bacteraemia, a retrospective study comparing 54 SM with 167 *P. aeruginosa* and 69 *Acinetobacter* species bacteraemic patients showed SM isolation within 30 days prior to infection onset as an independent risk factor for SM bacteraemia, with earlier SM isolation in 66.7%. Nearly half of these patients were considered to have secondary bacteraemia. The thirty-day all-cause mortality of 33.3% among the SM group was significantly higher than that of the other NFGNB groups, and catheter-related infections were associated with survival [16].

Likewise, the outcomes of SM infections acquired during ICU stay have prompted clinical physicians to consider antimicrobial treatment. In a prospective observational case-control study among immunocompetent cases with ICU-acquired infection related to SM (2% of overall incidence), 80% of patients had prior colonisation related to this microorganism [6]. The study reported a significantly higher mortality rate in cases with ICU-acquired SM infection than those with ICU-acquired SM colonisation (70% vs. 25%, OR = 2.5 [1.2 to 4.9], $p = 0.029$). Furthermore, ICU-acquired SM infection was independently associated with ICU mortality. Despite evidence suggesting that clinicians should consider the importance of the predictive value of proven colonisation by SM in critically ill patients, there is no evidence supporting the benefit of antimicrobial use; instead, it likely incurs an ecological cost in this scenario. Therefore, close monitoring of these colonised patients should be considered a daily best practice.

2.1.2. Why and When Should We Consider SM as a Real-Life Pathogen in the ICU? The Importance of VAP Cases in the Critically Ill

SM can cause serious infections, including bacteremia, tracheobronchitis, pneumonia, meningitis, endocarditis, endophthalmitis, skin and soft tissue, urinary tract, and oral cavity infections. Although this bacterium is normally nosocomial, community-onset infections have also been reported [3]. Worldwide, the most common clinically observed specimen is blood, with a frequency of 36.84%, followed by the eye and respiratory tract (19.29% and 15.78%, respectively) [11]. In the classic multicentre case-control study from the GAEI group, the authors underline a difference between ICU and cancer patients, with the most frequent infections being respiratory (especially VAP) in the former and primary or catheter-related bacteriemia in the latter [9].

From a global perspective, according to CHINET bacterial resistance surveillance data, in 2020, SM accounted for 2.98% of all strains and ranked third among NFGNB [5]. In the same way, in the recently published European surveillance, SM accounted for 0.8% of all healthcare-associated infections, rising to 1.9% in cases of pneumonia/lower respiratory infections [22]. Likewise, it is noteworthy that SM is usually linked to pulmonary infections in critically ill patients. In fact, in a 2021 CDC/NHSN updated national summary of pathogens distributions, SM appeared among the most frequently possible VAP pathogens not usually reported from other device-associated infections, accounting for 4% in hospital ICUs and ranking ninth for this type of healthcare infection. Similarly, in the Spanish national surveillance programme of ICU-acquired infection (ENVIN-HELICS registry) in 2023, SM represented 2.68% of isolated microorganisms among the main ICU-acquired infections. SM was especially important in the case of VAP (5.88%), ranking fourth after *P. aeruginosa*, *Klebsiella pneumoniae*, and *Staphylococcus aureus* [23].

Besides the above-mentioned risk factors for SM infections in critically ill patients, some evidence points to the length of ICU stay as associated with acquiring SM during hospitalisation, suggesting that empiric treatment should be considered for this microorganism in this setting. The GAEI group described a median duration of 17 days (range 0–180) before SM isolation [9]. A subsequent study reported a mean time of 14 ± 11 days between ICU admission and the first ICU-acquired SM [6]. The duration of invasive procedures (such as mechanical ventilation >14 days) also seems important, having been identified as an independent risk factor for ICU-acquired SM infection in a neurological ICU [24].

In a recently published retrospective bi-centre study including 103 ICU patients with SM infection, pneumonia (hospital-acquired pneumonia [HAP] and VAP) was the predominant clinical syndrome (72.8%), while 22% of cases were in haemato-oncology patients. In multivariable analysis, only increasing age and haemato-oncologic disease were shown to be independent risk factors for 28-day mortality SM infection, which was as high as 54.8% despite initial clinical and laboratory response after targeted therapy [13].

The possibility of developing fatal haemorrhagic pneumonia caused by SM has also been observed in the population with hematologic malignancies with SM bacteraemia. It is a rare presentation, with only 91 reported cases worldwide from 1990 to 2023, but with a very high associated 30-day mortality of 90.1%, even after prompt antibiotic treatment [25–27]. Due to its severity and rapid progression, after analysing the few survival cases, some authors emphasise the importance of early suspicion and suggest combination therapy, including TMP-SMX, for this clinical picture in this specific population, although no clinical studies are available [25,26]. The exact mechanism by which SM causes haemorrhage is unknown. Windhorst et al. propose pathogenic factors such as StmPr1, a protease with broad specificity secreted by SM, leading to tissue invasion, destruction, and haemorrhage [28]. Moreover, neutropenia ($<500/\text{mm}^3$) and thrombocytopenia ($<50{,}000/\text{mm}^3$) have been identified as risk factors for haemorrhagic pneumonia, which could partly explain the bleeding progression in patients with haematologic malignancies with SM bacteraemia [25].

2.2. Antibiotic Resistance Traits and Microbiological Diagnostic Challenges: Clinical Impact on the ICU Population

2.2.1. Basis of SM Antibiotic Resistance

Numerous intrinsic and acquired resistance traits make SM-caused infections notoriously difficult to treat. This bacterium is intrinsically resistant to a wide range of antibiotics, including most β-lactams, fluoroquinolones, tetracycline derivatives (except for doxycycline, minocycline, or tigecycline), chloramphenicol, all aminoglycosides (including kanamycin, tobramycin, amikacin, and neomycin) and trimethoprim [29]. SM employs a wide spectrum of antibiotic resistance mechanisms, which include overexpression/mutation of multidrug resistance efflux pumps, reduced membrane permeability, the chromosomally encoded Sm*qnr* gene (that protects both gyrase and topoisomerase IV from quinolones), and the production of beta-lactamase, carbapenemase, and aminoglycoside-modifying enzymes [11,29]. It is noteworthy that the high carbapenem resistance of SM is primarily caused by the expression of two chromosomally encoded extracellular ß-lactamases, bla_{L1} (a class B metallo-β-lactamase which is not inactivated by aztreonam) and bla_{L2} (a class A clavulanic acid susceptible cephalosporinase, which is susceptible to inhibition by serine-β-lactamase inhibitors such as clavulanic acid and avibactam), which would explain the clinical benefit of combined ceftazidime–avibactam if administered in combination with aztreonam [30].

Among its acquired resistance mechanisms, SM can develop cefiderocol resistance through different genetic pathways, such as mutations in the *tonB* gene or in the *smeT* promoter [29]. An increasing presence has also been noted of *sul*1, *sul*2, and *dfrA* genes that have been found both chromosomally and in plasmids, which contribute to SM resistance to trimethoprim-sulfamethoxazole (TMP/SMX). These genes are often associated with Class 1 integrons, which favour their mobility and even carry multiple resistance genes, which are conducive to multi-resistance.

2.2.2. Considerations for Empirical Antimicrobial Decision-Making

This nosocomial pathogen shows low susceptibility to many antibiotics commonly used to empirically treat hospital-acquired infections. In contrast, antimicrobials with a priori in vitro susceptibility, such as TMP/SMX, quinolones, and tetracyclines derivatives (minocycline and tigecycline), are not covered in usual clinical practice in the ICU setting. Gram-negative bacteria are the organisms most commonly responsible for serious infections in the ICU; however, dual empirical coverage usually includes *P. aeruginosa* and *Enterobacteriaceae* as the organisms most frequently involved, whereas SM is responsible for only a minority of cases. SM is, therefore, not typically covered and is likely to be subject to initial inappropriate treatment (ITT). Quinolone is sometimes suggested as an option in empiric combination therapy, such as in the PANNUCI algorithm for nosocomial pneumonia management in the ICU, in which cases SM may be covered [31]. However, quinolones are not always recommended for severe nosocomial infections with sepsis and septic shock, especially given that the resistance rate to ciprofloxacin and levofloxacin in *P. aeruginosa* currently exceeds 30% in most Spanish hospitals [32]. In a large retrospective analysis of ICU patients with bacteraemia and severe sepsis/septic shock caused by a Gram-negative organism, IIT was a key determinant of short-term mortality with a three-fold increase, and MDR was strongly associated with IIT [33]. Notably, SM was specifically identified as a predictor of IIT in this study population.

SM has been associated with infections after various prolonged antimicrobial treatments, especially with carbapenems, which probably would be selected for SM because of its intrinsic resistance to most of them [9,11]. As well as its prior use perse, cumulative exposure to meropenem has been associated with increased infection risk (hazard ratio, 1.17; 95% CI, 1.01–1.35; $p = 0.03$) in non-critically ill patients, resulting in a 17% increased risk of SM infection with each additional day of meropenem use [14]. Furthermore, a study by Xu et al. concluded that the use of three antibiotics for more than one week was an independent risk factor for SM pneumonia in ICU patients [34]. It seems that not only the type but also the time of exposure and the number of antimicrobials can impact SM infection development.

Interestingly, SM has been identified as the most frequent carbapenem-resistant (CR) Gram-negative species in hospitalised patients with HAP and VAP [35]. In this retrospective cohort study, which included 8969 patients, a total of 11.8% of isolates were CR, with nearly 60% of this requiring ICU admission. *P. aeruginosa* was the most common Gram-negative pathogen overall (21.1%) but was second to SM (16.8 vs. 38.7%) among CR species. In terms of clinical impact, it is noteworthy that CR was associated with an excess of 3.0 days (95% CI, 1.4–4.6) in overall length of stay and an excess of $8921 (95% CI, 3864–13,977) in hospital costs [35].

SM production of inducible carbapenemase, which hydrolyses and detoxifies antibiotics, is also involved in polymicrobial infections, especially among SM and *P. aeruginosa*, although the pathogenic role of SM is difficult to ascertain in this scenario. There is limited understanding of the way antimicrobial resistance evolves in the presence of non-targeted microbial species and how ecological interactions likely alter the effectiveness of antibiotic treatment. CF represents the paradigm of this co-infection, which affects up to a quarter of patients and is often associated with increased mortality [36]. A 24-day-long in vitro experimental study with two-species model CF communities highlighted some aspects related to bacterial eco-evolutionary dynamics in the absence of and under clinically relevant β-lactam imipenem concentrations. Firstly, they found that a clinical SM strain protected sensitive *P. aeruginosa* from imipenem. Secondly, the presence of SM led to an equal or increased rate of imipenem resistance development via parallel loss of function mutations in the OprD porin gene. Finally, and unexpectedly, they observed that resistant *P. aeruginosa* drove SM into extinction due to increased production of pyocyanin in the presence of imipenem, which was cytotoxic to SM [37]. Interestingly, there is some clinical evidence illustrating the way interactions between members can affect the prognosis of this specific polymicrobial infection. SM and *P. aeruginosa* can produce biofilm in the lungs, creating a thriving environment for both. In a Chinese retrospective analysis including severe pneumonia patients, a higher mortality rate and longer hospital stay were reported for those co-infected with *P. aeruginosa* and SM compared with those infected with only one or not infected [38].

2.2.3. Related Microbiological Diagnostic Challenges

Caution should be applied when considering in vitro results of SM susceptibility based on antimicrobial susceptibility testing (AST) guidelines (the Clinical and Laboratory Standards Institute [CLSI], the European Committee on Antimicrobial Susceptibility Testing [EUCAST], and Food and Drug Administration [FDA]), which are not standardised. CLSI has established minimum inhibitory concentration (MIC) interpretation criteria for seven antibiotics, including TMP-SMX, ticarcillin–clavulanate, ceftazidime, cefiderocol, levofloxacin, minocycline, and chloramphenicol. In contrast, the EUCAST has defined MIC and disc breakpoints only for TMP-SMX (an antimicrobial with nearly identical breakpoints for EUCAST (>4 mg/L) and CLSI ($\geq$4 mg/L)). The FDA only recognises ceftazidime breakpoints for SM. In real life, only five agents with interpretable antibiotic MIC data are available to clinicians for clinically relevant application in AST (TMP-SMX, ceftazidime, cefiderocol, levofloxacin and minocycline) [29,39]. As a result, differences among SM resistance rates to these antimicrobials become apparent among prevalence studies, and most importantly, the lack of adequate information available may have a considerable impact on patient treatment.

Accordingly, a recent report including 223 studies in which CLSI recommendations were used evaluated the prevalence of antibiotic resistance in clinical isolates of SM worldwide. The authors observed that the most frequent antibiotic resistance worldwide was against levofloxacin (14.4%) among prevalence studies, with an increased resistance especially in China, and against TMP/SMX (36.84%) among case reports/case series studies, with the highest resistance rate reported in Asia [11]. A more recent worldwide meta-analysis showed a low global prevalence of resistance to TMP-SMX (14.7%), suggesting that this antimicrobial remained effective as a first-line treatment for SM. Other findings were a relatively low resistance rate to levofloxacin (16%), a significant increase in resistance to tigecycline, and the lowest resistance rates documented for minocycline (3%) and cefiderocol (4%) [39]. Regarding the ICU population, the above-mentioned ENVIN-HELICS registry showed a trend towards increased SM resistance to TMP/SMX during the last two years (2022–2023) compared with the pre-pandemic period (2018) (6.2% and 13.5% vs. 0%, respectively), similar to tigecycline (60% and 80% vs. 0%), in contrast to levofloxacin that has remained the same or even decreased (13.65 and 13.3% vs. 15.38%, respectively). Moreover, this report showed an SM resistance of 53.8% to ceftazidime/avibactam and 50% to cefiderocol among 13 and 4 out of 113 tested strains, respectively, within 2022 and 2023 in the participating Spanish ICUs [23].

Despite the MDR profile of SM, clinicians should be aware of the epidemiologic and previous colonisation situation in their local institutions to ensure appropriate treatment. Familiarity with microbiological tests, from the simple Gram stain microscopy to new methods for rapid SM identification (such as Matrix-assisted laser desorption ionisation–time of flight [MALDI-TOF] mass spectrometry), as well as a deeper understanding of the value of syndromic panels to detect causative pathogens by molecular methods, are also essential to avoid ITT in the ICU setting (see Table 1). Regarding molecular detection, there are currently few methods that allow the detection of SM directly from biological samples. For the diagnosis of bacterial infections in the lower respiratory tract, the only platform that allows this detection from a direct sample is Unyvero. Furthermore, a recent randomised control trial involving patients with pneumonia in the ICU observed that the growth of 'off-panel' pathogens was unusual and most commonly due to *Citrobacter* species and SM. The lack of detection of these organisms by the pneumonia panel did not adversely affect patients' antimicrobial treatment in this trial [40]. Accordingly, a stewardship strategy for guiding an adjustment of empirical antimicrobial therapy based on the results of rapid microbiological testing like Biofire® Filmarray® Pneumonia Panel plus (BioFire Diagnostics, LLC, Salt Lake City, UT, USA) seems imperative in the management of critically ill patients [41]. Likewise, next-generation metagenomic sequencing (mNGS) has emerged as a promising tool in the field of medicine. Although it shows promising diagnostic performance for severe pneumonia in critically ill patients, facilitating precise diagnoses and treatments, the clinical value of this technology remains controversial due to challenges such as the lack of common standards and guidelines. Continued research and the development of standardized protocols are necessary to maximise its potential and ensure its clinical applicability [42].

Table 1. New microbiological diagnostic methods for rapid SM identification.

Diagnostic Test	Pathogen/ Resistance	Sample Type	Time Required to Detection (Hours)	Detection Limit	Sensitivity (%)	Specificity (%)	Robustness	Reference
Unyvero A50 System HPN (Curetis, Holzgerlingen, Germany)	21 Gram-negative and Gram-positive bacteria/17 antibiotic-resistant markers	Sputum, bronchoalveolar lavage, tracheal and bronchial secretions	<5 h	NR	84	98	NR	Sun et al., 2021 [43]
Unyvero A50 System BCU (Curetis)	34 Pathogens, 16 antibiotic resistance markers	Positive blood culture	<5 h	NR	96.8	99.8	NR	Burrack-Lange et al., 2018 [44]
Biofire®Filmarray® BCID2 (bioMeriéux, Craponne, France)	33 Gram-negative, Gram-positive bacteria, Candida spp., and 10 antibiotic-resistant markers	Positive blood culture	1 h	NR	>80 for SM	99.8	NR	Peri et al., 2022 [45]
Sepsis Flow Chip (VITRO Master Diagnóstica, Granada, Spain)	17 Gram-negative and Gram-positive bacteria, 1 yeast, and 19 antibiotic-resistant markers	Positive blood culture	3 h	NR	100 for SM	100	NR	Galiana et al., 2017 [46]
hemoFISH (Miacom Diagnostics, Düsseldorf, Germany)	19 Gram-negative and Gram-positive bacteria	Positive blood culture	>5 h	NR	<80–90 for SM	>95	NR	Reitz et al., 2018 [47]
Magicplex Sepsis Real-Time (Seegene, Seoul, Republic of Korea)	73 Gram-positive, 12 Gram-negative, 6 fungal, and 3 antibiotic-resistant markers	Whole blood	3–6 h	NR	65	92	NR	Carrara et al., 2013 [48]
MALDI Biotyper System (Bruker, Billerica, MA, USA)	Bacterial and fungal species or species groups	A single colony from isolate positive culture or positive whole blood cultures	minutes	-	73 for SM	99	NR	Gautam et al., 2017 [49]
LiDia-SEQ NGS (DNA Electronics Ltd., Carlsbad, CA, USA)	Bacterial and fungal pathogens	Whole blood	>4 h	1 CFU/mL	NR	NR	NR	Not found

Note: SM: *Stenothophomonas maltophilia*; NR: not reported; CFU: colony forming unit.

2.3. Best Evidence-Based Approach to SM Severe Infections. Antimicrobial Stewardship in the Critically Ill

As mentioned above, SM infection management can be hampered either by high-level intrinsic resistance to many antibiotic classes and the increasing occurrence of acquired resistance to the first-line drug cotrimoxazole (TMP/SMX) [3] or by a lack of coverage by the most used empirical antimicrobial strategies for ICU infections, which in turn can cast a shadow over its prognosis.

Different treatment guidelines for infections caused by multidrug-resistant Gram-negative microorganisms have recently been published, including recommendations on SM treatment in guidelines by the Infectious Diseases Society of America (IDSA) and the Society of Infectious Diseases and Clinical Microbiology (SEIMC) [30,50,51]. Published data on the optimal treatment for SM infections are limited. Despite the lack of randomised controlled trials comparing TMP/SMX with any other available treatment for SM infections, it is still currently considered the drug of choice based on high in vitro susceptibility rates [52].

For severe infection, the Spanish Society recommends considering combination therapy in immunocompromised patients (strength of recommendation B and quality of evidence II), preferably including TMX/SMX [50]. Likewise, IDSA recommendations from 2022 were recently updated in the 2023 guidelines on the treatment of antimicrobial-resistant Gram-negative infections [53]. The authors directly suggested two approaches: (1) combined use of two of the following agents: TMP-SMX, minocycline/tigecycline, cefiderocol, or levofloxacin, at least until clinical improvement is observed, primarily because of limited and conflicting in vitro and clinical data (limited to observational studies) supporting any individual agent and the need to increase the likelihood of appropriate treatment. (2) The combination of ceftazidime–avibactam plus aztreonam in situations of significant clinical instability following clinical failure with or intolerance to other agents.

It is noteworthy that the authors recommend a second approach, including ceftazidime–avibactam and aztreonam, in situations of significant clinical instability. This has been considered a reasonable treatment option for severe infections despite limited available clinical data and few case reports, based on the above-mentioned explanation that this combination can overcome the activity of both β-lactamases intrinsic to SM. The IDSA panel expressly advised avoiding ceftazidime as a treatment option because of the presence of β-lactamase genes intrinsic to SM that are expected to render this antimicrobial inactive. The panel also changed the aztreonam regimen in terms of suggested antibiotics dosing from the previous publication [30,53]. Regarding the ICU population, in an Italian case series of 26 COVID-19 ICU patients with VAP due to difficult-to-treat NFGNB, with SM isolated in six of these patients (mostly as part of polymicrobial infection), ceftazidime–avibactam was employed in different regimen combinations. The authors suggest that SM appears as a true pathogen in this patient population, promoting the development of haemorrhagic pneumonia or bacteraemia. A surprising finding was a 30-day overall mortality of 60.8% vs. 16% in an SM-specific subgroup [54].

The 2023 American guidelines proposed TMX-SMX and minocycline as the preferred components for combination. Minocycline has slightly more favourable in vitro data, availability of CLSI breakpoints, oral formulation, and likely improved tolerability compared with tigecycline. Moreover, minocycline has been associated with lower adverse effects and mortality than TMP/SMX in a retrospective study dealing with severe patients based on the APACHE-II score [55]. However, tigecycline is also a treatment option for SM infections [30], with extensive penetration into lung tissue at high doses, as demonstrated in critically ill patients [56]. In several series, moreover, the reported MICs for eravacycline are two- to four-fold lower than for tigecycline and frequently mirror minocycline for SM.

Fluoroquinolones are commonly used as an alternative for cases with TMP/SMX-resistant SM or with intolerance due to adverse side effects, especially in HIV-infected patients. Several retrospective observational studies comparing monotherapy with fluoroquinolones and TMP/SMX (with a quarter of patients in the ICU at the time of culture) have suggested that levofloxacin had similar efficacy [57] or even lower OR of death and length of hospital stay than TMP/SMX in patients with lower respiratory tract infections [50,58]. However, because of suboptimal results with fluoroquinolone monotherapy in in vitro studies, known mechanisms of resistance of SM to fluoroquinolones, the emergence of resistance during therapy, and inherent biases in the observational data, the IDSA panel suggests levofloxacin be used only as a component of combination therapy when prescribed for treatment of SM infections [53]. It is noteworthy that treatments (e.g., quinolones) that select mutants leading to multidrug efflux pump overexpression, such as SmeDEF, can reduce SM susceptibility to several antimicrobials simultaneously. This would explain co-resistance to quinolone and cotrimoxazole. However, it does not appear to affect susceptibility to either minocycline or tigecycline, which could thus be candidate antimicrobials in this context [29,52,59]. This could also be the rationale behind the use of antimicrobial combinations in severe infections.

Regarding second-line agents against SM infections, SEIMC experts have recommended their use for their in vitro activity against the isolate (B-II) [50]. In particular, the IDSA proposes cefiderocol because, despite the limited availability of clinical data, in vitro data and animal models are encouraging for its use in treating SM infections, initially in combination with a second active agent [51,53,60]. Clinically, a Spanish retrospective observational study [61] and a French case series [62] assessing the effect of cefiderocol treatment for severe infections due to difficult-to-treat resistant Gram-negative bacilli in critically ill patients reported a 30-day overall mortality rate of nearly 30%. Among the few patients infected with SM (5 and 4, respectively), mortality increased to 80%, although most were immunosuppressed, and related mortality was not specified. Lastly, the ongoing international retrospective medical chart review PROVE study, with a higher sample size regarding SM infections and with more than 70% of patients admitted to ICU, will soon shed further light on the real-life situation.

2.4. Preventive Measures: Theoretical Basis for Clinical Formulation of Prevention and Control Strategies to Reduce the Morbidity and Mortality of SM Infection in the ICU

SM is widely distributed in natural environments, such as soil, water, and hospital environments, and can also parasite the human skin, respiratory and digestive tracts. Since environmental and clinical strains are genetically closely related, soil might be a likely source for community-acquired infections [2]. Moreover, sink drains, faucets, water, and sponges have also been identified as environmental sources of SM in hospitals, reflecting the ability of this pathogen to survive on any humid surfaces and colonise them over the long term by forming biofilm and resisting commonly used biocides [2,29,36,63]. SM possesses multiple virulence factors that allow it to colonise and produce infection, and among the most important of these is the production of pili, flagella, fimbria structures, and adhesins, which contribute to adherence, auto-aggregation, and colonisation of biotic and abiotic surfaces. This scenario allows SM to become a potentially important pathogen in the ICU setting, where healthcare-associated infections are a global challenge.

Guided by whole genome sequencing analysis, there is provided evidence that sink drains serve as antibiotic-resistant organism persistent reservoirs (in particular, SM and *P. aeruginosa* but not *Enterobacterales* species) in ICUs, and moreover that this was associated with human clinical infections, specifically bacteriemia by some *P. aeruginosa* clones [64]. In another previously published study, patients with SM pneumonia were associated with clones originating from sinks and medical devices in a Swedish ICU outbreak [65]. Therefore, disinfection of all possible sources is imperative to avoid healthcare-associated infections with this pathogen [29]. In addition, SM can be transferred via healthcare providers by hand contact. This reinforces the fact that healthcare personnel need to improve infection control practices and keep a close surveillance system [17,66].

Finally, a hospital-acquired BSI has been observed that is seasonal with summer spikes. A national Belgian cohort study on this infection showed associations between ambient climate variables and hospital-acquired BSI incidence rates per microorganism, with Gram-negative but not Gram-positive incidence increasing by 13% for every 5 °C increase in temperature. Stenotrophomonas, Acinetobacter, and Klebsiella spp. demonstrated the highest correlation with increased temperature, and Stenotrophomonas and Bacteroides spp. had higher relative humidity. These factors also warrant further examination to improve patient safety in our units [67].

3. Discussion and Future Directions

SM has been identified as a novel nosocomial pathogen associated with life-threatening invasive infections and a high mortality rate in some patient populations, especially those who are severely ill or immunocompromised [10,25]. Clinicians should be made aware of the implications of isolating this organism and should interpret their findings considering clinical settings.

The ICU population is especially vulnerable to this pathogen because of patients' conditions and an environment conducive to SM colonisation and subsequent patient transmission. As mentioned above, SM can often be recovered from the oropharynx of hospitalised and CF patients. We could hypothesise that critically ill mechanically ventilated patients can mimic CF status, as in both cases, SM causes chronic infection of the airways, which contributes to inflammation and lung damage. Moreover, prolonged ICU stays are accompanied by numerous antimicrobial rounds: these induce ecological effects on microbiota that condition the emergence and frequently the coexistence of MDRB. CF represents the paradigm of bacterial–bacterial community interactions, including Pseudomonas spp. and SM, whose prevalence can be correlated with or sometimes be independent of the use of antimicrobials such as carbapenems [7]. Moreover, poor clinical outcomes in co-infected cases warrant further research to find better antibiotic treatment strategies and case management to reduce co-infection mortality [38].

SM diagnosis also raises many challenges. It is imperative to establish a reproducible, accurate, sensitive, and predictive standard method to detect clinically important susceptibility profiles in contemporary isolates. Moreover, molecular rapid methods should be included in guidelines, but these should preferentially be universal and available for all centres.

As previously mentioned, the use of carbapenem in daily practice in the ICU represents one of the most important risk factors for SM infections from a different perspective. Classically, Del Toro MD et al. hypothesised that antimicrobials would select for SM because of its intrinsic resistance to most antibiotics, thus making colonisation easier to detect with clinical cultures and favouring the possibility of infection in patients debilitated by invasive procedures [9]. Therefore, implementing an antimicrobial stewardship program (ASP) in the ICU attending to a combination of measures related to antimicrobial selection, PK/PD optimisation, and short time duration, is one of the main keys to optimising and dealing with the healthcare problem of increasing antibiotic resistance [68]. Furthermore, ASPs are widely accepted in the ICU, and it has been demonstrated that antimicrobials can be administered without compromising patient safety [69].

It is noteworthy that although TMP-SMX is the treatment of choice for SM infections, it is not routinely included in empirical treatment regimens due both to its adverse event profile and the relative rarity of SM infections in comparison to other Gram-negative bacilli. Consequently, a risk stratification strategy seems important. The use of clinical scoring tools while awaiting final culture results may help identify patients at increased risk for a particular infection, with the intent of reducing time to appropriate antimicrobial therapy. Accordingly, a risk score has been developed that predicts hematologic malignancy patients at increased risk for SM BSI to guide early TMP-SMX therapy [70]. Twenty percent of the 337 patients included were admitted to the ICU. The StenoSCORE, incorporating five variables (AML, absolute neutrophil counts, mucositis, central venous catheter, and carbapenem receipt for $\geq$3 days), performed moderately well in predicting this infection. Afterward, it was externally validated with a single-centre cohort study with hematologic malignancy, including 36 patients with SM BSI [71]. The authors also evaluated alternative variables that better predicted SM BSI and ICU admission within 12 h of index culture included in the so-called StenoSCORE2. ROC curve analysis of the StenoSCORE2 performance produced an AUC of 0.84 (95% CI 0.76–0.92), which was higher than the previously published StenoSCORE. A StenoSCORE2 ≥ 4 had a sensitivity of 86%, specificity of 76%, and accurately identified 77% of SM BSIs.

Overall, combination therapy with effective antibiotics has been suggested when SM infections are suspected [53]. Unlike the current recommendation of combination therapy for empiric treatment of suspected or proven septic shock in ICU patients and monotherapy for definitive treatment when culture results and susceptibility tests are available, even for NFGNB, combination therapy could be discussed in patients with proven difficult-to-treat pathogens such as SM or carbapenem-resistant *Enterobacteriaceae* during ASP in the ICU, following clinical practice guidelines [68,72].

Opening further lines of research may help control the spread of SM in the ICU setting, with the optimisation of infection control policies deserving special attention [17].

Table 2 shows the most relevant findings and evidence-based key messages regarding severe SM infections in the critically ill population.

Table 2. Most relevant findings and key messages regarding severe SM infections in the critically ill population.

Scenario	Clinical Evidence
Epidemiology	Recent surveillance data indicate that SM accounts for less than 3% of all strains of healthcare-associated infections, a percentage that doubles in the case of VAP [5,22,23]. Crude 28-day mortality is 54.8% [13], increasing to 90% if hemorrhagic pneumonia is present [25], and it is further increased with co-infection by *Pseudomonas aeruginosa* [38]
Risk factors	Importance of stratification strategy: pre-existing medical conditions (COPD, malignancy); length of ICU stay; invasive procedures and antimicrobial agents, especially CP [15]. StenoSCORE2 for SM bacteriemia prediction [71]
Colonisation	Oral SM relative abundance of 36% predicts infection [14]. Previous SM colonisation was found in 80% of patients with pneumonia and 67% of patients with bacteremia caused by SM [6,16]
Antibiotic resistance	SM is intrinsically resistant to a wide range of commonly used antibiotics [29]. The resistance surveillance data reflect an increase, especially for cotrimoxazole and tigecycline [11,23,39]
Diagnostic challenges	There is no consensus among antimicrobial susceptibility testing guidelines [29,39]. An ICU-ASP for guiding an adjustment of empirical antimicrobial therapy based on rapid microbiological testing seems imperative [41,68]
Empirical therapy	SM predicts initially inappropriate antibiotic therapy [33]
Directed therapy	Combination therapy is recommended until clinical improvement [51,53]
Prevention measures	SM establishes ambiental ICU reservoirs and is related to patient infection [64,65]. Optimisation of infection control policies deserves special attention [17]

Note: SM: *Stenothophomonas maltophilia*; VAP: ventilator-associated pneumonia; COPD: chronic obstructive pulmonary disease; ICU: intensive care unit; CP: carbapenems; ASP: antimicrobial stewardship program.

This paper has several limitations inherent to narrative review methodology, such as potential incomplete coverage, lack of quantitative analysis, and positive results bias. Heterogeneity in study designs and the lack of explicit criteria for study selection may have also introduced some bias. Nevertheless, to our knowledge, no previous study has comprehensively evaluated evidence on Stenotrophomonas maltophilia infections in critical patients. However, data are limited, and relevant clinical questions remain outstanding, such as the microbiological diagnostic challenges, proper antimicrobial stewardship in the critically ill, and concrete preventive measures in these settings.

4. Conclusions

SM infection remains a challenge for critical care physicians. A high index of suspicion and deep knowledge of both the local epidemiological situation and the new rapid diagnostic tools linked to the implementation of an ICU-ASP in daily practice, as well as control measures, would improve the ominous prognosis of this bacterium's presence in the ICU setting.

Author Contributions: N.C.: writing—original draft preparation and editing; M.R.O. and M.Á.C.: review and editing. All authors have read and agreed to the published version of the manuscript.

Funding: This research received no external funding.

Conflicts of Interest: The authors declare no conflicts of interest.

References

1. Ryan, R.; Monchy, S.; Cardinale, M.; Taghavi, S.; Crossman, L.; Avison, M.; Berg, G.; van der Lelie, D.; Dow, J.M. The versatility and adaptation of bacteria from the genus Stenotrophomonas. *Nat. Rev. Microbiol.* **2009**, *7*, 514–525. [CrossRef] [PubMed]
2. Brooke, J.S. Stenotrophomonas maltophilia: An emerging global opportunistic pathogen. *Clin. Microbiol. Rev.* **2012**, *25*, 2–41. [CrossRef] [PubMed]
3. Looney, W.J.; Narita, M.; Mühlemann, K. *Stenotrophomonas maltophilia*: An emerging opportunist human pathogen. *Lancet Infect. Dis.* **2009**, *9*, 312–323. [CrossRef] [PubMed]
4. Fihman, V.; Le Monnier, A.; Corvec, S.; Jaureguy, F.; Tankovic, J.; Jacquier, H.; Carbonnelle, E.; Bille, E.; Illiaquer, M.; Cattoir, V.; et al. *Stenotrophomonas maltophilia*—The most worrisome threat among unusual non-fermentative gram-negative bacilli from hospitalized patients: A prospective multicenter study. *J. Infect.* **2012**, *64*, 391–398. [CrossRef] [PubMed]
5. Fupin, H.; Yan, G.; Demei, Z.; Fu, W.; Xiaofei, J. CHINET surveillance of bacterial resistance: Results of 2020. *Chin J Infect Chemother.* **2021**, *21*, 377–387. [CrossRef]
6. Nseir, S.; Pompeo, C.; Brisson, H.; Dewavrin, F.; Tissier, S.; Diarra, M.; Boulo, M.; Durocher, A. Intensive care unit-acquired Stenotrophomonas maltophilia: Incidence, risk factors, and outcome. *Crit. Care.* **2006**, *10*, R143. [CrossRef] [PubMed]
7. Koulenti, D.; Vandana, K.E.; Rello, J. Current viewpoint on the epidemiology of nonfermenting Gram-negative bacterial strains. *Curr. Opin. Infect. Dis.* **2023**, *36*, 545–554. [CrossRef] [PubMed]
8. Horan, T.C.; Andrus, M.; Dudeck, M.A. CDC/NHSN surveillance definition of health care-associated infection and criteria for specific types of infections in the acute care setting. *Am. J. Infect. Control* **2008**, *36*, 309e32. [CrossRef] [PubMed]
9. Del Toro, M.D.; Rodríguez-Bano, J.; Herrero, M.; Rivero, A.; García-Ordoñez, M.A.; Corzo, J.; Pérez-Cano, R.; Grupo Andaluz para el Estudio de las Enfermedades Infecciosas. Clinical epidemiology of Stenotrophomonas maltophilia colonization and infection: A multicenter study. *Medicine* **2002**, *81*, 228–239. [CrossRef] [PubMed]
10. Falagas, M.; Kastoris, A.; Vouloumanou, E.; Rafailidis, P.; Kapaskelis, A.; Dimopoulos, G. Attributable mortality of Stenotrophomonas maltophilia infections: A systematic review of the literature. *Future Microbiol.* **2009**, *4*, 1103–1109. [CrossRef] [PubMed]
11. Dadashi, M.; Hajikhani, B.; Nazarinejad, N.; Noorisepehr, N.; Yazdani, S.; Hashemi, A.; Hashemizadeh, Z.; Goudarzi, M.; Fatemeh, S. Global prevalence and distribution of antibiotic resistance among clinical isolates of Stenotrophomonas maltophilia: A systematic review and meta-analysis. *J. Glob. Antimicrob. Resist.* **2023**, *34*, 253–267. [CrossRef] [PubMed]
12. Laing, F.P.Y.; Ramotar, K.; Read, R.R.; Alfieri, N.; Kureishi, A.; Henderson, E.A.; Louie, T.J. Molecular epidemiology of Xanthomonas maltophilia colonization and infection in the hospital environment. *J. Clin. Microbiol.* **1995**, *33*, 513–518. [CrossRef] [PubMed]
13. Dimopoulos, G.; Garnacho-Montero, J.; Paramythiotou, E.; Gutierrez-Pizarraya, A.; Gogos, C.; Adriansen-Pérez, M.; Diakaki, C.; Matthaiou, D.K.; Poulakou, G.; Akinosoglou, K. Upraising Stenotrophomonas maltophilia in Critically Ill Patients: A New Enemy? *Diagnostics* **2023**, *13*, 1106. [CrossRef] [PubMed]
14. Aitken, S.L.; Sahasrabhojane, P.V.; Kontoyiannis, D.P.; Savidge, T.C.; Arias, C.A.; Ajami, N.J.; Shelburne, S.A.; Galloway-Peña, J.R. Alterations of the Oral Microbiome and Cumulative Carbapenem Exposure Are Associated With Stenotrophomonas maltophilia Infection in Patients With Acute Myeloid Leukemia Receiving Chemotherapy. *Clin. Infect. Dis.* **2021**, *72*, 1507–1513. [CrossRef] [PubMed]
15. Wang, N.; Tang, C.; Wang, L. Risk Factors for Acquired Stenotrophomonas maltophilia Pneumonia in Intensive Care Unit: A Systematic Review and Meta-Analysis. *Front Med.* **2022**, *8*, 808391. [CrossRef] [PubMed]

16. Hotta, G.; Matsumura, Y.; Kato, K.; Nakano, S.; Yunoki, T.; Yamamoto, M.; Nagao, M.; Ito, Y.; Takakura, S.; Ichiyama, S. Risk factors and outcomes of Stenotrophomonas maltophilia bacteraemia: A comparison with bacteraemia caused by Pseudomonas aeruginosa and Acinetobacter species. *PLoS ONE.* **2014**, *9*, e112208. [CrossRef] [PubMed]
17. Álvarez-Lerma, F.; Catalán-González, M.; Álvarez, J.; Sánchez-García, M.; Palomar-Martínez, M.; Fernández-Moreno, I.; Garnacho-Montero, J.; Barcenilla-Gaite, F.; García, R.; Aranaz-Andrés, J.; et al. Impact of the "Zero Resistance" program on acquisition of multidrug-resistant bacteria in patients admitted to Intensive Care Units in Spain. A prospective, intervention, multimodal, multicenter study. *Med. Intensiv.* **2023**, *47*, 193–202. [CrossRef] [PubMed]
18. Detsis, M.; Karanika, S.; Mylonakis, E. ICU Acquisition Rate, Risk Factors, and Clinical Significance of Digestive Tract Colonization With Extended-Spectrum Beta-Lactamase-Producing Enterobacteriaceae: A Systematic Review and Meta-Analysis. *Crit. Care Med.* **2017**, *45*, 705–714. [CrossRef] [PubMed]
19. Torres, I.; Huntley, D.; Tormo, M.; Calabuig, M.; Hernández-Boluda, J.C.; Terol, M.J.; Carretero, C.; de Michelena, P.; Pérez, A.; Piñana, J.L.; et al. Multi-body-site colonization screening cultures for predicting multi-drug resistant Gram-negative and Gram-positive bacteremia in hematological patients. *BMC Infect. Dis.* **2022**, *22*, 172. [CrossRef] [PubMed]
20. Scheich, S.; Koenig, R.; Wilke, A.C.; Lindner, S.; Reinheimer, C.; Wichelhaus, T.A.; Hogardt, M.; Kempf, V.A.J.; Kessel, J.; Weber, S.; et al. Stenotrophomonas maltophilia colonization during allogeneic hematopoietic stem cell transplantation is associated with impaired survival. *PLoS ONE.* **2018**, *13*, e0201169. [CrossRef] [PubMed]
21. Ishikawa, K.; Nakamura, T.; Kawai, F.; Uehara, Y.; Mori, N. Stenotrophomonas maltophilia Infection Associated with COVID-19: A Case Series and Literature Review. *Am. J. Case Rep.* **2022**, *23*, e936889. [CrossRef] [PubMed]
22. European Centre for Disease Prevention and Control. *Point Prevalence Survey of Healthcare-Associated Infections and Antimicrobial Use in European Acute Care Hospitals*; ECDC: Stockholm, Sweden, 2024.
23. ENVIN-HELICS. Available online: http://hws.vhebron.net/envin-helics/ (accessed on 19 May 2024).
24. Guo, L.; Li, H.; Li, Q.; Juan, J. Antimicrobial drug-sensitivity and clinical risk factors of stenotro-phomnas maltophilia in the neurological intensive care unit. *J. Xiangnan Univ. (Med. Sci.)* **2014**, *16*, 21–24.
25. Huang, C.; Kuo, S.; Lin, L. Hemorrhagic Pneumonia Caused by Stenotrophomonas maltophilia in Patients with Hematologic Malignancies-A Systematic Review and Meta-Analysis. *Medicina* **2024**, *15*, 162. [CrossRef] [PubMed]
26. Gutierrez, C.; Pravinkumar, E.; Balachandran, D.; Schneider, V. Fatal hemorrhagic pneumonia: Don't forget Stenotrophomonas maltophilia. *Respir. Med. Case Rep.* **2016**, *19*, 12–14. [CrossRef] [PubMed]
27. Imoto, W.; Yamada, K.; Yamairi, K.; Shibata, W.; Namikawa, H.; Yukawa, S.; Yoshii, N.; Nakaie, K.; Hirose, A.; Koh, H.; et al. Clinical Characteristics of Rapidly Progressive Fatal Hemorrhagic Pneumonia Caused by Stenotrophomonas maltophilia. *Intern. Med.* **2020**, *59*, 193–198. [CrossRef] [PubMed]
28. Windhorst, S.; Frank, E.; Georgieva, D.N.; Genov, N.; Buck, F.; Borowski, P.; Weber, W. The major extracellular protease of the nosocomial pathogen Stenotrophomonas maltophilia: Characterization of the protein and molecular cloning of the gene. *J. Biol. Chem.* **2022**, *277*, 11042–11049. [CrossRef] [PubMed]
29. Mojica, M.F.; Humphries, R.; Lipuma, J.J.; Mathers, A.J.; Rao, G.G.; Shelburne, S.A.; Fouts, D.E.; Van Duin, D.; Bonomo, R.A. Clinical challenges treating Stenotrophomonas maltophilia infections: An update. *JAC Antimicrob. Resist.* **2022**, *4*, dlac040. [CrossRef] [PubMed]
30. Tamma, P.D.; Aitken, S.L.; Bonomo, R.A.; Mathers, A.J.; van Duin, D.; Clancy, C.J. Infectious Diseases Society of America Guidance on the Treatment of AmpC beta-Lactamase-Producing Enterobacterales, Carbapenem-Resistant Acinetobacter baumannii, and Stenotrophomonas maltophilia Infections. *Clin. Infect. Dis.* **2022**, *74*, 2089–2114. [CrossRef] [PubMed]
31. Zaragoza, R.; Vidal-Cortés, P.; Aguilar, G.; Borges, M.; Diaz, E.; Ferrer, R.; Maseda, E.; Nieto, M.; Nuvials, F.X.; Ramirez, P.; et al. Update of the treatment of nosocomial pneumonia in the ICU. *Crit. Care.* **2020**, *24*, 383. [CrossRef] [PubMed]
32. Mensa, J.; Barberán, J.; Ferrer, R.; Borges, M.; Rascado, P.; Maseda, E.; Oliver, A.; Marco, F.; Adalia, R.; Aguilar, G.; et al. Recommendations for antibiotic selection for severe nosocomial infections. *Rev. Esp. Quimioter.* **2021**, *34*, 511–524. [CrossRef] [PubMed]
33. Zilberberg, M.D.; Shorr, A.F.; Micek, S.T.; Vazquez-Guillamet, C.; Kollef, M.H. Multi-drug resistance, inappropriate initial antibiotic therapy and mortality in Gram-negative severe sepsis and septic shock: A retrospective cohort study. *Crit. Care.* **2014**, *18*, 596. [CrossRef] [PubMed]
34. Xu, N.L.; Shi, S.J.; Lai, Z.S.; Li, H.R.; Lian, S.Q.; Chen, Y.S. A case-control study on the risk factors for lower respiratory tract infection by Stenotrophomonas maltophilia in a medical intensive care unit. *Chin. J. Tuberc. Respir. Dis.* **2011**, *34*, 735–738. [PubMed]
35. Zilberberg, M.D.; Nathanson, B.H.; Sulham, K.; Fan, W.; Shorr, A.F. A novel algorithm to analyze epidemiology and outcomes of carbapenem resistance among patients with hospital-acquired and ventilator-associated pneumonia: A retrospective cohort study. *Chest* **2019**, *155*, 1119–1130. [CrossRef] [PubMed]
36. Sherrard, L.J.; Tunney, M.M.; Elborn, J.S. Antimicrobial resistance in the respiratory microbiota of people with cystic fibrosis. *Lancet* **2014**, *384*, 703–713. [CrossRef] [PubMed]
37. Quinn, A.M.; Bottery, M.J.; Thompson, H.; Friman, V.P. Resistance evolution can disrupt antibiotic exposure protection through competitive exclusion of the protective species. *ISME J.* **2022**, *16*, 2433–2447. [CrossRef] [PubMed]

38. Yin, C.; Yang, W.; Meng, J.; Lv, Y.; Wang, J.; Huang, B. Co-infection of Pseudomonas aeruginosa and Stenotrophomonas maltophilia in hospitalised pneumonia patients has a synergic and significant impact on clinical outcomes. *Eur. J. Clin. Microbiol. Infect. Dis.* **2017**, *36*, 2231–2235. [CrossRef] [PubMed]
39. Bostanghadiri, N.; Sholeh, M.; Navidifar, T.; Dadgar-Zankbar, L.; Elahi, Z.; van Belkum, A.; Darban-Sarokhalil, D. Global mapping of antibiotic resistance rates among clinical isolates of Stenotrophomonas maltophilia: A systematic review and meta-analysis. *Ann. Clin. Microbiol. Antimicrob.* **2024**, *23*, 26. [CrossRef] [PubMed]
40. Poole, S.; Tanner, A.R.; Naidu, V.V.; Borca, F.; Phan, H.; Saeed, K.; Grocott, M.P.W.; Dushianthan, A.; Moyses, H.; Clark, T.W. Molecular point-of-care testing for lower respiratory tract pathogens improves safe antibiotic de-escalation in patients with pneumonia in the ICU: Results of a randomised controlled trial. *J. Infect.* **2022**, *85*, 625–633. [CrossRef] [PubMed]
41. Clari, M.A.; Carbonell, N.; Albert, E.; Navarro, D. Proposal for antimicrobial therapy stewardship of lower respiratory tract infection in mechanically-ventilated patients based upon the Biofire® Filmarray® Pneumonia Plus panel results. *Enfermedades Infecc. Microbiol. Clin.* **2023**, *41*, 521–523. [CrossRef] [PubMed]
42. Lv, M.; Zhu, C.; Zhu, C.; Yao, J.; Xie, L.; Zhang, C.; Huang, J.; Du, X.; Feng, G. Clinical values of metagenomic next-generation sequencing in patients with severe pneumonia: A systematic review and meta-analysis. *Front. Cell Infect. Microbiol.* **2023**, *13*, 1106859. [CrossRef] [PubMed]
43. Sun, L.; Li, L.; Du, S.; Liu, Y.; Cao, B. An evaluation of the Unyvero pneumonia system for rapid detection of microorganisms and resistance markers of lower respiratory infections-a multicenter prospective study on ICU patients. *Eur. J. Clin. Microb. Infect. Dis.* **2021**, *40*, 2113–2121. [CrossRef] [PubMed]
44. Burrack-Lange, S.C.; Personne, Y.; Huber, M.; Winkler, E.; Weile, J.; Knabbe, C.; Görig, J.; Rohde, H. Multicenter assessment of the rapid Unyvero Blood Culture molecular assay. *J. Med. Microbiol.* **2018**, *67*, 1294–1301. [CrossRef] [PubMed]
45. Peri, A.M.; Ling, W.; Furuya-Kanamori, L.; Harris, P.N.A.; Paterson, D.L. Performance of BioFire Blood Culture Identification 2 Panel (BCID2) for the detection of bloodstream pathogens and their associated resistance markers: A systematic review and meta-analysis of diagnostic test accuracy studies. *BMC Infect. Dis.* **2022**, *22*, 794. [CrossRef] [PubMed]
46. Galiana, A.; Coy, J.; Gimeno, A.; Guzman, N.M.; Rosales, F.; Merino, E.; Royo, G.; Rodríguez, J.C. Evaluation of the Sepsis Flow Chip assay for the diagnosis of blood infections. *PLoS ONE.* **2017**, *12*, e0177627. [CrossRef] [PubMed]
47. Reitz, A.; Poppert, S.; Rieker, M.; Frickmann, H. Evaluation of FISH for Blood Cultures under Diagnostic Real-Life Conditions. *Eur. J. Microbiol. Immunol.* **2018**, *8*, 135–141. [CrossRef] [PubMed]
48. Carrara, L.; Navarro, F.; Turbau, M.; Seres, M.; Morán, I.; Quintana, I.; Martino, R.; González, Y.; Brell, A.; Cordon, O.; et al. Molecular diagnosis of bloodstream infections with a new dual-priming oligonucleotide-based multiplex PCR assay. *J. Med. Microbiol.* **2013**, *62 (Pt. 11)*, 1673–1679. [CrossRef] [PubMed]
49. Gautam, V.; Sharma, M.; Singhal, L.; Kumar, S.; Kaur, P.; Tiwari, R.; Ray, P. MALDI-TOF mass spectrometry: An emerging tool for unequivocal identification of non-fermenting Gram-negative bacilli. *Indian. J. Med. Res.* **2017**, *145*, 665–672. [CrossRef] [PubMed]
50. Pintado, V.; Ruiz-Garbajosa, P.; Aguilera-Alonso, D.; Baquero-Artigao, F.; Bou, G.; Cantón, R.; Grau, S.; Gutiérrez-Gutiérrez, B.; Larrosa, N.; Machuca, I.; et al. Executive summary of the consensus document of the Spanish Society of Infectious Diseases and Clinical Microbiology (SEIMC) on the diagnosis and antimicrobial treatment of infections due to carbapenem-resistant Gram-negative bacteria. *Enfermedades Infecc. Microbiol. Clin.* **2023**, *41*, 360–370. [CrossRef] [PubMed]
51. Cantón, R.; Ruiz-Garbajosa, P. Treatment guidelines for multidrug-resistant Gram-negative microorganisms. *Rev. Esp. Quimioter.* **2023**, *36* (Suppl. S1), 46–51. [CrossRef] [PubMed]
52. Wei, C.; Ni, W.; Cai, X.; Zhao, J.; Cui, J. Evaluation of Trimethoprim/Sulfamethoxazole (SXT), Minocycline, Tigecycline, Moxifloxacin, and Ceftazidime Alone and in Combinations for SXT-Susceptible and SXT-Resistant Stenotrophomonas maltophilia by In Vitro Time-Kill Experiments. *PLoS ONE.* **2016**, *11*, e0152132. [CrossRef] [PubMed]
53. Tamma, P.D.; Aitken, S.L.; Bonomo, R.A.; Mathers, A.J.; van Duin, D.; Clancy, C.J. Infectious Diseases Society of America 2023 Guidance on the Treatment of Antimicrobial Resistant Gram-Negative Infections. *Clin. Infect. Dis.* **2023**, *18*, ciad428. [CrossRef] [PubMed]
54. Burastero, G.J.; Orlando, G.; Santoro, A.; Menozzi, M.; Franceschini, E.; Bedini, A.; Cervo, A.; Faltoni, M.; Bacca, E.; Biagioni, E.; et al. Ceftazidime/Avibactam in Ventilator-Associated Pneumonia Due to Difficult-to-Treat Non-Fermenter Gram-Negative Bacteria in COVID-19 Patients: A Case Series and Review of the Literature. *Antibiotics* **2022**, *11*, 1007. [CrossRef] [PubMed]
55. Junco, S.J.; Bowman, M.C.; Turner, R.B. Clinical outcomes of Stenotrophomonas maltophilia infection treated with trimethoprim/sulfamethoxazole, minocycline, or fluoroquinolone monotherapy. *Int. J. Antimicrob. Agents.* **2021**, *58*, 106367. [CrossRef] [PubMed]
56. De Pascale, G.; Lisi, L.; Pia Ciotti, G.M.; Vallecoccia, M.S.; Cutuli, S.L.; Cascarano, L.; Gelormini, C.; Bello, G.; Montini, L.; Carelli, S.; et al. Pharmacokinetics of high-dose tigecycline in critically ill patients with severe infections. *Ann. Intensive Care.* **2020**, *10*, 94. [CrossRef] [PubMed]
57. Wang, Y.L.; Scipione, M.R.; Dubrovskaya, Y.; Papadopoulos, J. Monotherapy with fluoroquinolone or trimethoprim-sulfamethoxazole for treatment of Stenotrophomonas maltophilia infections. *Antimicrob. Agents Chemother.* **2014**, *58*, 176–182. [CrossRef] [PubMed]

58. Sarzynski, S.H.; Warner, S.; Sun, J.; Matsouaka, R.; Dekker, J.P.; Babiker, A.; Li, W.; Lai, Y.L.; Danner, R.L.; Fowler, V.G., Jr.; et al. Trimethoprim-Sulfamethoxazole Versus Levofloxacin for Stenotrophomonas maltophilia Infections: A Retrospective Comparative Effectiveness Study of Electronic Health Records from 154 US Hospitals. *Open Forum Infect. Dis.* **2022**, *9*, ofab644. [CrossRef] [PubMed]
59. Sánchez, M.B.; Martínez, J.L. The efflux pump SmeDEF contributes to trimethoprim-sulfamethoxazole resistance in Stenotrophomonas maltophilia. *Antimicrob. Agents Chemother.* **2015**, *59*, 4347–4348. [CrossRef] [PubMed]
60. Gijón, D.; García-Castillo, J.; Fernández-López, M.C.; Bou, G.; Siller, M.; Calvo-Montes, J.; Pitart, C.; Vila, J.; Torno, N.; Gimeno, C.; et al. In vitro activity of cefiderocol and other newly approved antimicrobials against multi-drug resistant Gram-negative pathogens recovered in intensive care units in Spain and Portugal. *Rev. Esp. Quimioter.* **2024**, *37*, 69–77. [CrossRef] [PubMed]
61. Balandín, B.; Pintado, V.; Pérez-Pedrero, M.J.; Martínez-Sagasti, F.; Sancho-González, M.; Soriano-Cuesta, C.; Gesso, C.M.; Chicot, M.; de Luna, R.R.; Asensio-Martín, M.J.; et al. Multicentre study of cefiderocol for treatment of Gram-negative bacteria infections in critically ill patients. *Int. J. Antimicrob. Agents.* **2024**, *63*, 107121. [CrossRef] [PubMed]
62. Wicky, P.H.; Poiraud, J.; Alves, M.; Patrier, J.; d'Humières, C.; Lê, M.; Kramer, L.; de Montmollin, É.; Massias, L.; Armand-Lefèvre, L.; et al. Cefiderocol Treatment for Severe Infections due to Difficult-to-Treat-Resistant Non-Fermentative Gram-Negative Bacilli in ICU Patients: A Case Series and Narrative Literature Review. *Antibiotics* **2023**, *12*, 991. [CrossRef] [PubMed]
63. Guyot, A.; Turton, J.F.; Garner, D. Outbreak of Stenotrophomonas maltophilia on an Intensive Care Unit. *J. Hosp. Infect.* **2013**, *85*, 303–307. [CrossRef] [PubMed]
64. Sukhum, K.V.; Newcomer, E.P.; Cass, C.; Wallace, M.A.; Johnson, C.; Fine, J.; Sax, S.; Barlet, M.H.; Burnham, C.D.; Dantas, G.; et al. Antibiotic-resistant organisms establish reservoirs in new hospital built environments and are related to patient blood infection isolates. *Commun Med.* **2022**, *2*, 62. [CrossRef] [PubMed]
65. Gideskog, M.; Welander, J.; Melhus, Å. Cluster of S. maltophilia among patients with respiratory tract infections at an intensive care unit. *Infect. Prev. Pract.* **2020**, *2*, 100097. [CrossRef] [PubMed]
66. Baidya, A.; Kodan, P.; Fazal, F.; Tsering, S.; Menon, P.R.; Jorwal, P.; Chowdhury, U.K. Stenotrophomonas maltophilia: More than just a colonizer! Indian. *J. Crit. Care Med.* **2019**, *23*, 434. [CrossRef] [PubMed]
67. Blot, K.; Hammami, N.; Blot, S.; Vogelaers, D.; Lambert, M.L. Seasonal variation of hospital-acquired bloodstream infections: A national cohort study. *Infect. Control Hosp. Epidemiol.* **2022**, *43*, 205–211. [CrossRef] [PubMed]
68. Mokrani, D.; Chommeloux, J.; Pineton de Chambrun, M.; Hékimian, G.; Luyt, C.E. Antibiotic stewardship in the ICU: Time to shift into overdrive. *Ann. Intensive Care.* **2023**, *13*, 39. [CrossRef] [PubMed]
69. Pérez-Torres, D.; Tamayo-Lomas, L.M.; Domínguez-Gil González, M.; Almendros-Muñoz, R.; Sacristán-Salgado, M.A.; González-González, E.; Berezo-García, J.A.; Díaz-Rodríguez, C.; Canas-Pérez, I.; Lorenzo-Vidal, B.; et al. Antimicrobial stewardship program in an Intensive Care Unit: A retrospective observational analysis of the results 15 months after its implementation. *Rev. Esp. Quimioter.* **2023**, *36*, 477–485. [CrossRef] [PubMed]
70. Karaba, S.M.; Goodman, K.E.; Amoah, J.; Cosgrove, S.E.; Tamma, P.D. StenoSCORE: Predicting Stenotrophomonas maltophilia Bloodstream Infections in the Hematologic Malignancy Population. *Antimicrob. Agents Chemother.* **2021**, *65*, e0079321. [CrossRef] [PubMed]
71. Gill, E.L.; Gill, C.M.; McEvoy, C. Validation of a Stenotrophomonas maltophilia bloodstream infection prediction score in the hematologic malignancy population. *Ann. Hematol.* **2024**, *103*, 1745–1752. [CrossRef] [PubMed]
72. Torres, A.; Niederman, M.S.; Chastre, J.; Ewig, S.; Fernandez-Vandellos, P.; Hanberger, H.; Kollef, M.; Li Bassi, G.; Luna, C.M.; Martin-Loeches, I.; et al. International ERS/ESICM/ESCMID/ALAT guidelines for the management of hospital-acquired pneumonia and ventilator associated pneumonia: Guidelines for the management of hospital acquired pneumonia (HAP)/ventilator-associated pneumonia (VAP) of the European Respiratory Society (ERS), European Society of Intensive Care Medicine (ESICM), European Society of Clinical Microbiology and Infectious Diseases (ESCMID) and Asociacion Latinoamericana del Torax (ALAT). *Eur. Respir. J.* **2017**, *50*, 1700582. [CrossRef] [PubMed]

antibiotics

MDPI

Article

Real-Time TDM-Based Expert Clinical Pharmacological Advice Program for Attaining Aggressive Pharmacokinetic/Pharmacodynamic Target of Continuous Infusion Meropenem in the Treatment of Critically Ill Patients with Documented Gram-Negative Infections Undergoing Continuous Veno-Venous Hemodiafiltration

Milo Gatti [1,2,*], Matteo Rinaldi [1,3], Tommaso Tonetti [1,4], Antonio Siniscalchi [5], Pierluigi Viale [1,3] and Federico Pea [1,2]

1 Department of Medical and Surgical Sciences, Alma Mater Studiorum University of Bologna, 40138 Bologna, Italy; mat.rinaldi1989@gmail.com (M.R.); tommaso.tonetti@unibo.it (T.T.); pierluigi.viale@unibo.it (P.V.); federico.pea@unibo.it (F.P.)

2 Clinical Pharmacology Unit, Department for Integrated Infectious Risk Management, IRCCS Azienda Ospedaliero-Universitaria of Bologna, 40138 Bologna, Italy

3 Infectious Disease Unit, Department for Integrated Infectious Risk Management, IRCCS Azienda Ospedaliero-Universitaria of Bologna, 40138 Bologna, Italy

4 Division of Anesthesiology, Department of Anesthesia and Intensive Care, IRCCS Azienda Ospedaliero-Universitaria di Bologna, 40138 Bologna, Italy

5 Anesthesia and Intensive Care Medicine, IRCCS Azienda Ospedaliero-Universitaria di Bologna, 40138 Bologna, Italy; antonio.siniscalchi@aosp.bo.it

* Correspondence: milo.gatti2@unibo.it

Abstract: (1) Objectives: to describe the pharmacokinetic/pharmacodynamic (PK/PD) profile of continuous infusion (CI) meropenem in critical patients with documented Gram-negative infections undergoing continuous veno-venous hemodiafiltration (CVVHDF) and to assess the relationship with microbiological outcome. (2) Methods: Data were retrospectively retrieved for patients admitted to the general and the post-transplant intensive care units in the period October 2022–May 2023 who underwent CVVHDF during treatment with CI meropenem optimized by means of a real-time therapeutic drug monitoring (TDM)-based expert clinical pharmacological advice (ECPA) program for documented Gram-negative infections. Steady-state meropenem plasma concentrations were measured, and the free fractions (fC_{ss}) were calculated. Meropenem total clearance (CL_{tot}) was calculated at each TDM assessment, and the impact of CVVHDF dose intensity and of residual diuresis on CL_{tot} was investigated by means of linear regression. Optimal meropenem PK/PD target attainment was defined as an fC_{ss}/MIC ratio > 4. The relationship between meropenem PK/PD target attainment and microbiological outcome was assessed. (3) Results: A total of 24 critical patients (median age 68 years; male 62.5%) with documented Gram-negative infections were included. Median (IQR) meropenem fC_{ss} was 19.9 mg/L (17.4–28.0 mg/L). Median (IQR) CL_{tot} was 3.89 L/h (3.28–5.29 L/h), and median (IQR) CVVHDF dose intensity was 37.4 mL/kg/h (33.8–44.6 mL/kg/h). Meropenem dosing adjustments were provided in 20 out of 24 first TDM assessments (83.3%, all decreases) and overall in 26 out of the 51 total ECPA cases (51.0%). Meropenem PK/PD target attainment was always optimal, and microbiological eradication was achieved in 90.5% of assessable cases. (4) Conclusion: the real-time TDM-guided ECPA program was useful in attaining aggressive PK/PD targeting with CI meropenem in critically ill patients undergoing high-intensity CVVHDF and allowed microbiological eradication in most cases with dosing regimens ranging between 125 and 500 mg q6h over 6 h.

Keywords: meropenem; continuous infusion; continuous veno-venous hemodiafiltration; continuous renal replacement therapy; Gram-negative infections; PK/PD target attainment; microbiological outcome

1. Introduction

Sepsis and septic shock are major life-threatening infection-related conditions affecting critically ill patients, which may often cause multiorgan failure and may account for high mortality rates and massive antibiotic consumption [1].

The *Enterobacterales* and some non-fermenting pathogens like *P. aeruginosa* and *A. baumannii* are the Gram-negatives responsible for the majority of the cases of sepsis/septic shock reported among critically ill patients admitted to the intensive care unit (ICU) [2–4]. Unfortunately, nowadays the presence of carbapenem resistance (CR) is rapidly growing among Gram-negatives in the ICU setting [5]. Consequently, meropenem is being progressively superseded by novel beta-lactam/beta-lactamase inhibitors showing valuable activity against CR-Gram-negative infections [6]. According to recent guidelines and guidance, meropenem still remains the first-line option for treating infections caused by extended-spectrum beta-lactamase (ESBL)- and/or by AmpC-producing *Enterobacterales*, and is a valuable option for treating those caused by carbapenem-susceptible *P. aeruginosa* or *A. baumannii* [7–9]. Referring to antimicrobial resistance in the EU/EEA (EARS-Net), according to the last ECDC annual epidemiological report, ESBL- and/or AmpC-producing *Enterobacterales* and *P. aeruginosa* strains resistant to ceftazidime and/or to piperacillin–tazobactam accounted for 23.8–55.3% and 19.1–23.4% of isolates, respectively [10].

Notably, it was shown that attaining an aggressive pharmacokinetic/pharmacodynamic (PK/PD) target of $100\% fT_{>4-8\times MIC}$ with continuous infusion (CI) beta-lactams, including meropenem, was associated in critically ill ICU patients with both maximization of clinical efficacy and suppression of resistance development [11–13]. Unfortunately, achieving this goal in septic patients may be hampered by the need for continuous renal replacement therapy (CRRT). CRRT is needed in up to 70% of cases of sepsis-related acute kidney injury (AKI) [14,15], and may consistently increase meropenem clearance [16]. In critically ill patients undergoing CRRT, selecting proper meropenem dosing regimens for attaining aggressive PK/PD targets may be hindered by the CRRT operative conditions (i.e., modality for solute removal, type of filter material, effluent flow rate), by the patient's specific pathophysiological conditions (i.e., residual renal function and/or capillary leak syndrome), and by poor susceptibility of the bacterial pathogen to meropenem (i.e., high minimum inhibitory concentrations [MIC]) [16].

Unfortunately, guidance for choosing proper antimicrobial dosing regimens focused on aggressive PK/PD targets during CRRT is currently lacking [17,18]. In this challenging scenario, implementing a real-time therapeutic drug monitoring (TDM)-based expert clinical pharmacological advice (ECPA) program may be helpful in personalizing the CI meropenem dosing regimen for each critically ill patient undergoing CRRT, according to the so-called antimicrobial therapy puzzle concept [19].

The aim of this study was to assess retrospectively the usefulness of a real-time TDM-based ECPA program for attaining aggressive PK/PD targeting by CI meropenem in the treatment of critically ill patients with documented Gram-negative infections undergoing continuous veno-venous hemodiafiltration (CVVHDF).

2. Results

Overall, 24 critically ill patients had CI meropenem dosing regimens personalized by means of the TDM-based ECPA for treating documented Gram-negative infections while undergoing CVVHDF. Demographics and clinical features of the patients are summarized in Table 1. Case-by-case features of the included patients are described in Table 2.

Table 1. Demographics and clinical characteristics of included patients.

Demographics and Clinical Variables	Patients (N = 24)
Patient demographics	
Age (years) [median (IQR)]	68 (61–74)
Gender (male/female) [n (%)]	15/9 (62.5/37.5)

Table 1. *Cont.*

Demographics and Clinical Variables	Patients (N = 24)
Caucasian [n (%)]	23 (95.8)
Body weight (Kg) [median (IQR)]	67.5 (60.0–80.0)
Body mass index (Kg/m^2) [median (IQR)]	24.0 (22.0–27.6)
Charlson Comorbidity Index [median (IQR)]	5 (3–6)
Underlying diseases [n (%)]	
Bowel perforation	7 (29.2)
OLTx	6 (25.0)
Acute-on-chronic liver failure	3 (12.5)
Cholangitis/cholecystitis	3 (12.5)
Acute pulmonary edema	2 (8.3)
Others *	3 (12.5)
Severity of infections	
SOFA score at infection onset [median (IQR)]	14 (10.75–17)
Mechanical ventilation [n (%)]	21 (87.5)
Vasopressors [n (%)]	20 (83.3)
CVVHDF settings	
Total effluent flow rate (mL/h) [median (IQR)]	2800 (2615–2900)
CVVHDF dose intensity (mL/kg/h) [median (IQR)]	37.4 (33.8–44.6)
Blood flow rate (mL/min) [median (IQR)]	150 (150–150)
Net removal (mL/h) [median (IQR)]	90 (50–120)
Residual diuresis (mL/24 h) [median (IQR)]	140 (40.0–417.5)
Site of infection [n (%)]	
VAP	9 (37.5)
BSI	7 (29.2)
cIAI + BSI	3 (12.5)
cIAI	2 (8.3)
cIAI + VAP	2 (8.3)
VAP + BSI	1 (4.2)
Gram-negative clinical isolates [1] [n (%)]	
Escherichia coli	7 (25.9)
Klebsiella pneumoniae	7 (25.9)
Enterobacter cloacae	5 (18.5)
Proteus mirabilis	3 (11.2)
Pseudomonas aeruginosa	2 (7.4)
Klebsiella oxytoca	1 (3.7)
Klebsiella aerogenes	1 (3.7)
Acinetobacter baumannii	1 (3.7)
Antibiotic treatment	
Meropenem daily dose (mg) [median (IQR)]	500 q8h over 8 h (250–1000 q6h over 6 h)
Meropenem fC_{ss} (mg/L) [median (IQR)]	19.9 (17.4–28.0)
Meropenem CL_{tot} (L/h) [median (IQR)]	3.89 (3.28–5.29)
Combination therapy [n (%)]	10 (41.7)
Tigecycline	9
Ciprofloxacin	1
Treatment duration (days) [median (IQR)]	10.5 (6–17)
PK/PD target attainment	
Meropenem fC_{ss}/MIC [median (IQR)]	147.2 (48.5–196.9)
fC_{ss}/MIC > 4 [n (%)]	24 (100.0)
fC_{ss}/MIC = 1–4 [n (%)]	0 (0.0)
fC_{ss}/MIC < 1 [n (%)]	0 (0.0)
TDM-based ECPA	
Overall TDM-based ECPA	51
N. of TDM-based ECPA per patient [median (IQR)]	1 (1–3)
N. of dosage confirmations at first TDM assessment [n (%)]	4 (16.7)
N. of dosage increases at first TDM assessment [n (%)]	0 (0.0)
N. of dosage decreases at first TDM assessment [n (%)]	20 (83.3)

Table 1. *Cont.*

Demographics and Clinical Variables	Patients (N = 24)
Overall n. of dosage confirmations [n (%)]	25 (49.0)
Overall n. of dosage increases [n (%)]	1 (2.0)
Overall n. of dosage decreases [n (%)]	25 (49.0)
Clinical outcome	
Microbiological eradication [2] [n (%)]	19 (90.5)
Resistance development [2] [n (%)]	0 (0.0)
Clinical cure [n (%)]	13 (54.2)
30-day mortality rate [n (%)]	12 (50.0)

* including obstructive acute kidney injury (n = 1), DRESS syndrome (n = 1), and febrile neutropenia (n = 1). [1] A total of 27 pathogens were isolated. [2] Assessable in 21 out of 24 cases. BSI: bloodstream infection; cIAI: complicated intrabdominal infection; CL_{tot}: total clearance; C_{ss}: steady-state concentration; CVVHDF: continuous veno-venous hemodiafiltration; ECPA: expert clinical pharmacological advice; IQR: interquartile range; MIC: minimum inhibitory concentration; OLTx: orthotopic liver transplant; PK/PD: pharmacokinetic/pharmacodynamic; SOFA: sequential organ failure assessment; TDM: therapeutic drug monitoring; VAP: ventilator-associated pneumonia.

Median [interquartile range (IQR)] age was 68 years (61–74 years), with a male preponderance (62.5%). Median (IQR) Charlson Comorbidity Index (CCI) score was 5 (3–6). Bowel perforation (7 cases; 29.2%) and orthotopic liver transplant (6 cases; 25.0%) were the most frequent underlying diseases. Median (IQR) sequential organ failure assessment (SOFA) score at infection onset was 14 (10.75–17). In total, 21 out of 24 patients (87.5%) underwent invasive mechanical ventilation, and cardiovascular support with vasopressors was required in 83.3% of cases.

CVVHDF was always performed by means of a Prisma flex system equipped with an AN69 high-flux ST-150 filter membrane, and regional anticoagulation was achieved by means of citrate. Median (IQR) blood flow rate (Q_b) and total effluent flow rate were 150 mL/min (150–150 mL/min) and 2800 mL/h (2615–2900 mL/h), respectively. Median (IQR) CVVHDF dose was 37.4 mL/kg/h (33.8–44.6 mL/kg/h). Replacement solution was always delivered post-filter. In total, 18 out of 24 patients (75.0%) had residual 24-h urinary output with a median (IQR) of 140 mL (40.0–417.5 mL), and values higher than 500 mL were reported in three cases (12.5%).

Infection types were ventilator-associated pneumonia (VAP) in 9/24 cases (37.5%), bloodstream infection (BSI) in 7/24 cases (29.2%), complicated intrabdominal infection (cIAI) plus BSI in 3/24 cases (12.5%), cIAI and cIAI plus VAP in 2/24 cases each (8.3%), and VAP plus BSI in one case (4.2%). Overall, 27 Gram-negative pathogens were isolated, with *Escherichia coli* (25.9%), *Klebsiella pneumoniae* (25.9%), *Enterobacter cloacae* (18.5%), and *Proteus mirabilis* (11.2%) being the most frequent. ESBL and/or AmpC producers accounted for 17 out of 24 (70.8%) *Enterobacterales* clinical isolates. MIC values of meropenem ranged from 0.12 mg/L to 1 mg/L.

Median (IQR) daily CI maintenance dose (MD) of meropenem was 500 q8h over 8 h (250–1000 q6h over 6 h). Combination therapy was implemented in 10 out of 24 patients (41.7%), with tigecycline and with ciprofloxacin in 9 and in 1 case, respectively. Median (IQR) treatment duration was 10.5 days (6–17 days). Median (IQR) free steady-state concentrations (fC_{ss}) of meropenem were 19.9 mg/L (17.4–28.0 mg/L), and meropenem total CL (CL_{tot}) was 3.89 L/h (3.28–5.29 L/h). Meropenem CL_{tot} correlated poorly both with CVVHDF dose intensity ($r = 0.22$; $p = 0.13$) and with residual diuresis ($r = 0.02$; $p = 0.87$).

A total of 51 TDM-based ECPA recommendations for meropenem were carried out, with a median (IQR) of 1 (1–3) per patient. Dosing adjustments were recommended in 20 out of 24 first TDM assessments (83.3%, all decreases), and overall in 26 out of 51 total ECPA cases (51.0%, of which 2.0% increases and 49.0% decreases). Meropenem PK/PD target attainment was optimal in all of the cases (100.0%) with a median (IQR) fC_{ss}/MIC ratio of 147.2 (48.5–196.9).

Table 2. Case-by-case demographic and clinical features of 24 critically ill patients with documented Gram-negative infections treated with CI meropenem according to a TDM-guided ECPA program during CVVHDF support.

ID Case	Age/Gender	Underlying Disease	CCI	MV/ Vasopressors	Baseline SOFA Score	Type of Infection	Pathogen	MIC (mg/L)	Initial Meropenem MD	Average *f*Css (mg/L)	Average *f*Css/MIC Ratio	PK/PD Target Attainment	Combination Therapy	Microbiological Eradication	Clinical Cure	30-Day Mortality Rate
#1	54/M	ACLF	5	Yes/Yes	19	BSI	ESBL-producing *Escherichia coli*	0.12	500 mg q6h over 6 h	19.11	159.25	Optimal	None	Yes	No *	Yes
#2	77/F	Cholangitis	3	Yes/Yes	15	cIAI + BSI	*Enterobacter cloacae*	0.12	1000 mg q6h over 6 h	22.91	190.94	Optimal	Tigecycline	No	No	No
#3	67/F	OLTx	5	Yes/Yes	16	VAP	*Enterobacter cloacae*	1	1000 mg q6h over 6 h	44.59	44.59	Optimal	Tigecycline	No	No	Yes
#4	70/F	Bowel perforation	3	Yes/Yes	17	BSI	ESBL-producing *Escherichia coli*	0.12	1000 mg q6h over 6 h	75.66	630.47	Optimal	None	NA	No	Yes
#5	67/F	OLTx	5	Yes/Yes	16	VAP	*Enterobacter cloacae*	1	1000 mg q6h over 6 h	30.02	30.02	Optimal	None	Yes	No *	Yes
#6	77/F	Cholangitis	3	Yes/Yes	16	cIAI + BSI	*Enterobacter cloacae*	0.12	250 mg q6h over 6 h	8.43	70.23	Optimal	Tigecycline	Yes	Yes	No
#7	63/M	OLTx	6	Yes/Yes	17	cIAI + BSI	*Klebsiella oxytoca*	0.12	1000 mg q6h over 6 h	18.54	148.31	Optimal	Tigecycline	Yes	Yes	No
#8	62/M	Acute pulmonary oedema	6	Yes/No	6	VAP	ESBL-producing *Klebsiella pneumoniae*	0.5	500 mg q6h over 6 h	20.91	41.81	Optimal	Ciprofloxacin	Yes	Yes	No
#9	63/M	OLTx	6	Yes/Yes	17	VAP	*Acinetobacter baumannii*	1	1000 mg q6h over 6 h	27.59	27.59	Optimal	Tigecycline	Yes	Yes	No
#10	57/F	OLTx	5	Yes/No	12	VAP	*Proteus mirabilis*	0.12	1000 mg q6h over 6 h	18.69	155.78	Optimal	None	Yes	Yes	No
#11	81/M	Acute pulmonary oedema	5	Yes/Yes	11	VAP	ESBL-producing *Klebsiella pneumoniae*	0.12	1000 mg q6h over 6 h	42.24	351.98	Optimal	None	Yes	No *	Yes
#12	58/M	ACLF	7	No/Yes	15	BSI	*Klebsiella pneumoniae*	0.12	1000 mg q6h over 6 h	30.09	250.72	Optimal	None	Yes	Yes	Yes
#13	62/M	Bowel perforation	2	Yes/Yes	18	cIAI	ESBL-producing *Escherichia coli*	0.12	250 mg q6h over 6 h	5.98	48.92	Optimal	None	Yes	No *	Yes
#14	41/M	ACLF	3	No/No	8	BSI	ESBL-producing *Escherichia coli* ESBL-producing *Klebsiella pneumoniae*	0.12 0.12	750 mg q6h over 6 h	25.77	214.78	Optimal	None	Yes	Yes	No

Table 2. *Cont.*

ID Case	Age/Gender	Underlying Disease	CCI	MV/Vasopressors	Baseline SOFA Score	Type of Infection	Pathogen	MIC (mg/L)	Initial Meropenem MD	Average *f*Css (mg/L)	Average *f*Css/MIC Ratio	PK/PD Target Attainment	Combination Therapy	Microbiological Eradication	Clinical Cure	30-Day Mortality Rate
#15	73/M	Bowel perforation	4	Yes/Yes	9	cIAI + VAP	ESBL-producing *Proteus mirabilis*	0.12	1000 mg q6h over 6 h	29.20	233.63	Optimal	Tigecycline	Yes	No *	Yes
#16	74/M	Bowel perforation	6	Yes/Yes	12	cIAI + VAP	*Escherichia coli* *Proteus mirabilis*	0.12	1000 mg q6h over 6 h	27.34	218.74	Optimal	None	NA	No	Yes
#17	71/M	Obstructive AKI	9	Yes/Yes	18	VAP	ESBL-producing *Klebsiella pneumoniae*	0.12	1000 mg q6h over 6 h	8.82	70.56	Optimal	None	NA	No	Yes
#18	71/M	Bowel perforation	5	Yes/Yes	9	BSI	ESBL-producing *Klebsiella pneumoniae*	1	1000 mg q6h over 6 h	16.82	16.82	Optimal	None	Yes	Yes	Yes
#19	69/M	Dress syndorme	9	Yes/Yes	11	VAP	AmpC-producing *Klebsiella aerogenes*	0.12	500 mg q6h over 6 h	14.70	122.50	Optimal	Tygeciccline	Yes	Yes	No
#20	83/F	Bowel perforation	7	Yes/Yes	20	VAP + BSI	ESBL-producing *Escherichia coli*	0.12	1000 mg q6h over 6 h	17.54	146.18	Optimal	None	Yes	No *	Yes
#21	50/F	OLT	4	Yes/Yes	12	BSI	*Pseudomonas aeruginosa*	0.25	250 mg q6h CI	20.04	80.16	Optimal	Tygeciccline	Yes	Yes	No
#22	77/M	Bowel perforation	7	Yes/No	9	cIAI	*Escherichia coli* *Enterobacter cloacae*	0.12 0.12	1000 mg q6h over 6 h	17.95	149.61	Optimal	Tygeciccline	Yes	Yes	No
#23	56/M	Febrile neutropenia	3	No/Yes	13	BSI	ESBL-producing *Escherichia coli*	0.12	1000 mg q6h over 6 h	19.83	158.63	Optimal	None	Yes	Yes	No
#24	74/F	Cholecistitis	3	Yes/Yes	10	VAP	*Pseudomonas aeruginosa*	1	500 mg q6h over 6 h	14.80	14.80	Optimal	None	Yes	Yes	No

* case #1: ESBL-producing *E. coli* was eradicated from follow-up blood culture, but signs and symptoms of the infection persisted, resulting in clinical failure and subsequent implementation of compassionate care; case #5: *Enterobacter cloacae* was eradicated from follow-up BAL, but signs and symptoms of the infection persisted, resulting in clinical failure and mortality; case #11: ESBL-producing *K.pneumoniae* was eradicated from follow-up BAL, but signs and symptoms of infection persisted, resulting in clinical failure and subsequent implementation of compassionate care; case #13: ESBL-producing *E. coli* was eradicated from peritoneal fluid, but fever and need for vasopressors persisted; case #15: ESBL-producing *P. mirabilis* was eradicated from peritoneal fluid, but fever and need for vasopressors persisted, resulting in implementation of compassionate care due to inoperability; case #20: ESBL-producing *E. coli* was eradicated from peritoneal fluid, but fever and need for vasopressors persisted, resulting in implementation of compassionate care due to underlying conditions. ACLF: acute-on-chronic liver failure; AKI: acute kidney injury; BSI: bloodstream infection; CCI: Charlson Comorbidity Index; cIAI: intrabdominal infection; Css: steady-state concentrations; ECPA: expert clinical pharmacological advice; ESBL: extended-spectrum beta-lactamase; MD, maintenance dose; MIC: minimum inhibitory concentration; MV: mechanical ventilation; NA: not assessed; OLTx: orthotopic liver transplant; PK/PD: pharmacokinetic/pharmacodynamic; SOFA: sequential organ failure assessment; TDM: therapeutic drug monitoring; VAP: ventilator-associated pneumonia. PK/PD target column: green box: optimal PK/PD target; yellow box: quasi-optimal PK/PD target; red box: suboptimal PK/PD target. Microbiological eradication column: green box: microbiological eradication; red box: microbiological failure; grey box: not assessable.

Microbiological outcome was assessable in 21/24 cases. Microbiological eradication was achieved in 19/21 cases (90.5%). Microbiological failure occurred in two cases (9.5%), namely in one with bacteraemic cIAI due to *Enterobacter cloacae*, and in another with VAP caused by *Enterobacter cloacae*. No cases of resistance developed. Clinical cure was achieved in 54.2% of patients, and the 30-day mortality rate was 50.0%.

The TDM-based meropenem dosing ECPA provided in our study is summarized in Table 3.

Table 3. Meropenem dosing ECPA provided in our study.

Optimal PK/PD Target	MIC of Isolated Pathogen (mg/L)	TDM-Based Meropenem Dosing ECPA Recommendation
fC_{ss}/MIC > 4	0.12	125 mg q6h over 6 h
fC_{ss}/MIC > 4	0.25–1	250 mg q6h over 6 h
fC_{ss}/MIC > 4	2	500 mg q6h over 6 h

CI: continuous infusion; C_{ss}: steady-state concentration; MIC: minimum inhibitory concentration; PK/PD: pharmacokinetic/pharmacodynamic

3. Discussion

Our study described the attainment of aggressive PK/PD targeting by CI meropenem by means of a real-time TDM-based ECPA program in a cohort of critically ill patients with documented severe Gram-negative infections undergoing high-intensity CVVHDF.

Several studies have assessed the population PK of meropenem in critical patients undergoing CRRT, and were recently meta-analyzed [20]. Interestingly, median meropenem CL_{tot} was approximately 25% higher in our study than in previous studies (3.89 L/h vs. 3.03 L/h) [20]. This finding could be explained by the high dose intensity of CVVHDF applied, which was approximately two-thirds higher than reported in previous studies (median 37.4 vs. 25.0 mL/kg/h). Meropenem CL_{tot} was far lower in our cohort compared with healthy subjects (15.54 L/h) [21]. This is in agreement with the severity of the sepsis-related AKI and the multi-organ failure affecting these patients, as witnessed by the relevant proportion of cases having anuria and high SOFA scores at infection onset.

The lack of correlation between CVVHDF dose intensity and meropenem CL_{tot} is not unexpected, being consistent with what has been previously reported [22–26]. In our study, this could be explained on the one hand by wide intra- and interindividual differences regarding filter age and/or drug adsorption [22], and on the other hand by the fact that the almost homogeneous dose intensity of CVVHDF applied in all of the patients precluded the possibility of showing consistent differences of meropenem CL_{tot} among cases.

The lack of significant correlation between meropenem CL_{tot} and residual diuresis is inconsistent with previous studies [22,27]. This might be explained by the fact that only approximately 10% of our patients had residual diuresis, but we should also recognize that measuring 24 h urinary creatinine clearance rather than residual diuresis might have enabled more reliable assessment of residual renal function [28].

The most interesting finding of our study was that CI meropenem doses ranging from 125 to 500 mg q6h over 6 h attained aggressive PK/PD targets in all of the cases undergoing high-intensity CVVHDF and allowed microbiological eradication in the vast majority of these. CI may be the best administration mode for attaining aggressive PK/PD targets with beta-lactams under the same daily dose [29,30]. In this scenario, adopting a real-time TDM-guided ECPA program could be very valuable in allowing prompt dose reduction whenever clinical isolates have wild-type MICs, as occurred in more than 80% of first TDM assessments in the current study, thus also minimizing potential adverse events associated with drug overexposure [31,32].

This may further support the role that a "patient-centered" approach may have in selecting antimicrobial dosing regimens for critically ill patients undergoing CRRT, by taking into account all of the potential variables hindering the aggressive PK/PD target attainment of a specific agent [16].

We believe that our findings could also provide some useful suggestions for attaining aggressive PK/PD targeting with CI meropenem in patients with documented Gram-negative infections susceptible to meropenem requiring CVVHDF support with dose intensity similar to ours, for intensive care physicians in centers where real-time TDM is unfeasible. Specifically, the suggested dosing regimens could range from 125 mg q6h over 6 h in cases of clinical isolates with an MIC value $\leq$ 0.12 mg/L, up to 250 mg q6h over 6 h in cases of clinical isolates with MIC values ranging 0.25–1 mg/L, and 500 mg q6h over 6 h in cases of clinical isolates with MIC values at the clinical breakpoint of 2 mg/L.

We recognize that our study has some limits. The retrospective monocentric study design and the limited sample size should be acknowledged. Only total meropenem concentrations were measured, and the free fractions were estimated by means of the plasma protein binding reported in healthy subjects; with these values being low, the bias should be only marginal. Residual renal function was not assessed by means of 24 h measured urinary creatinine clearance. The role of combo-therapy on microbiological outcome could not be ruled out. Finally, our findings may not be reliable enough in cases of low-intensity CVVHDF or other CRRT modalities.

4. Materials and Methods

4.1. Study Design

This retrospective study investigated critically ill patients who, in the period between 1 October 2022 and 31 May 2023, were admitted to the general ICU or the post-transplant ICU of the IRCCS Azienda Ospedaliero-Universitaria of Bologna, Italy, and were treated with CI meropenem optimized by means of real-time TDM-guided ECPA for documented Gram-negative infections while undergoing CVVHDF. Patients affected by COVID-19 were excluded.

4.2. Data Collection

Demographic (age, sex weight, height, body mass index [BMI]) and clinical/laboratory data (CCI, underlying disease, SOFA score at infection onset, need for mechanical ventilation and/or for vasopressor support) were retrieved for each patient. Clinical isolates, MIC values for meropenem, type/site of infection, treatment duration, meropenem dosage and average plasma C_{ss}, eventual co-administration of other anti-Gram-negative active antimicrobial agents, overall number of ECPAs, ECPA-recommended dosing adjustments at first and subsequent TDM assessment, microbiological and clinical outcomes, and 30-day mortality rate were also collected.

CVVHDF operative conditions were retrieved at each TDM assessment. Specifically, data concerning type of filter, selected anticoagulant, Q_b, pre-blood pump (PBP) fluid rate, dialysate flow rate (Q_d), percentage of pre-/post-dilution, replacement fluid rate, and net removal rate per hour were collected. Furthermore, data on 24 h residual diuresis on the day of TDM assessment were also extracted. The total effluent flow rate was defined according to the following equation: pre-filter replacement fluid rate + post-filter replacement fluid rate + net removal rate + PBP fluid rate + Q_d, as previously reported [33]. CVVHDF dose intensity was calculated as the total effluent flow rate normalized to body weight.

Site of infection was defined according to the Centers for Disease Control and Prevention (CDC) criteria [34]. Documented BSI was defined as the isolation of a Gram-negative pathogen from at least one blood culture [34]. Documented VAP was defined as the isolation of one or more Gram-negative pathogens with a bacterial load $\geq 10^4$ CFU/mL in the bronchoalveolar lavage (BAL) fluid culture after > 48 h from endotracheal intubation and initiation of mechanical ventilation in patients showing new or progressive lung infiltrates [35,36]. cIAI was defined as the isolation of one or more Gram-negative pathogens from the peritoneal fluid in patients with infection extended to multiple organs into the peritoneal space [36,37].

The MIC values for meropenem against Gram-negative clinical isolates (*Enterobacterales* and/or *Pseudomonas aeruginosa*) were measured by means of a semi-automated broth microdilution method (Microscan Beckman NMDRM1) and interpreted according to the European Committee on Antimicrobial Susceptibility Testing (EUCAST) clinical breakpoints [38]. Pathogens were considered as meropenem-susceptible whenever the MIC value was ≤2 mg/L.

4.3. Meropenem Administration and Sampling Procedure

Meropenem was prescribed by the treating intensive care physicians and/or the infectious disease consultant as first- or second-line therapy according to results of antimicrobial susceptibility tests. Therapy was always started with a loading dose (LD) of 2 g over 2 h infusion, followed by an initial MD administered by CI. Aqueous solutions were reconstituted every 6–8 h and infused over 6–8 h in order to prevent meropenem degradation, as recommended [39,40].

The initial MD regimen was defined on a case-by-case basis in relation to CVVHDF conditions, presence/absence of residual diuresis, site of infection, and underlying clinical conditions. Dosing was subsequently optimized by means of a real-time TDM-guided ECPA program. For this purpose, blood samples for measuring meropenem C_{ss} were first collected after at least 24 h from starting therapy, and then reassessed every 48–72 h whenever feasible. Total meropenem plasma concentrations were determined by means of a validated liquid chromatography–tandem mass spectrometry method [12]. Precision and accuracy were assessed by replicate analysis of quality control samples against calibration standards. The intra- and inter-assay coefficients of variations were <±15%, as required by the EMA guidelines. The lower limit of quantification was 0.3 mg/L. The assay was linear in the range from 0.3 to 84.4 mg/L. At each TDM assessment, meropenem CL_{tot} was calculated by means of the following formula: CL_{tot} (L/h) = infusion rate (mg/h)/C_{ss} (mg/L).

Real-time expert interpretation of meropenem TDM results was performed by well-trained MD clinical pharmacologists (ECPA) with long-standing expertise who suggested dosing adaptation whenever needed. The TDM-guided ECPA was structured as previously reported [19].

4.4. Relationship between Meropenem Aggressive PK/PD Target and Microbiological Outcome

The percentage of time of CI meropenem fC_{ss} above the MIC was selected as the best PK/PD parameter for efficacy and defined as the fC_{ss}/MIC ratio (equivalent to $\%fT_{>MIC}$). Considering that only total meropenem concentrations were measured, the f fraction was calculated by multiplying total meropenem C_{ss} by 0.98, according to a 2% plasma protein binding [41].

Aggressive PK/PD target attainment was defined as optimal when the fC_{ss}/MIC ratio was >4 (equivalent to $100\%fT_{>4\times MIC}$), and quasi-optimal or suboptimal when fC_{ss}/MIC ratio was 1–4 or <1 (equivalent to $100\%fT_{1-4\times MIC}$ and to $<100\%fT_{1\times MIC}$), respectively, as previously reported [42]. Specifically, a $fC_{ss}/MIC > 4$ is equal to $fC_{ss} > 4 \times MIC$. Considering that meropenem was administered by CI in all included patients, it may be supposed that C_{ss} were stable and constant throughout the 24 h. Consequently, the $fC_{ss} > 4 \times MIC$ may be expressed as $100\%fT_{>4\times MIC}$, as previously reported [12].

In patients undergoing more than one TDM-guided ECPA recommendation, average meropenem fC_{ss} was considered by calculating the mean of all of the observed C_{ss} values (the first one before any dosage adjustment and the subsequent ones after eventual dosage adjustments).

This threshold was selected according to in vitro, experimental animal, and clinical studies showing that attaining aggressive PK/PD targets of C_{ss}/MIC ratios ≥ 4 (equivalent to $100\%f_{>4\times MIC}$) with beta-lactams may be associated both with maximization of clinical efficacy and with microbiologic eradication and prevention of resistance development against Gram-negative pathogens [11–13,43].

Optimization of meropenem dosing was performed as previously reported [19]. Specifically, a 25% or 50% dosing decrease was adopted whenever the C_{ss}/MIC ratio was equal to 8–10 or above 10, respectively; dosing was confirmed whenever the C_{ss}/MIC ratio was equal to 4–8; and 25% or 50% dosing increase was implemented whenever the C_{ss}/MIC ratio was equal to 2–4 or below 2, respectively.

Microbiological eradication and clinical outcome were assessed for each patient and correlated with meropenem PK/PD target attainment. Microbiological eradication or failure was defined, respectively, as the absence or the persistence of the same Gram-negative pathogen isolated in the index cultures in at least one subsequent assessment after starting meropenem therapy. Resistance development was defined as an increase in the meropenem MIC value against the original clinical isolate beyond the EUCAST clinical breakpoint of susceptibility. Primary outcome was microbiological eradication, whereas clinical cure (defined as the complete resolution of signs and symptoms of the infection coupled with documented microbiological eradication at the end of treatment and absence of recurrence or relapse at 30-day follow-up and/or resistance development) and 30-day mortality rate represented the secondary outcomes.

4.5. Statistical Analysis

Continuous data are expressed as median and interquartile range (IQR), whereas categorical variables are presented as counts or percentages. The relationships between CVVHDF dose intensity or residual diuresis and meropenem CL_{tot} were assessed by linear regression, and the Pearson's r value was calculated. p values < 0.05 were considered statistically significant. Statistical analysis was performed by using MedCalc for Windows (MedCalc statistical software, version 19.6.1, MedCalc Software Ltd., Ostend, Belgium).

5. Conclusions

In conclusion, our findings suggested that a real-time TDM-guided ECPA program may be useful in attaining aggressive PK/PD targeting with CI meropenem in critically ill patients undergoing high-intensity CVVHDF and that dosing regimens ranging between 125 and 500 mg q6h over 6 h may allow microbiological eradication in most cases. The profile of the susceptibility test results of the Gram-negative isolates to meropenem may be a major factor affecting the magnitude of the CI meropenem dosing regimen needed when very homogeneous operative conditions for CVVHDF are applied. Large prospective studies are warranted to confirm our findings.

Author Contributions: Conceptualization, M.G. and F.P.; methodology, M.G.; formal analysis, M.G.; data curation, M.G. and M.R.; writing—original draft preparation, M.G.; writing—review and editing, T.T., A.S., P.V. and F.P. All authors have read and agreed to the published version of the manuscript.

Funding: This research received no external funding.

Institutional Review Board Statement: The study was conducted according to the guidelines of the Declaration of Helsinki and approved by the local ethical committee [No. 442/2021/Oss/AOUBo, approved on 28 June 2021].

Informed Consent Statement: Signed informed consent was waived due to the retrospective and observational nature of the investigation, according to hospital agreements.

Data Availability Statement: The data presented in this study are available on request from the corresponding author. The data are not publicly available due to privacy concerns.

Conflicts of Interest: M.G. received personal fees from Angelini; P.V has served as a consultant for Biomerieux, Gilead, Merck Sharp & Dohme, Nabriva, Nordic Pharma, Pfizer, Thermo-Fisher, and Venatorx, and received payment for serving on the speaker's bureau for Correvio, Gilead, Merck Sharp & Dohme, Nordic Pharma and Pfizer; F.P participated in speaker bureau for Angelini, Basilea Pharmaceutica, Gilead, Hikma, Merck Sharp & Dohme, Nordic Pharma, Pfizer, and Sanofi Aventis, and in advisory board for Angelini, Basilea Pharmaceutica, Correvio, Gilead, Merck Sharp & Dohme, Nordic Pharma, Novartis, Pfizer, and Thermo-Fisher. The authors report no other conflict of interest in this work.

References

1. Angus, D.C.; van der Poll, T. Severe Sepsis and Septic Shock. *N. Engl. J. Med.* **2013**, *369*, 840–851. [CrossRef] [PubMed]
2. Vincent, J.-L.; Sakr, Y.; Singer, M.; Martin-Loeches, I.; Machado, F.R.; Marshall, J.C.; Finfer, S.; Pelosi, P.; Brazzi, L.; Aditianingsih, D.; et al. Prevalence and Outcomes of Infection Among Patients in Intensive Care Units in 2017. *JAMA* **2020**, *323*, 1478–1487. [CrossRef] [PubMed]
3. MacVane, S.H. Antimicrobial Resistance in the Intensive Care Unit: A Focus on Gram-Negative Bacterial Infections. *J. Intensive Care Med.* **2017**, *32*, 25–37. [CrossRef] [PubMed]
4. Sader, H.S.; Farrell, D.J.; Flamm, R.K.; Jones, R.N. Antimicrobial Susceptibility of Gram-Negative Organisms Isolated from Patients Hospitalized in Intensive Care Units in United States and European Hospitals (2009–2011). *Diagn. Microbiol. Infect. Dis.* **2014**, *78*, 443–448. [CrossRef]
5. Martín-Loeches, I.; Diaz, E.; Vallés, J. Risks for Multidrug-Resistant Pathogens in the ICU. *Curr. Opin. Crit. Care* **2014**, *20*, 516–524. [CrossRef] [PubMed]
6. Yahav, D.; Giske, C.G.; Grāmatniece, A.; Abodakpi, H.; Tam, V.H.; Leibovici, L. New β-Lactam-β-Lactamase Inhibitor Combinations. *Clin. Microbiol. Rev.* **2020**, *34*, 10–1128. [CrossRef]
7. Tamma, P.D.; Aitken, S.L.; Bonomo, R.A.; Mathers, A.J.; van Duin, D.; Clancy, C.J. Infectious Diseases Society of America 2022 Guidance on the Treatment of Extended-Spectrum β-Lactamase Producing Enterobacterales (ESBL-E), Carbapenem-Resistant Enterobacterales (CRE), and Pseudomonas Aeruginosa with Difficult-to-Treat Resistance (DTR-P. Aeruginosa). *Clin. Infect. Dis.* **2022**, *75*, 187–212. [CrossRef]
8. Tamma, P.D.; Aitken, S.L.; Bonomo, R.A.; Mathers, A.J.; van Duin, D.; Clancy, C.J. Infectious Diseases Society of America Guidance on the Treatment of AmpC β-Lactamase-Producing Enterobacterales, Carbapenem-Resistant Acinetobacter Baumannii, and Stenotrophomonas Maltophilia Infections. *Clin. Infect. Dis.* **2022**, *74*, 2089–2114. [CrossRef]
9. Paul, M.; Carrara, E.; Retamar, P.; Tängdén, T.; Bitterman, R.; Bonomo, R.A.; de Waele, J.; Daikos, G.L.; Akova, M.; Harbarth, S.; et al. European Society of Clinical Microbiology and Infectious Diseases (ESCMID) Guidelines for the Treatment of Infections Caused by Multidrug-Resistant Gram-Negative Bacilli (Endorsed by European Society of Intensive Care Medicine). *Clin. Microbiol. Infect.* **2022**, *28*, 521–547. [CrossRef] [PubMed]
10. ECDC Antimicrobial Resistance in the EU/EEA (EARS-Net)—Annual Epidemiological Report for 2019. Available online: https://www.ecdc.europa.eu/en/about-us/networks/disease-networks-and-laboratory-networks/ears-net-data (accessed on 25 August 2023).
11. Sumi, C.D.; Heffernan, A.J.; Lipman, J.; Roberts, J.A.; Sime, F.B. What Antibiotic Exposures Are Required to Suppress the Emergence of Resistance for Gram-Negative Bacteria? A Systematic Review. *Clin. Pharmacokinet* **2019**, *58*, 1407–1443. [CrossRef]
12. Gatti, M.; Cojutti, P.G.; Pascale, R.; Tonetti, T.; Laici, C.; Dell'Olio, A.; Siniscalchi, A.; Giannella, M.; Viale, P.; Pea, F. Assessment of a PK/PD Target of Continuous Infusion Beta-Lactams Useful for Preventing Microbiological Failure and/or Resistance Development in Critically Ill Patients Affected by Documented Gram-Negative Infections. *Antibiotics* **2021**, *10*, 1311. [CrossRef]
13. Alshaer, M.H.; Maranchick, N.; Alexander, K.M.; Manigaba, K.; Shoulders, B.R.; Felton, T.W.; Mathew, S.K.; Peloquin, C.A. Beta-Lactam Target Attainment and Associated Outcomes in Patients with Bloodstream Infections. *Int. J. Antimicrob. Agents* **2023**, *61*, 106727. [CrossRef] [PubMed]
14. Hoste, E.A.J.; Lameire, N.H.; Vanholder, R.C.; Benoit, D.D.; Decruyenaere, J.M.A.; Colardyn, F.A. Acute Renal Failure in Patients with Sepsis in a Surgical ICU: Predictive Factors, Incidence, Comorbidity, and Outcome. *J. Am. Soc. Nephrol.* **2003**, *14*, 1022–1030. [CrossRef] [PubMed]
15. Uchino, S.; Kellum, J.A.; Bellomo, R.; Doig, G.S.; Morimatsu, H.; Morgera, S.; Schetz, M.; Tan, I.; Bouman, C.; Macedo, E.; et al. Acute Renal Failure in Critically Ill Patients: A Multinational, Multicenter Study. *JAMA* **2005**, *294*, 813–818. [CrossRef] [PubMed]
16. Gatti, M.; Pea, F. Antimicrobial Dose Reduction in Continuous Renal Replacement Therapy: Myth or Real Need? A Practical Approach for Guiding Dose Optimization of Novel Antibiotics. *Clin. Pharmacokinet* **2021**, *60*, 1271–1289. [CrossRef]
17. Hoff, B.M.; Maker, J.H.; Dager, W.E.; Heintz, B.H. Antibiotic Dosing for Critically Ill Adult Patients Receiving Intermittent Hemodialysis, Prolonged Intermittent Renal Replacement Therapy, and Continuous Renal Replacement Therapy: An Update. *Ann. Pharmacother* **2020**, *54*, 43–55. [CrossRef]
18. Li, L.; Li, X.; Xia, Y.; Chu, Y.; Zhong, H.; Li, J.; Liang, P.; Bu, Y.; Zhao, R.; Liao, Y.; et al. Recommendation of Antimicrobial Dosing Optimization During Continuous Renal Replacement Therapy. *Front. Pharmacol.* **2020**, *11*, 786. [CrossRef]
19. Gatti, M.; Cojutti, P.G.; Bartoletti, M.; Tonetti, T.; Bianchini, A.; Ramirez, S.; Pizzilli, G.; Ambretti, S.; Giannella, M.; Mancini, R.; et al. Expert Clinical Pharmacological Advice May Make an Antimicrobial TDM Program for Emerging Candidates More Clinically Useful in Tailoring Therapy of Critically Ill Patients. *Crit. Care* **2022**, *26*, 178. [CrossRef]
20. Peng, Y.; Cheng, Z.; Xie, F. Population Pharmacokinetic Meta-Analysis and Dosing Recommendation for Meropenem in Critically Ill Patients Receiving Continuous Renal Replacement Therapy. *Antimicrob. Agents Chemother.* **2022**, *66*, e0082222. [CrossRef] [PubMed]
21. Moon, Y.S.; Chung, K.C.; Gill, M.A. Pharmacokinetics of Meropenem in Animals, Healthy Volunteers, and Patients. *Clin. Infect. Dis.* **1997**, *24* (Suppl. 2), S249–S255. [CrossRef] [PubMed]
22. Petersson, J.; Giske, C.G.; Eliasson, E. Poor Correlation between Meropenem and Piperacillin Plasma Concentrations and Delivered Dose of Continuous Renal Replacement Therapy. *Antimicrob. Agents Chemother.* **2021**, *65*, e02029-20. [CrossRef] [PubMed]

23. Jamal, J.-A.; Udy, A.A.; Lipman, J.; Roberts, J.A. The Impact of Variation in Renal Replacement Therapy Settings on Piperacillin, Meropenem, and Vancomycin Drug Clearance in the Critically Ill: An Analysis of Published Literature and Dosing Regimens*. *Crit. Care Med.* **2014**, *42*, 1640–1650. [CrossRef]
24. Roberts, D.M.; Liu, X.; Roberts, J.A.; Nair, P.; Cole, L.; Roberts, M.S.; Lipman, J.; Bellomo, R. RENAL Replacement Therapy Study Investigators A Multicenter Study on the Effect of Continuous Hemodiafiltration Intensity on Antibiotic Pharmacokinetics. *Crit. Care* **2015**, *19*, 84. [CrossRef]
25. Roberts, J.A.; Joynt, G.; Lee, A.; Choi, G.; Bellomo, R.; Kanji, S.; Mudaliar, M.Y.; Peake, S.L.; Stephens, D.; Taccone, F.S.; et al. The Effect of Renal Replacement Therapy and Antibiotic Dose on Antibiotic Concentrations in Critically Ill Patients: Data from the Multinational SMARRT Study. *Clin. Infect. Dis.* **2020**, *72*, 1369–1378. [CrossRef]
26. Valtonen, M.; Tiula, E.; Backman, J.T.; Neuvonen, P.J. Elimination of Meropenem during Continuous Veno-Venous Haemofiltration and Haemodiafiltration in Patients with Acute Renal Failure. *J. Antimicrob. Chemother.* **2000**, *45*, 701–704. [CrossRef] [PubMed]
27. Ulldemolins, M.; Soy, D.; Llaurado-Serra, M.; Vaquer, S.; Castro, P.; Rodríguez, A.H.; Pontes, C.; Calvo, G.; Torres, A.; Martín-Loeches, I. Meropenem Population Pharmacokinetics in Critically Ill Patients with Septic Shock and Continuous Renal Replacement Therapy: Influence of Residual Diuresis on Dose Requirements. *Antimicrob. Agents Chemother.* **2015**, *59*, 5520–5528. [CrossRef] [PubMed]
28. Sangla, F.; Marti, P.E.; Verissimo, T.; Pugin, J.; de Seigneux, S.; Legouis, D. Measured and Estimated Glomerular Filtration Rate in the ICU: A Prospective Study. *Crit. Care Med.* **2020**, *48*, e1232–e1241. [CrossRef]
29. Gatti, M.; Pea, F. Continuous versus Intermittent Infusion of Antibiotics in Gram-Negative Multidrug-Resistant Infections. *Curr. Opin. Infect. Dis.* **2021**, *34*, 737–747. [CrossRef] [PubMed]
30. Roberts, J.A.; Croom, K.; Adomakoh, N. Continuous Infusion of Beta-Lactam Antibiotics: Narrative Review of Systematic Reviews, and Implications for Outpatient Parenteral Antibiotic Therapy. *Expert Rev. Anti Infect. Ther.* **2023**, *21*, 375–385. [CrossRef] [PubMed]
31. Roger, C.; Louart, B. Beta-Lactams Toxicity in the Intensive Care Unit: An Underestimated Collateral Damage? *Microorganisms* **2021**, *9*, 1505. [CrossRef]
32. Vardakas, K.Z.; Kalimeris, G.D.; Triarides, N.A.; Falagas, M.E. An Update on Adverse Drug Reactions Related to β-Lactam Antibiotics. *Expert Opin. Drug Saf.* **2018**, *17*, 499–508. [CrossRef] [PubMed]
33. Gatti, M.; Rinaldi, M.; Gaibani, P.; Siniscalchi, A.; Tonetti, T.; Giannella, M.; Viale, P.; Pea, F. A Descriptive Pharmacokinetic/Pharmacodynamic Analysis of Continuous Infusion Ceftazidime-Avibactam for Treating DTR Gram-Negative Infections in a Case Series of Critically Ill Patients Undergoing Continuous Veno-Venous Haemodiafiltration (CVVHDF). *J. Crit. Care* **2023**, *76*, 154301. [CrossRef] [PubMed]
34. Horan, T.C.; Andrus, M.; Dudeck, M.A. CDC/NHSN Surveillance Definition of Health Care-Associated Infection and Criteria for Specific Types of Infections in the Acute Care Setting. *Am. J. Infect. Control* **2008**, *36*, 309–332. [CrossRef] [PubMed]
35. Chastre, J.; Fagon, J.-Y. Ventilator-Associated Pneumonia. *Am. J. Respir. Crit. Care Med.* **2002**, *165*, 867–903. [CrossRef]
36. Miller, J.M.; Binnicker, M.J.; Campbell, S.; Carroll, K.C.; Chapin, K.C.; Gilligan, P.H.; Gonzalez, M.D.; Jerris, R.C.; Kehl, S.C.; Patel, R.; et al. A Guide to Utilization of the Microbiology Laboratory for Diagnosis of Infectious Diseases: 2018 Update by the Infectious Diseases Society of America and the American Society for Microbiology. *Clin. Infect. Dis.* **2018**, *67*, e1–e94. [CrossRef] [PubMed]
37. Silva-Nunes, J.; Cardoso, T. Intra-Abdominal Infections: The Role of Different Classifications on the Selection of the Best Antibiotic Treatment. *BMC Infect. Dis.* **2019**, *19*, 980. [CrossRef]
38. EUCAST—European Committee on Antimicrobial Susceptibility Testing. *European Committee on Antimicrobial Susceptibility Testing Breakpoint Tables for Interpretation of MICs and Zone Diameters Version 12.0, Valid from 2022-01-01*; EUCAST: Basel, Switzerland, 2022.
39. Carlier, M.; Stove, V.; Verstraete, A.G.; De Waele, J.J. Stability of Generic Brands of Meropenem Reconstituted in Isotonic Saline. *Minerva Anestesiol.* **2015**, *81*, 283–287.
40. Fawaz, S.; Barton, S.; Whitney, L.; Swinden, J.; Nabhani-Gebara, S. Stability of Meropenem After Reconstitution for Administration by Prolonged Infusion. *Hosp. Pharm.* **2019**, *54*, 190–196. [CrossRef]
41. Craig, W.A. The Pharmacology of Meropenem, a New Carbapenem Antibiotic. *Clin. Infect. Dis.* **1997**, *24* (Suppl. 2), S266–S275. [CrossRef]
42. Sanz Codina, M.; Gatti, M.; Troisi, C.; Fornaro, G.; Pasquini, Z.; Trapani, F.; Zanoni, A.; Caramelli, F.; Viale, P.; Pea, F. Relationship between Pharmacokinetic/Pharmacodynamic Target Attainment and Microbiological Outcome in Critically Ill COVID-19 Patients with Documented Gram-Negative Superinfections Treated with TDM-Guided Continuous-Infusion Meropenem. *Pharmaceutics* **2022**, *14*, 1585. [CrossRef] [PubMed]
43. Tam, V.H.; Chang, K.-T.; Zhou, J.; Ledesma, K.R.; Phe, K.; Gao, S.; Van Bambeke, F.; Sánchez-Díaz, A.M.; Zamorano, L.; Oliver, A.; et al. Determining β-Lactam Exposure Threshold to Suppress Resistance Development in Gram-Negative Bacteria. *J. Antimicrob. Chemother.* **2017**, *72*, 1421–1428. [CrossRef] [PubMed]

antibiotics

MDPI

Systematic Review

Cefiderocol Versus Best Available Therapy in the Treatment of Critically Ill Patients with Severe Infections Due to Resistant Gram-Negative Bacteria: A Systematic Review and Meta-Analysis

Carlos Risco-Risco [1,*], César Henriquez-Camacho [2,3], Marta Herrera-Rueda [2], José Barberán [4,5] and David Andaluz-Ojeda [6,7,8,*]

1 Internal Medicine Department, University Hospital HM Sanchinarro, HM Hospitales, 28015 Madrid, Spain
2 Internal Medicine Department, Móstoles University Hospital, 28935 Madrid, Spain; cesaraugusto.henriquez@salud.madrid.org (C.H.-C.)
3 Faculty of Medicine, Francisco de Vitoria University, 28223 Madrid, Spain
4 Internal Medicine Department, University Hospital HM Monteprincipe, HM Hospitales, Boadilla del Monte, 28660 Madrid, Spain
5 HM Faculty of Health Sciences, Camilo Jose Cela University, 28692 Madrid, Spain
6 Intensive Care Department, Palencia University Hospital Complex, 34004 Palencia, Spain
7 Critical Care Area, University Hospital HM Sanchinarro, HM Hospitales, 28015 Madrid, Spain
8 Group of Biomedical Research on Critical Care (BioCritic), Valladolid University, 47003 Valladolid, Spain
* Correspondence: carlosriscorisco@yahoo.es (C.R.-R.); davidandaluz78@yahoo.es (D.A.-O.)

Abstract: Background: This study aims to assess the effectiveness and safety of cefiderocol in treating severe infections caused by multidrug-resistant Gram-negative bacteria (MDR-GNB) in critically ill patients, particularly those in intensive care units (ICUs). Methods: A meta-analysis of studies, including randomized clinical trials and observational studies in adult patients, was performed. Studies with at least 50% of critically ill patients were included. Studies with small sample size or without comparison groups were excluded. Sources included PubMed, Scopus, or Google Scholar, up to 14 August 2024. Risk of bias was assessed according to the Cochrane tool. The main outcome examined was 30-day mortality, while secondary outcomes assessed included clinical cure rates and adverse effects. Results were expressed with odds ratios. No funding was received for this study. It was registered in the International Prospective Register of Systematic Reviews (PROSPERO) with reference CRD42024563041. Results: eight studies, with 1339 patients were included in the meta-analysis. Cefiderocol treatment was associated with a lower 30-day mortality rate than other available therapies (pooled OR 0.47; 95% CI: 0.23–0.97, $p = 0.04$), particularly in cases of carbapenem-resistant *A. baumannii* infections (pooled OR 0.29; 95% CI: 0.14–0.60, $p < 0.001$). Although there was a non-significant trend toward higher clinical cure rates in the cefiderocol group (OR 1.59; 95% CI: 0.96–2.62, $p = 0.07$), the drug demonstrated at least non-inferiority when compared to other treatment options. Study limitations included moderate heterogeneity between studies, and a high risk of bias in non-RCT studies. (Five cohort studies were included). Another limitation is that five of the eight studies compared cefiderocol versus colistine, an antibiotic with known toxicity. Conclusions: The findings suggest that cefiderocol is a promising therapeutic option for managing severe MDR-GNB infections in critically ill patients, offering a potential global benefit on mortality and at least non-inferiority in the cure rate when compared with other therapies.

Keywords: severe infections; cefiderocol; *Acinetobacter baumannii*; critically ill; ICU; MDR; Gram-negative bacteria

1. Introduction

The rise of multidrug-resistant (MDR) Gram-negative bacteria (GNB) stands as a significant global health challenge in the 21st century, making the treatment of infections caused by these microorganisms more difficult [1]. These microorganisms are difficult to treat because of their ability to develop resistance to multiple classes of antibiotics [2,3]. Non-fermenting Gram-negative bacteria, such as *Acinetobacter baumannii* and *Pseudomonas aeruginosa*, and carbapenem-resistant *Enterobacteriaceae* (CRE) are among the most concerning MDR pathogens due to their association with elevated rates of morbidity and mortality among hospitalized patients, especially those in intensive care unit (ICU) settings [4]. Among these pathogens, *Acinetobacter* has emerged as a particularly formidable foe because of its resistance to multiple antibiotics, including carbapenems. Recent research has revealed that carbapenem-resistant *A. baumannii* (CRAB) rates reach or exceed 50% in 21 countries across Southern and Eastern Europe [5]. When these microorganisms cause infections in more severe patients, such as those in the ICU setting, the problem is severely exacerbated because limited therapeutic options lead to high morbidity and mortality rates. Cefiderocol, a siderophore cephalosporin, has garnered attention because of its unique mechanism of action and potent activity against a wide range of MDR-GNB, including carbapenem-resistant strains [6].

Cefiderocol operates via a unique mechanism that distinguishes it from the other antibiotics. As a siderophore cephalosporin, in addition to passive diffusion through porin-mediated channels, it exploits the bacterial iron uptake system to penetrate bacterial cells, which allows high concentrations of the drug to be delivered to the site of cephalosporin action [2]. This mechanism not only enhances its uptake but also circumvents many traditional resistance mechanisms (porin deficiency, upregulation of efflux pump expression, and production of β-lactamases, including carbapenemases) employed by Gram-negative bacteria that limit the efficacy of other antibiotics. Its spectrum of activity encompasses a variety of problematic pathogens, MDR-GNB, such as *Pseudomonas aeruginosa, Acinetobacter baumannii, Stenotrophomonas maltophilia, and Enterobacterales*, which are commonly associated with nosocomial infections in ICU settings.

Several studies have demonstrated the clinical efficacy of cefiderocol against a variety of MDR-GNB [7–9]. However, most pivotal trials of cefiderocol have focused on patients with moderate or non-severe infections. Most studies on cefiderocol in ICU settings are limited to case series and a few retrospective cohort studies, making it difficult to draw robust conclusions regarding drug outcomes in this scenario [4,10]. Critically ill patients present different characteristics than other patients, which can alter the pharmacokinetics/pharmacodynamics (pK/pD) of many antibiotics. Situations, such as immunosuppression, increased volume of distribution, hypoalbuminemia, renal failure, and organ support measures, including continuous renal replacement therapy and extracorporeal membrane oxygenation, are frequently used in critically ill patients and may lead to both interpatient and intrapatient variabilities in drug pharmacokinetics, which can significantly alter antibiotic concentrations, thereby affecting their effectiveness [11,12]. This highlights the need for a further investigation into cefiderocol efficacy in the ICU setting. This meta-analysis aimed to systematically review and analyze the existing literature on the effectiveness and safety of cefiderocol in treating severe infections, paying special attention to critically ill patients. By consolidating data from various studies, we seek to provide a robust assessment of the role of cefiderocol in managing these challenging infections, thereby aiding clinicians in making evidence-based decisions.

2. Results

We screened 1590 original works, of which 1325 articles were excluded after reviewing the titles and abstracts; 265 papers were obtained for full-text review. Following the exclusion of 257 papers that did not meet the inclusion criteria, eight studies were ultimately included in the analysis [13–20]. The process of article selection is illustrated in Figure 1.

Three studies were multicenter RCTs [13–15], four were single-center retrospective cohort studies [16,17,19,20], and the remaining study corresponded to a single-center prospective cohort [18]. The sample sizes varied between 73 and 371 patients, amounting to a total of 1339 participants. Five of the studies were carried out in Italy [16–20], while the others were multinational, involving centers from the US, Europe, and Asia [13–15].

Lower respiratory tract infections were the most frequently reported, with five studies including cases of ventilator-associated pneumonia (VAP) or hospital-acquired pneumonia (HAP) [15,18–20]. One study included bloodstream infections [17], another included complicated UTI or acute pyelonephritis [13], and the rest of the studies included different types of severe infections in ICU settings. It is worth noting that most studies (5/8) included selectively severe CRAB infections, regardless of the infection site [16–20]. A total of 702 patients were treated with cefiderocol, whereas 637 received other therapies. Cefiderocol was compared with colistin-containing regimens in four studies [16–19] all on severe CRAB infections. In two studies, cefiderocol was compared with carbapenems [13,15], and in the other two studies [14,20], with best available therapy (BAT).

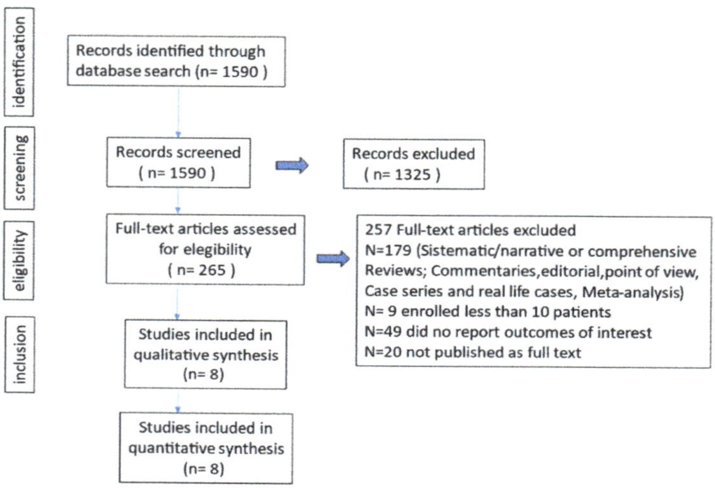

Figure 1. PRISMA flow diagram of the process of identification and selection of articles included in the meta-analysis.

With respect to the outcomes assessed, 30-day mortality was examined in seven studies, with the exception of one [13]. Tables 1 and 2 present the description of the studies, together with the overall 30-day mortality rate for the entire population studied, encompassing all treatment protocols, while in four studies the clinical cure rate was compared [13–15,18].

Table 1. General Information of Studies and Populations. RCT: Randomized clinical trials, BAT: Best available therapy, PI: Principal investigator, ICU: Intensive care unit, HAP: Hospital acquired pneumonia; HCAP: Health care-associated pneumonia, VAP: Ventilator associated pneumonia CRAB: Carbapenem resistant *Acinetobacter baumannii*; UTI: Urinary tract infection; BSI: Blood stream infections.

Reference	Settings	Study Period (Follow-Up)	Study Design	N. Patients	Median Age (Years)	Male (%)
Portsmouth 2018 [13]	International (PI: USA)	Feb 2015–Aug 2016 (14 days)	RCT multicenter (67 centers) double blind	371	Cefiderocol:62.3 Imipenem-Cilastatin: 61.3	Cefiderocol:47 Imipenem-Cilastatin:48
Basetti 2020 [14]	International (PI: Italy)	Sep 2016–Apr 2019 (14 days)	RCT multicenter (95 centres) open label	150	Cefiderocol:63.1 BAT:63	Cefiderocol:65 BAT:29
Wunderink 2021 [15]	International (PI: USA)	Oct 2017–Apr 2019 (14–21 days)	RCT multicenter (17 centers) double blind	291	Cefiderocol:64.6 Meropenem:65.4	Cefiderocol:68 Meropenem:69
Falcone 2022 [16]	Italy	Jan 2020–Aug 2021 (30 days)	Single-center retrospective cohort	124	Cefiderocol:63 Colistin:68	Cefiderocol:61.7 Colistin:81.8

Table 1. *Cont.*

Reference	Settings	Study Period (Follow-Up)	Study Design	N. Patients	Median Age (Years)	Male (%)
Bavaro 2023 [17]	Italy	Jan 2020–Dec 2022 (90 days)	Single-center retrospective cohort	118	Cefiderocol:69 Colistin:71	Cefiderocol:60 Colistin:59
Dalfino 2023 [18]	Italy	Mar 2021–Dec 2022 (28 days)	Single-center prospective	90	Cefiderocol:67 Non-Cefiderocol: 64	Cefiderocol:86 Colistin:38
Russo 2023 [19]	Italy	Mar 2020–Aug 2022 (30 days)	Single-center retrospective cohort adjusted by propensity score	73	Cefidercol:67 Colistin:60	Cefiderocol:26.3 Colistin regimen:24
Rando 2023 [20]	Italy	Sep 2020–Dec 2022 (28 days)	Single-center retrospective cohort	121	Cefiderocol:64 BAT:68	Cefiderocol: 76 BAT:77

Table 2. Treatments, Type of Infection, and Clinical Outcomes. BAT: Best available therapy, PI: Principal investigator, ICU: Intensive care unit, HAP: Hospital acquired pneumonia; HCAP: Health care-associated pneumonia, VAP: Ventilator associated pneumonia CRAB: Carbapenem resistant *Acinetobacter baumannii*; UTI: Urinary tract infection; BSI: Blood stream infection.

Reference	Type of Infection	Treatments	Mortality (%)	Cure Rate (%)
Portsmouth 2018 [13]	Complicated UTI or acute pyelonephritis	Cefiderocol vs. Imipenem-Cilastatin	Not reported	Cefiderocol:72.6% Imipenem: 54.6%
Basetti 2020 [14]	HAP, VAP, HCAP, BSI, or complicated UTI (carbapenem-resistant GNB)	Cefiderocol vs. Best Available Therapy (BAT)	Cefiderocol: 34% BAT: 18%	Cefiderocol:52.5%, BAT: 44.9%
Wunderink 2021 [15]	VAP, HAP, or HCAP (Gram-negative)	Cefiderocol vs. Meropenem	Cefiderocol: 21%, Meropenem: 20%	Cefiderocol: 64.8% Meropenem: 66.6%
Falcone 2022 [17]	Severe CRAB infections	Cefiderocol vs. Colistin	Cefiderocol: 34%, Colistin: 55%	Not reported
Bavaro 2023 [17]	BSI caused by CRAB	Cefiderocol vs. Colistin	Cefiderocol: 40%, Colistin: 59%	Not reported
Dalfino 2023 [18]	VAP due to CRAB	Cefiderocol + inhaled colistin vs. Colistin	Cefiderocol: 35% Colistin: 52%	Cefiderocol: 75% Colistin: 52%
Russo 2023 [19]	VAP and BSI in COVID-19 ICU patients	Cefiderocol vs. Colistin	Cefiderocol: 32% Colistin: 98%	Not reported
Rando 2023 [20]	CRAB-VAP in critically ill COVID patients	Cefiderocol vs. BAT	Cefiderocol: 44% BAT: 67%	Not reported

2.1. Quality Appraisal of Studies Included in the Analysis

The three RCTs that included all but one were judged to have a low risk of bias for at least three domains, while the remaining study (Basetti, 2020 only provided information in the text to evaluate one domain (performing bias). Five observational studies, including a comparator group, were judged to have a high risk of bias according to the Newcastle–Ottawa scale. Finally, among the eight studies, six were deemed to have a high risk of bias, one had an intermediate risk [13], and only Wunderink et al. [15] showed a low risk of bias. The quality assessment of the included studies is shown in Figure 2.

Publication bias was explored using a sensible test (Egger) combined with a specific test (Peters). Both tests showed no evidence for publication bias: Egger test $p = 0.658$, Peters test $p = 0.385$.

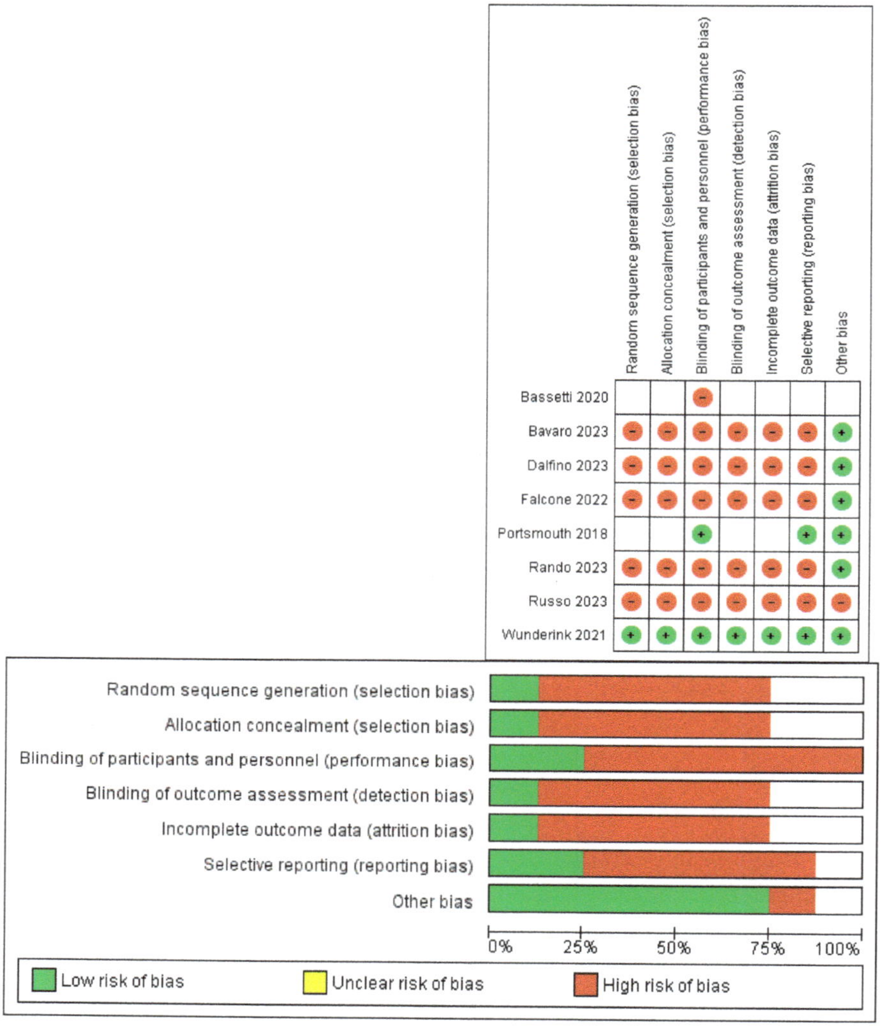

Figure 2. Risk of bias summary and bias graph.

2.2. Meta-Analysis of Studies Evaluating Mortality

When we compared cefiderocol monotherapy versus other therapies among the seven studies that analyzed mortality [14–20], we observed a 28-day mortality rate of 31% among 702 patients receiving cefiderocol versus 48.2% among the 637 patients treated with other therapeutic regimens ($p < 0.001$). In the random effects model, the cumulative OR was 0.47(95% CI: 0.23–0.97, $p = 0.04$), in favor of cefiderocol.

Moderate heterogeneity was detected between the studies ($I^2 = 48.25\%$, $p = 0.07$). These findings were more robust in a sub-analysis of studies that enrolled only patients with CRAB infections [16–20]. In this scenario, we observed a significantly lower cumulative OR for a 30 day-mortality rate among the 204 patients receiving cefiderocol compared to 277 patients treated with BAT (OR 0.29; 95% CI: 0.14–0.60; $p < 0.001$) (Figure 3b). Moderate heterogeneity was observed between the groups ($I^2 = 51\%$, $p = 0.08$).

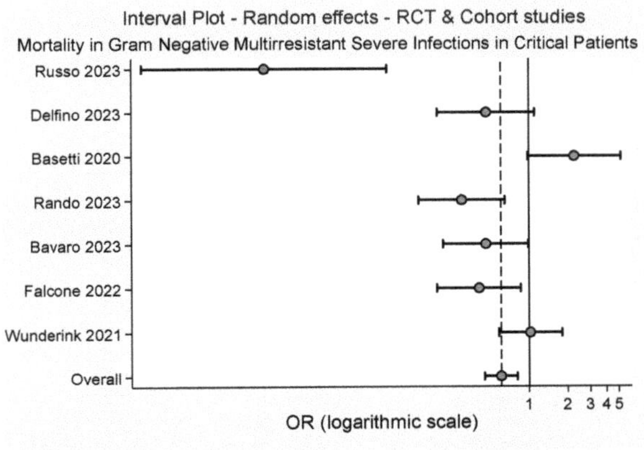

Study	OR	95% Conf.Interval		IoV Weighted OR	I^2
Russo 2023	0.009	0.001	0.08		
Delfino 2023	0.46	0.19	1.11		
Basetti 2020	2.26	0.98	5.19		
Rando 2023	0.29	0.14	0.65	**0.47 (0.23-0.97)**	48.25%
Bavaro 2023	0.46	0.21	0.99		
Falcone 2022	0.41	0.19	0.87		
Wunderink 2021	1.03	0.58	1.81		
Global	**0.48**	**0.37**	**0.63**		
			p	**0.04**	**0.07**

(**a**) Overall population

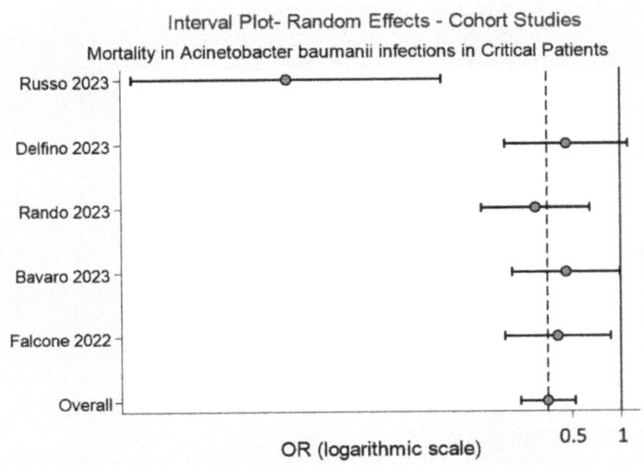

Study	OR	95% Conf.Interval		IoV Weighted OR	I^2
Russo 2023	**0.009**	**0.001**	**0.08**		
Delfino 2023	0.46	0.19	1.11		
Rando 2023	0.29	0.14	0.65	**0.29 (0.15-0.60)**	**57.75%**
Bavaro 2023	0.46	0.21	0.99		
Falcone 2022	0.41	0.19	0.87		
Global	**0.30**	**0.21**	**0.44**		
			p	**<0.001**	**0.08**

(**b**) CRAB infection population

Figure 3. *Cont.*

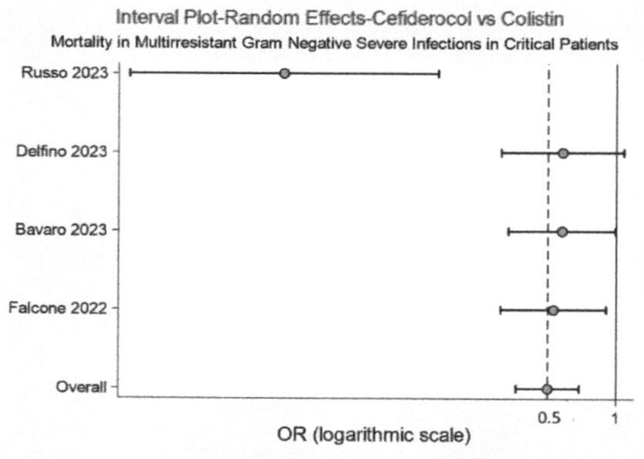

Study	OR	95% Conf.Interval		IoV Weighted OR	I^2
Falcone 2022	0.41	0.19	0.87	0.27 (0.10-0.81)	57.22
Bavaro 2023	0.46	0.21	0.99		
Russo 2023	0.09	0.001	0.08		
Delfino 2023	0.46	0.19	1.11		
Global	**0.29**	**0.19**	**0.45**		
			p	0.008	0.07

(**c**) Cefiderocol vs. Colistin based therapies

Figure 3. Meta-analysis of studies evaluating the 30-day mortality rate in patients treated with cefiderocol.

Four out of seven studies reported mortality using colistin as a comparator. We performed a sub-analysis comparing cefiderocol- and colistin-based therapies and found a cumulative OR for 30-day mortality of 0.27 (95% CI: 0.19–0.81, $p = 0.008$), with moderate heterogeneity between studies ($I^2 = 57\%$, $p = 0.07$) (Figure 3c).

2.3. *Meta-Analysis of Studies Evaluating Microbiological Failure and Clinical Cure*

Only four of the eight studies [13–15,18] included in this meta-analysis (three RCTs and one cohort study) described the composite of clinical and microbiological outcomes at the test of cure (i.e., 7 days after treatment cessation) as the primary or secondary endpoint, which was used to establish the non-inferiority of cefiderocol versus the other available therapies. Considering these four studies globally, the meta-analysis of the cure rate showed a percentage of cure in the cefiderocol group of 66.91% versus 57.81% in the BAT group ($p = 0.005$). On the random effects model, the cumulative OR of cure was 1.59 (95% CI: 0.96–2.62, p-value = 0.07), in favor of cefiderocol with low heterogeneity between the studies [$I^2 = 2.77\%$, $p = 0.44$] (Figure 4a).

The superiority of cefiderocol was not evidenced in the sub-analysis, which included only patients enrolled in the three RCTs (lower risk of bias). In this case, the cumulative OR was 1.41 (95% CI: 0.81–2.47, p-value = 0.23) without showing significant differences in the rates of cure between both groups, and with low heterogeneity between the studies ($I^2 = 0.0$, $p = 0.43$) (Figure 4b).

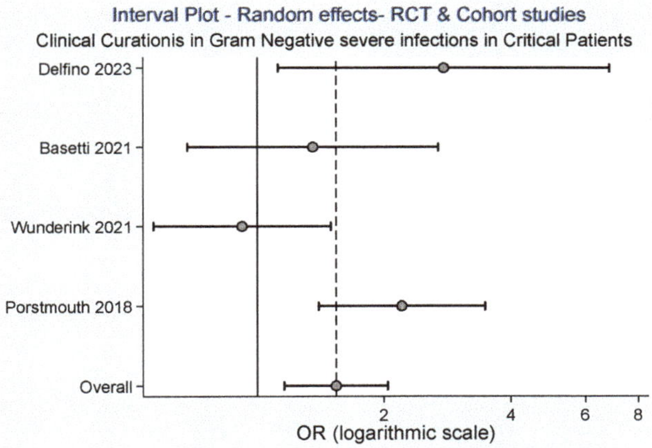

Study	OR	95% Conf.Interval		IoV Weighted OR	Chi Square Homogeneity
Delfino 2023	2.77	1.12	6.84	1.59 (0.96-2.62)	2.7
Basetti 2021	1.36	0.68	2.69		
Wunderink 2021	0.92	0.57	1.49		
Portsmouth 2018	2.2	1.89	3.47		
Global	**1.47**	**1.12**	**1.94**		
			p	0.07	0.44

(**a**) Overall population

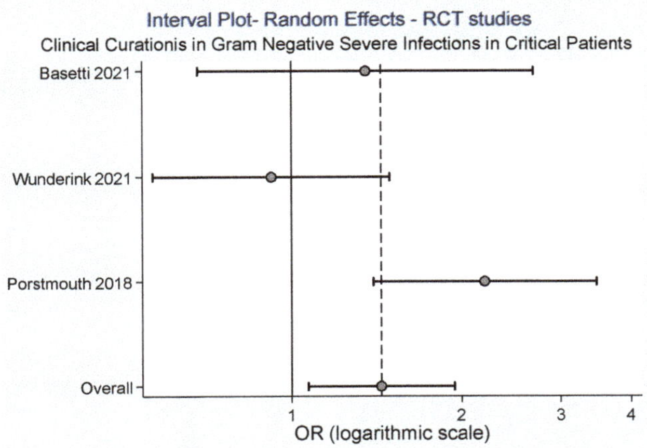

Study	OR	95% Conf.Interval		IoV Weighted OR	I^2
Basetti 2021	1.36	0.68	2.69	1.41 (0.81-2.47)	0.00
Wunderink 2021	0.92	0.57	1.49		
Portsmouth 2018	2.2	1.39	3.47		
Global	**1.38**	**1.03**	**1.85**		
			p	0.23	0.43

(**b**) RCTs population

Figure 4. Meta-analysis of studies evaluating the curation rate in patients treated with cefiderocol vs. best available therapy.

3. Discussion

The findings from this meta-analysis indicate that patients receiving cefiderocol for severe MDR-GNB infections experience more favorable clinical outcomes compared to those treated with best available therapy (BAT). Our results show a notably reduced 30-day mortality rate in the cefiderocol group and a non-significant trend towards a higher clinical cure rate in this group, with at least non-inferiority compared to the other treatments. Among the eight studies included in this systematic review, only three were RCTs, and five were observational studies. The risk of bias was considered high in all studies except for two of the three RCTs [13,14].

The overall mortality results of our meta-analysis were favorable for cefiderocol. We found a significantly favorable effect, with greater survival in the cefiderocol group, regardless of the pathogen type or site of infection. The lower mortality in the cefiderocol group was consistent both in the overall population and in studies that included only severe CRAB infections. However, neither of the two RCTs [14,15] that evaluated 30-day mortality showed a benefit in favor of cefiderocol. The CREDIBLE-CR study [15] was a phase 3, multicenter trial focused on the efficacy and safety of cefiderocol for treating severe carbapenem-resistant Gram-negative infections. It demonstrated that cefiderocol had clinical and microbiological effectiveness comparable to that of best available therapy (BAT). However, in cases involving *Acinetobacter* spp. infections, the study found a higher overall mortality rate with cefiderocol compared to BAT (49% vs. 18%, respectively), particularly among patients with pneumonia, bloodstream infections, or severe sepsis due to CRAB. This disparity might be attributed to an uneven distribution of patients, as those on cefiderocol had a higher incidence of septic shock (26% vs. 6% in the BAT group) and longer ICU stays at the time of randomization (81% vs. 47%), indicating a greater baseline risk for mortality. Another randomized controlled trial, the APEKS-NP study [14], was a multicenter, double-blind, parallel-group phase 3 trial involving adult patients with hospital-acquired or ventilator-associated Gram-negative pneumonia. Participants were randomly assigned to receive either 3-hour intravenous infusions of cefiderocol (2 g) or meropenem (2 g) every 8 h for 7–14 days. This study concluded that cefiderocol was non-inferior to meropenem, with mortality rates of 12.4% and 11.6%, respectively.

Thus, the overall mortality results in favor of cefiderocol in our meta-analysis can be attributed to the remaining studies included. Although these were all observational studies, most of them had a retrospective design, and all found a lower mortality rate in the cefiderocol group than in the control group. It is important to emphasize that most of these studies were conducted entirely in ICU settings [16,18–20] and mainly included patients with a diagnosis of VAP due to CRAB. However, none of the RCTs analyzed in this meta-analysis exclusively included critically ill patients. In fact, Bassetti et al. [14] and Wunderink et al. [15] included 52% and 68% of critically ill patients at randomization, respectively, which likely suggests a lower or overall disease severity in these studies and therefore a better prognosis than those included in the aforementioned observational studies. Another circumstance that may influence our results is that in most of the observational studies included in this meta-analysis, the control arm used therapeutic regimens based on colistin as BAT. This drug has known harmful side effects and an unfavorable PK/PD profile, which could impact clinical outcomes. Nevertheless, a significant body of recent preclinical data from in vitro and in vivo studies indicates a potential clinical benefit of polymyxin-based treatments, either as monotherapy or in combination. These therapies have demonstrated synergistic activity against extensively drug-resistant (XDR) and difficult-to-treat resistant (DTR) strains of *P. aeruginosa, Klebsiella pneumoniae, and A. baumannii,* supporting their use in such cases. [21,22].

Regarding clinical cure, our meta-analysis showed a trend towards a higher cure rate (not statistically significant) in the cefiderocol group; however, this trend was not observed when considering only the RCTs, although cefiderocol still demonstrated non-inferiority in this outcome compared to BAT. Only four of the eight studies [13–15,18] included in the meta-analysis reported cure rates, which significantly limits the observation of this finding.

Of the four aforementioned studies, two (Basetti et al. and Wunderink et al.) [14,15] did not find any difference in the cure rate in favor of cefiderocol. The previously mentioned limitations in these two trial studies, particularly those in the CREDIBLE-CR study [15], may also significantly influence the findings at this endpoint. Recent in vitro studies and real-world case series have shown a high rate of microbiological eradication and clinical cure when using cefiderocol to treat MDR-GNB in the ICU setting. In a recent study by Fendian et al., involving a cohort of critically ill patients with severe infections caused by MDR- or XDR-GNB, clinical cure was achieved in 90% of patients, while microbiological cure was seen in 80% [4]. Other studies have reported similar results [10,23]. Recent narrative reviews and expert commentaries have analyzed preclinical data, case series, and specific real-life scenarios in the ICU setting, such as continuous renal replacement therapy, ECMO, and immunosuppression, suggesting a benefit of cefiderocol over other treatments [24–29].

Notably, the findings of this meta-analysis align with the data recently reported by the authors of the PERSEUS study [30]. This retrospective, multicenter observational study was designed to evaluate the efficacy and safety of cefiderocol in real-world settings for adult patients with GNB infections. It included 261 critically ill adult patients with limited treatment options, all of whom received cefiderocol for ≥72 h for confirmed GNB infections. Of these patients, 64.8% were resistant to all tested antibiotics, and 44.4% had failed prior antibiotic treatments. The cohort was severely ill, with 63.2% in the ICU, 47.1% on mechanical ventilation, and 28% suffering from septic shock. The study found that patients treated with cefiderocol achieved an overall clinical success rate (defined as a combination of clinical cure and/or survival at day 28) of 84.3%, with a 28-day all-cause mortality rate of 21.5% [30]. The majority of patients had respiratory tract infections (47.9%) primarily caused by pathogens such as *Pseudomonas aeruginosa* (66.7%), *Klebsiella pneumoniae* (10.0%), and *Stenotrophomonas maltophilia* (7.7%).

These findings, including those concerning mortality and clinical cure, are in line with the results of our study. As far as we know, no other meta-analysis has specifically explored the role of cefiderocol in critically ill patients with MDR-GNB infections. Hsueh et al. [31] conducted a meta-analysis that included one phase 2 and two phase 3 trials, with the primary outcome focused on clinical response at the test of cure. Cefiderocol achieved clinical and microbiological responses comparable to those of the comparator agents. However, this work did not specifically focus on infections caused by MDR-GNB or on critically ill patients. In two recent meta-analyses, Onorato et al. [32] and Gatti et al. [8] analyzed cefiderocol-based regimens versus BAT in the treatment of CRAB infections. None of the studies focused on critically ill patients, but similar to our findings, they observed a significantly lower mortality rate [RR: 0.74 (95% CI: 0.57–0.95) and OR: 0.53 (95% CI: 0.39–0.71)] in the groups treated with cefiderocol compared to BAT. No differences were observed in the rates of microbiological and clinical failure.

Despite this, our meta-analysis has several limitations that should prompt cautious interpretation of our findings. Few high-quality studies have analyzed the role of cefiderocol in critically ill patients. Limited evidence is available on cohort studies with a high risk of bias. Many of these studies are limited to CRAB infections, and only a few address infections caused by other MDR-GNB, such as *Enterobacteriaceae* or other non-fermenting GNB. Additionally, in many cases, the comparator is colistin, and no studies have compared cefiderocol with newer antibiotics, including beta-lactamase inhibitors.

Under these circumstances, our conclusions should not be generalized because of the lack of additional trials to address these gaps. It is also necessary to investigate this drug further in a specific population of critically ill patients. However, based on our findings and recent evidence, cefiderocol has proven to be safe and effective, presenting a promising and viable option for treating MDR Gram-negative infections in the ICU setting.

4. Material and Methods

4.1. Search Strategy and Selection Criteria

We performed a systematic review and meta-analysis, including randomized controlled trials (RCTs) and observational cohort studies, comparing the mortality rate and other clinical outcomes (such as clinical cure rate) among patients with severe infections, preferably in ICU settings due to MDR-GNB, receiving cefiderocol or best available therapy. Our study adhered to the PRISMA guidelines [33] and was registered in the International Prospective Register of Systematic Reviews (PROSPERO) under the reference CRD42024563041.

Two authors (C.R.-R. and D.A.O.) conducted a search of original reports published up to August 2024 using MEDLINE, Scopus, and Google Scholar. The term 'cefiderocol' was used to identify studies for inclusion in the analysis. The following search strategy was used:

PubMed (last access 14 August 2024): ("Cefiderocol" AND "ICU") OR ("Cefiderocol" AND "Critical Care")) OR ("Cefiderocol" AND "Severe Infection") OR ("Cefiderocol" AND "critically ill") OR ("Cefiderocol" AND "nosocomial pneumonia") OR ("Cefiderocol" AND "ventilator associated pneumonia") OR ("Ceftiderocol" AND "sepsis") OR ("Cefiderocol" AND "bloodstream infection")

Google Scholar (last access 14 August 2024): "Cefiderocol" AND ("ICU" OR "Critical Care" OR "Severe Infection") AND ("RCT " OR "Cohort")

Scopus (last access 14 August 2024): "Cefiderocol" AND "Severe Infections" "Cefiderocol" AND "Critical Care", "Cefiderocol" AND "ICU", "Cefiderocol" AND "Critically ill patients"

The results of this search were assessed by two independent reviewers to choose the studies ultimately included in the systematic review and meta-analysis.

Studies referenced in the bibliographies of all relevant papers from the initial search were also considered for inclusion. Two researchers (C.R.-R. and D.A.O.) independently reviewed the titles and abstracts of all citations to select the articles for analysis, documenting the reasons for excluding each study. Thereafter, they retrieved articles previously selected to evaluate them for inclusion as full-text articles. In cases of disagreement, a third author (CJHC) made a definite decision.

4.2. Inclusion and Exclusion Criteria

Randomized controlled trials (RCTs) or observational cohort studies were selected if they included adult patients with severe infections caused by MDR-GNB admitted to the ICU, comparing treatment with cefiderocol versus other therapeutic alternatives. The selected studies must also provide data on mortality and/or clinical cure. Given the absence of RCTs exclusively involving critically ill patients, we decided to include those in which at least 50% of the study population were critically ill, with the remainder presenting severe infections meeting sepsis criteria.

Studies were excluded under the following conditions: (i) studies where less than 50% of the participants were critically ill; (ii) studies with fewer than 10 participants; (iii) studies lacking a comparison group; (iv) observational studies without multivariate analysis adjusting for potential confounders; (v) studies not published as full papers; (vi) meta-analyses, letters, reviews, meeting abstracts, or editorial comments; and (vii) studies not published in English.

4.3. Data Analysis

The quality of all studies was evaluated using established criteria, and the risk of bias for each study was assessed with RevMan tool, version 5.4.1, following Cochrane guidelines [34]. (CHC performed this assessment). We employed random effects models to estimate the combined effect from aggregate data due to heterogeneity between studies [35].

Most of the studies provided estimates of the risk of death or clinical cure. (ORs or 28–30 days HRs). We pooled these data based on raw data on mortality or clinical cure in different studies and obtained combined results with adjusted ORs (with 95% confidence intervals). Graphical representations of results were performed with the interval plot method. All data used in the meta-analyses were extracted from the published data included in the final selected articles.

Observational studies and RCTs were presented in separate interval plots categorized by study design. Heterogeneity between studies was evaluated using I^2 statistics, which indicate the percentage of variation across studies attributable to heterogeneity rather than random chance [36]. In order to overcome possible bias due to heterogeneity between groups, subgroup meta-analysis was performed: only RCT studies, only studies addressing *Acinetobacter baumanii*, or only studies with colistin treatment as the control group. Publication bias was assessed using a combination of a sensible test (Egger) and a specific test (Peters). Statistical analysis was performed using the software STATA v. 16.2.

5. Conclusions

The emergence of MDR-GNB represents a significant challenge in the management of severe infections in critically ill patients. Cefiderocol, with its unique mechanism of action, has demonstrated efficacy and is a promising option for treating these infections. Although the risk of bias was considered high, our data seem to strengthen the efficacy profile of cefiderocol in severe MDR-GNB infections, especially those occurring in ICU settings, with a global benefit on mortality and at least non-inferiority in the cure rate when compared with other available therapies. However, more randomized clinical trials focusing exclusively on critically ill patients are needed to compare the action of this drug with the other best available therapies for the treatment of this type of infection to better allocate this novel drug in the real-world practice.

Author Contributions: Conceptualization, C.R.-R. and D.A.-O.; methodology, C.R.-R. and C.H.-C.; software, C.R.-R. and C.H.-C.; validation, C.H.-C. and C.R.-R.; formal analysis, C.R.-R.; investigation, D.A.-O., C.R.-R. and M.H.-R.; resources, C.R.-R. and D.A.-O.; writing—original draft preparation, D.A.-O. and C.R.-R.; writing—review and editing, D.A.-O., C.R.-R., M.H.-R., J.B. and C.H.-C.; visualization, D.A.-O., C.R.-R., J.B., M.H.-R. and C.H.-C.; supervision, J.B.; project administration, D.A.-O., C.R.-R., C.H.-C. and J.B. All authors have read and agreed to the published version of the manuscript.

Funding: This research received no external funding.

Institutional Review Board Statement: Ethical approval was not required for this study.

Informed Consent Statement: Not applicable.

Data Availability Statement: Raw data are available upon reasonable request from the corresponding authors.

Conflicts of Interest: The authors declare no conflicts of interest.

References

1. World Health Organization. World Health Organization Publishes List of Bacteria for Which New Antibiotics Are Urgently Needed. Available online: https://www.who.int/news/item/27-02-2017-who-publishes-list-of-bacteria-for-which-new-antibiotics-are-urgently-needed (accessed on 14 August 2024).
2. Kazmierczak, K.M.; Tsuji, M.; Wise, M.G.; Hackel, M.; Yamano, Y.; Echols, R.; Sahm, D.F. In vitro activity of cefiderocol, a siderophore cephalosporin, against a recent collection of clinically relevant carbapenem-non-susceptible Gram-negative bacilli, including serine carbapenemase- and metallo-β-lactamase-producing isolates (SIDERO-WT-2014 Study). *Int. J. Antimicrob. Agents* **2019**, *53*, 177–184. [PubMed]
3. Wang, C.; Yang, D.; Wang, Y.; Ni, W. Cefiderocol for the Treatment of Multidrug-Resistant Gram-Negative Bacteria: A Systematic Review of Currently Available Evidence. *Front Pharmacol.* **2022**, *13*, 896971. [CrossRef] [PubMed]
4. Fendian, Á.M.; Albanell-Fernández, M.; Tuset, M.; Pitart, C.; Castro, P.; Soy, D.; Bodro, M.; Soriano, A.; Del Río, A.; Martínez, J.A. Real-Life Data on the Effectiveness and Safety of Cefiderocol in Severely Infected Patients: A Case Series. *Infect. Dis. Ther.* **2023**, *12*, 1205–1216. [CrossRef] [PubMed]
5. Barbier, F.; Hraiech, S.; Kernéis, S.; Veluppillai, N.; Pajot, O.; Poissy, J.; Roux, D.; Zahar, J.-R.; French Intensive Care Society. Rationale and evidence for the use of new beta-lactam/beta-lactamase inhibitor combinations and cefiderocol in critically ill patients. *Ann. Intensive Care* **2023**, *13*, 65. [CrossRef] [PubMed]

6. Bassetti, M.; Vena, A.; Giacobbe, D.R. Efficacy and safety of cefiderocol for the treatment of severe Gram-negative bacterial infections: A systematic review. *J. Antimicrob. Chemother.* **2023**, *76*, 1299–1302. [CrossRef]
7. Sajib, M.I.; Monteforte, M.; Go, R. Clinical Outcome of Cefiderocol for Infections with Carbapenem-Resistant Organisms. *Antibiotics* **2023**, *12*, 936. [CrossRef]
8. Gatti, M.; Cosentino, F.; Giannella, M.; Viale, P.; Pea, F. Clinical efficacy of cefiderocol-based regimens in patients with carbapenem-resistant Acinetobacter baumannii infections: A systematic review with meta-analysis. *Int. J. Antimicrob. Agents* **2024**, *63*, 107047. [CrossRef]
9. Kirsch, B.; Jensen, S. Efficacy of cefiderocol in treating multidrug-resistant *Acinetobacter baumannii* infections: A meta-analysis. *Infect. Dis. Ther.* **2023**.
10. Wicky, P.-H.; Poiraud, J.; Alves, M.; Patrier, J.; D'humières, C.; Lê, M.; Kramer, L.; de Montmollin, É.; Massias, L.; Armand-Lefèvre, L.; et al. Cefiderocol Treatment for Severe Infections due to Difficult-to-Treat-Resistant Non-Fermentative Gram-Negative Bacilli in ICU Patients: A Case Series and Narrative Literature Review. *Antibiotics* **2023**, *12*, 991. [CrossRef]
11. Morales Castro, D.; Dresser, L.; Granton, J.; Fan, E. Pharmacokinetic Alterations Associated with Critical Illness. *Clin. Pharmacokinet.* **2023**, *62*, 209–220. [CrossRef]
12. Katsube, T.; Echols, R.; Arjona Ferreira, J.C.; Krenz, H.K.; Berg, J.K.; Galloway, C. Cefiderocol, a Siderophore Cephalosporin for Gram-Negative Bacterial Infections: Pharmacokinetics and Safety in Subjects with Renal Impairment. *J. Clin. Pharmacol.* **2017**, *57*, 584–591. [CrossRef] [PubMed]
13. Portsmouth, S.; van Veenhuyzen, D.; Echols, R.; Machida, M.; Ferreira, J.C.A.; Ariyasu, M.; Tenke, P.; Nagata, T.D. Cefiderocol versus imipenem-cilastatin for the treatment of complicated urinary tract infections caused by Gram-negative uropathogens: A phase 2, randomised, double-blind, non-inferiority trial. *Lancet Infect. Dis.* **2018**, *18*, 1319–1328. [CrossRef] [PubMed]
14. Bassetti, M.; Echols, R.; Matsunaga, Y.; Ariyasu, M.; Doi, Y.; Ferrer, R.; Lodise, T.P.; Naas, T.; Niki, Y.; Paterson, D.L.; et al. Efficacy and safety of cefiderocol or best available therapy for the treatment of serious infections caused by carbapenem-resistant Gram-negative bacteria (CREDIBLE-CR): A randomised, open-label, multicentre, pathogen-focused, descriptive, phase 3 trial. *Lancet Infect. Dis.* **2021**, *21*, 226–240. [CrossRef] [PubMed]
15. Wunderink, R.G.; Matsunaga, Y.; Ariyasu, M.; Clevenbergh, P.; Echols, R.; Kaye, K.S.; Kollef, M.; Menon, A.; Pogue, J.M.; Shorr, A.F.; et al. Cefiderocol versus high-dose, extended-infusion meropenem for the treatment of Gram-negative nosocomial pneumonia (APEKS-NP): A randomised, double-blind, phase 3, non-inferiority trial. *Lancet Infect. Dis.* **2021**, *21*, 213–225. [CrossRef] [PubMed]
16. Falcone, M.; Tiseo, G.; Leonildi, A.; Della Sala, L.; Vecchione, A.; Barnini, S.; Farcomeni, A.; Menichetti, F. Cefiderocol- Compared to Colistin-Based Regimens for the Treatment of Severe Infections Caused by Carbapenem-Resistant *Acinetobacter baumannii*. *Antimicrob. Agents Chemother.* **2022**, *66*, e0214221. [CrossRef] [PubMed]
17. Bavaro, D.F.; Papagni, R.; Belati, A.; Diella, L.; De Luca, A.; Brindicci, G.; De Gennaro, N.; Di Gennaro, F.; Romanelli, F.; Stolfa, S.; et al. Cefiderocol Versus Colistin for the Treatment of Carbapenem-Resistant *Acinetobacter baumannii* Complex Bloodstream Infections: A Retrospective, Propensity-Score Adjusted, Monocentric Cohort Study. *Infect. Dis. Ther.* **2023**, *12*, 2147–2163. [CrossRef]
18. Dalfino, L.; Stufano, M.; Bavaro, D.F.; Diella, L.; Belati, A.; Stolfa, S.; Romanelli, F.; Ronga, L.; Di Mussi, R.; Murgolo, F.; et al. Effectiveness of First-Line Therapy with Old and Novel Antibiotics in Ventilator-Associated Pneumonia Caused by Carbapenem-Resistant *Acinetobacter baumannii*: A Real Life, Prospective, Observational, Single-Center Study. *Antibiotics* **2023**, *12*, 1048. [CrossRef]
19. Russo, A.; Bruni, A.; Gullì, S.; Borrazzo, C.; Quirino, A.; Lionello, R.; Serapide, F.; Garofalo, E.; Serraino, R.; Romeo, F.; et al. Efficacy of cefiderocol- vs. colistin-containing regimen for treatment of bacteraemic ventilator-associated pneumonia caused by carbapenem-resistant *Acinetobacter baumannii* in patients with COVID-19. *Int. J. Antimicrob. Agents* **2023**, *62*, 106825. [CrossRef]
20. Rando, E.; Cutuli, S.L.; Sangiorgi, F.; Tanzarella, E.S.; Giovannenze, F.; De Angelis, G.; Murri, R.; Antonelli, M.; Fantoni, M.; De Pascale, G. Cefiderocol-containing regimens for the treatment of carbapenem-resistant *A. baumannii* ventilator-associated pneumonia: A propensity-weighted cohort study. *JAC Antimicrob. Resist.* **2023**, *5*, dlad085. [CrossRef]
21. Dickstein, Y.; Lellouche, J.; Amar, M.B.D.; Schwartz, D.; Nutman, A.; Daitch, V.; Yahav, D.; Leibovici, L.; Skiada, A.; Antoniadou, A.; et al. Treatment Outcomes of Colistin- and Carbapenem-resistant *Acinetobacter baumannii* Infections: An Exploratory Subgroup Analysis of a Randomized Clinical Trial. *Clin. Infect. Dis.* **2019**, *69*, 769–776. [CrossRef]
22. Ardebili, A.; Izanloo, A.; Rastegar, M. Polymyxin combination therapy for multidrug-resistant, extensively-drug resistant, and difficult-to-treat drug-resistant gram-negative infections: Is it superior to polymyxin monotherapy? *Expert Rev. Anti Infect. Ther.* **2023**, *21*, 387–429. [CrossRef] [PubMed]
23. Bavaro, D.F.; Belati, A.; Diella, L.; Stufano, M.; Romanelli, F.; Scalone, L.; Stolfa, S.; Ronga, L.; Maurmo, L.; Dell'aera, M.; et al. Cefiderocol-Based Combination Therapy for "Difficult-to-Treat" Gram-Negative Severe Infections: Real-Life Case Series and Future Perspectives. *Antibiotics* **2021**, *10*, 652. [CrossRef]
24. Viale, P.; Sandrock, C.E.; Ramirez, P.; Rossolini, G.M.; Lodise, T.P. Treatment of critically ill patients with cefiderocol for infections caused by multidrug-resistant pathogens: Review of the evidence. *Ann. Intensive Care* **2023**, *13*, 52. [CrossRef] [PubMed]
25. Möhlmann, J.E.; van Luin, M.; Uijtendaal, E.V.; Zahr, N.; Sikma, M.A. Continuous infusion of cefiderocol in a critically ill patient with continuous venovenous haemofiltration. *Br. J. Clin. Pharmacol.* **2023**, *89*, 3753–3757. [CrossRef] [PubMed]

26. Gatti, M.; Rinaldi, M.; Tonetti, T.; Gaibani, P.; Siniscalchi, A.; Viale, P.; Pea, F. Pharmacokinetics/pharmacodynamics of cefiderocol administered by continuous infusion in a case series of critically ill patients with carbapenem-resistant *Acinetobacter baumannii* infections undergoing continuous venovenous haemodiafiltration (CVVHDF). *Int. J. Antimicrob. Agents* **2023**, *62*, 106852. [CrossRef]
27. Mercadante, S.; Tripiciano, C.; Romani, L.; Di Nardo, M.; Bottari, G.; Goffredo, B.M.; Simeoli, R.; Guzzo, I.; Lancella, L.; Antachopoulos, C.; et al. The Use of Cefiderocol as Salvage Therapy in an Infant Receiving ECMO and Continuous Renal Replacement Therapy. *Antibiotics* **2023**, *13*, 37. [CrossRef]
28. Berry, A.V.; Conelius, A.; Gluck, J.A.; Nicolau, D.P.; Kuti, J.L. Cefiderocol is Not Sequestered in an Ex Vivo Extracorporeal Membrane Oxygenation (ECMO) Circuit. *Eur. J. Drug Metab. Pharmacokinet.* **2023**, *48*, 437–441. [CrossRef]
29. de la Fuente, C.; Rodríguez, M.; Merino, N.; Carmona, P.; Machuca, I.; Córdoba-Fernández, M.; Guzmán-Puche, J.; Domínguez, A.; López-Viñau, T.; García, L.; et al. Real-life use of cefiderocol for salvage therapy of severe infections due to carbapenem-resistant Gram-negative bacteria. *Int. J. Antimicrob. Agents* **2023**, *62*, 106818. [CrossRef]
30. Ramirez, P.; Merino, E.; Sarda, J.; Gonzalez, A.J.; Verardi, S.; Fortun, J. Real-world effectiveness and safety of cefiderocol in patients with Gram-negative bacterial infections in the early access programme in Spain: Results of the PERSEUS study. In Proceedings of the ESCMID Global, Vienna, Austria, 11–15 April 2024.
31. Hsueh, S.C.; Chao, C.M.; Wang, C.Y.; Lai, C.C.; Chen, C.H. Clinical efficacy and safety of cefiderocol in the treatment of acute bacterial infections: A systematic review and meta-analysis of randomised controlled trials. *J. Glob. Antimicrob. Resist.* **2021**, *24*, 376–382. [CrossRef]
32. Onorato, L.; de Luca, I.; Monari, C.; Coppola, N. Cefiderocol either in monotherapy or combination versus best available therapy in the treatment of carbapenem-resistant *Acinetobacter baumannii* infections: A systematic review and meta-analysis. *J. Infect.* **2024**, *88*, 106113. [CrossRef]
33. Moher, D.; Liberati, A.; Tetzlaff, J.; Altman, D.G. Preferred reporting items for systematic reviews and meta-analyses: The PRISMA statement. *BMJ* **2009**, *339*, b2535. [CrossRef] [PubMed]
34. Sterne, J.A.C.; Savović, J.; Page, M.J.; Elbers, R.G.; Blencowe, N.S.; Boutron, I.; Cates, C.J.; Cheng, H.Y.; Corbett, M.S.; Eldridge, S.M.; et al. RoB 2: A revised Cochrane risk-of-bias tool for randomized trials. *BMJ* **2019**, *366*, l4898. [CrossRef] [PubMed]
35. DerSimonian, R.; Kacker, R. Random-effects model for meta-analysis of clinical trials: An update. *Contemp. Clin. Trials* **2007**, *28*, 105–114. [CrossRef] [PubMed]
36. Higgins, J.P.; Thompson, S.G. Quantifying heterogeneity in a meta-analysis. *Stat. Med.* **2002**, *21*, 1539–1558. [CrossRef] [PubMed]

antibiotics MDPI

Article

Challenges Facing Two Outbreaks of Carbapenem-Resistant *Acinetobacter baumannii*: From Cefiderocol Susceptibility Testing to the Emergence of Cefiderocol-Resistant Mutants

Montserrat Rodríguez-Aguirregabiria [1,*], Fernando Lázaro-Perona [2], Juana Begoña Cacho-Calvo [2], Mª Soledad Arellano-Serrano [1], Juan Carlos Ramos-Ramos [3], Eduardo Rubio-Mora [2], Mariana Díaz-Almirón [4] and Mª José Asensio-Martín [1]

1 Critical Care Department, Hospital Universitario La Paz, IdiPAZ, 28046 Madrid, Spain; mariasoledad.arellano@salud.madrid.org (M.S.A.-S.); mjose.asensio@salud.madrid.org (M.J.A.-M.)
2 Microbiology Department, Hospital Universitario La Paz, 28046 Madrid, Spain; juanabegona.cacho@salud.madrid.org (J.B.C.-C.); ermora@salud.madrid.org (E.R.-M.)
3 Internal Medicine Department, Infectious Diseases Unit, Hospital Universitario La Paz, CIBERINFEC, IdiPAZ, 28046 Madrid, Spain; juancarlos.ramos@salud.madrid.org
4 Research Unit, Hospital La Paz Institute for Health Research, IdiPAZ, 28046 Madrid, Spain; mariana.diaz@salud.madrid.org
* Correspondence: montserrat.rodriguez@salud.madrid.org

Abstract: Carbapenem-resistant *Acinetobacter baumannii* (CRAB) infections are associated with poor outcomes depending on patient's conditions, clinical severity and type of infection, and treatment is challenging given the limited therapeutic options available. The aim of this study was to describe the clinical and microbiological characteristics of two outbreaks caused by CRAB in an intensive care unit (ICU). In addition, the mechanisms of resistance detected in these strains and the treatment chosen according to the available therapeutic options were analyzed. Overall, 28 patients were included. Ten patients (35.71%) had ventilator-associated pneumonia (VAP), ten (35.71%) had a bloodstream infection (BSI), and eight (28.57%) were only colonized. Recurrent infection occurred in 25% (5/20) of infected patients. Two different strains of *A. baumannii* were isolated from the index patient of the first outbreak. The first strain belonged to the ST85 and carried the bla_{NDM-1} carbapenemase gene, while the second belonged to the ST2 and carried bla_{OXA-23}, and bla_{OXA-66} carbapenemase genes. The phylogenetic analysis revealed that the ST2 strain was the cause of the major outbreak, and mutations in the AmpC gene were related to progressive increasing minimum inhibitory concentration (MIC) and finally, cefiderocol-resistance in one strain. The CRAB isolates from the second outbreak were also identified as ST2. Cefiderocol-resistant strains tests identified by the disc diffusion method were involved in 24% (6/25) of nosocomial infections. Using broth microdilution (BMD) ComASP® only, 33.3% (2/6) of these strains were cefiderocol-resistant. All-cause ICU mortality was 21.4%. Conclusions: Cefiderocol is the first approved siderophore cephalosporin for the treatment of CRAB infections. Cefiderocol-resistant strains were related with bla_{NDM-1} carbapenemase and mutations in the AmpC gene. Cefiderocol-resistant strains or that cannot be properly interpreted by disk diffusion, should be retested using BMD for definitive categorization.

Keywords: *Acinetobacter baumannii*; carbapenem-resistant; outbreak; cefiderocol

1. Introduction

Acinetobacter baumannii complex is an opportunistic pathogen that has successfully developed multiple antibiotic resistance mechanisms and frequently causes outbreaks in healthcare institutions and hospitals [1]. *A. baumannii* poses a significant threat to immunocompromised or chronically ill patients, particularly in intensive care units (ICUs) due to high exposure to invasive procedures and prolonged antibiotic therapy [2,3].

A. baumannii can easily survive on both moist and dry surfaces. In addition, *A. baumannii* can also colonize the skin, respiratory tract, oral cavity, and other sections of the human body [4]. Differentiating between colonization and acute infection in critically ill patients is challenging [5].

Resistance mechanisms in *A. baumannii* include reduced membrane permeability, antibiotic efflux, genetic mutation, post-translational modifications, and antibiotic inactivation via beta-lactamases [6]. Carbapenem resistance is mainly due to OXA-type Class-D enzymes (OXA-27, OXA-49, OXA-25, OXA-26, and OXA-40) and less frequently to metallo-β-lactamases (MBLs) such as VIM, IMP, and NDM-1. Additionally, chromosomal cephalosporinase (e.g., AmpC, plasmid-mediated β-lactamases such as TEM-1, TEM-2, OXA-21, and OXA-37), and extended-spectrum b-lactamases (ESBLs) are frequently expressed [7].

The most common clinical manifestations of *A. baumannii* are nosocomial pneumonia and bloodstream infection (BSI). Although *A. baumannii* has been considered a pathogen with limited virulence, invasive infections, especially those caused by multi-drug resistant strains, are associated with increased morbidity and mortality in predisposed patients [8]. In the EUROBACT-II study, 11.9% of hospital-acquired BSI were caused by *A. baumannii* and 84.6% were resistant to carbapenems [9]. Falcone et al. recently reported a 43.2% thirty-day mortality in patients with CRAB bacteremia, and the attributable mortality rate was 16% [10]. *A. baumannii* is usually a cause of ventilator-associated pneumonia (VAP) with mortality ranging from 30 to 70% [11,12]. CRAB infections have become especially difficult to treat owing to the paucity of therapeutic options. There are no conclusive data regarding the optimal antibiotic therapy against CRAB infections [12,13].

The aim of this study was to describe the clinical and microbiological characteristics of two outbreaks caused by CRAB in an ICU. In addition, the mechanisms of resistance detected in these strains and the treatment chosen according to the available therapeutic options were analyzed.

2. Materials and Methods

2.1. Study Design and Patient Selection

This was a retrospective, observational study conducted in a major teaching hospital. Patients colonized or infected by CRAB who were admitted consecutively in the ICU from October 2022 to November 2023 were included.

The inclusion criteria were: (1) age $\geq$ 18 years; (2) positive surveillance cultures for CRAB; (3) blood culture or respiratory tract culture positive for CRAB. Polymicrobial etiology was not excluded. All episodes of CRAB infections were reported for each patient. All patients were managed by the same team of physicians. Antimicrobial therapies were selected according to the clinical judgement of the team of physicians and infectious disease specialists. All data were extracted retrospectively.

Medical records were reviewed to extract clinical information. The following data were recorded: demographics, reason for admission, Charlson comorbidity index, and comorbid conditions. Immunodepression included advanced solid cancer, solid organ transplantation, hemato-oncological patients, corticosteroid therapy or other chronic immunosuppressive therapies, and HIV infection. In addition, the following data were registered: Acute Physiology and Chronic Health Evaluation (APACHE) II score, CRAB colonization or infection, source of infection, the empirical and targeted antimicrobial therapy, severity with the Sequential Organ Failure Assessment score (SOFA) at the time of infection, development of septic shock, life-supporting therapies such as mechanical ventilation (MV), continuous renal replacement therapy (CRRT), and extracorporeal membrane oxygenation (ECMO) carried out during hospitalization, and length of stay in the intensive care unit (ICU) and hospital. The Abbreviated Burn Severity Index (ABSI) and Total Burned Body Surface area (TBSA), and early surgical intervention by escharotomy were recorded in burn patients. The development of resistance to antibiotic treatment was carefully monitored. The decision to withhold or withdraw life-sustaining treatment because of underlying conditions or the futility of invasive treatment was reviewed. The occurrence of adverse events during antibiotic treatment, especially nephrotoxicity, was noted. Acute kidney injury (AKI) was defined according to the Second International Consensus Conference of the Acute Dialysis Quality Initiative (ADQI) group [14]. Early mortality, within 7 days after the diagnosis and related to the infection, and all-cause mortality in ICU were assessed.

2.2. Definitions

According to CDC/NHSC criteria, infections were classified into the following categories: ventilator-associated pneumonia and bloodstream infections [15]. The onset of bacteriemia was defined as the day when the blood culture that eventually yielded *A. baumannii* was obtained. Episodes of bloodstream infections were considered acquired in the ICU if they appeared within 48 h after ICU admission. The severity of infections was assessed according to the Third International Consensus Definitions for Sepsis and Septic Shock [16]. The length of hospital and ICU stay was calculated as the number of days from the date of admission to the date of discharge or death. The Charlson Comorbidity Index was calculated based on previous definitions [17]. CRAB colonization was evaluated weekly through active surveillance in ICU patients [18]. Clinical cure was defined as the resolution of signs and symptoms of infection. Relapse or recurrence was defined as a subsequent CRAB infection requiring antimicrobial treatment. Progression, recurrence, or relapse of nosocomial pneumonia were considered treatment failure.

2.3. Bacterial Isolates Identification and Susceptibility Testing

2.3.1. Strain

All clinical isolates from patients were identified using MALDI TOF (Bruker Daltonics GmbH & Co. KG, Bremen, Germany). The MicroScan WalkAway plus System (Beckman Coulter, Brea, CA, USA) was used for routine antimicrobial susceptibility tests (AST). The results of AST were interpreted according to the European Committee on Antimicrobial Susceptibility Testing (EUCAST) breakpoints.

2.3.2. Cefiderocol Susceptibility Test

The first isolate of CRAB from each patient was tested for cefiderocol susceptibility. The cefiderocol susceptibility tests were performed by the disc diffusion method (Liofilchem, Roseto degli Abruzzi, Italy) on Mueller–Hinton medium plates (MH agar plates), and new broth microdilution (BMD) commercially available tests, ComASP® (Liofilchem, Roseto degli Abruzzi, Italy), in vitro according to the FDA drug approved label (https://www.accessdata.fda.gov/cdrh_docs/reviews/K230479.pdf, accessed on 14 July 2024). The results were interpreted according to the breakpoints proposed by EUCAST: zone diameters of $\geq$17 mm for the cefiderocol 30 µg disk correspond to minimum inhibitory concentration (MIC) values below the PK-PD breakpoint of $S \leq 2$ mg/L (https://www.eucast.org/clinical_breakpoints, accessed on 14 July 2024). BMD ComASP® was not available in our institution during the first outbreak and the strains were tested afterwards.

Synergy analyses were performed using the fixed proportion with the E-test method. The fractional inhibitory concentration (FIC) index (FICI) was calculated for the E-test by using the following formula: FICI = FIC of agent A + FIC B, where FIC A is the MIC of the combination/MIC of drug A alone, and FIC B is the MIC of the combination/MIC of drug B alone. FICI results were interpreted with the following criteria: synergy, FICI $\leq$ 0.5; independent interaction, FICI 0.5- $\leq$ 4; and antagonism, FICI > 4 [19].

2.4. Molecular Analysis

Most *A. baumannii* recovered from patients or the environment were subjected to whole genome sequencing during the outbreak. DNA was extracted with the DNeasy® blood&Tissue kit (Qiagen GmbH, Hilden, Germany) and sequenced in the Ion GeneStudio S5 system (Thermo Fisher Scientific, Waltham, MA, USA) using the NEBNext® Fast DNA Library Prep Set for Ion Torrent™ (New England Biolabs, Ipswich, MA, USA). Genome assembly was performed using spades v3.14.1 (https://github.com/ablab/spades, accessed on 14 July 2024) and single nucleotide polymorphisms (SNP) analysis with Snippy v4.6.0 (https://github.com/tseemann/snippy, accessed on 14 July 2024). Phylogenetic analysis was carried on using FastTree 2.0.0 (http://www.microbesonline.org/fasttree, accessed on 14 July 2024). Analysis of resistance genes and plasmids was performed using ABRicate v1.0.1 (https://github.com/tseemann/abricate, accessed on 21.8.24). MLST was determined with the mlst v.2.23.0 software (https://github.com/tseemann/mlst, accessed on 14 July 2024). Phylogenetic results were continuously reported to the Preventive Medicine department.

2.5. Statistical Analysis

A descriptive univariate analysis was carried out for all study variables. Frequency results were expressed as absolute and relative frequencies. Continuous variables were expressed with the main measures of dispersion (mean, standard deviation, median, and interquartile range). Comparative analysis was performed with the Pearson Chi-Square test (or Fisher's exact test for 2 × 2 tables or likelihood ratio in mXn tables, if necessary) or with non-parametric equivalents Mann–Whitney U test in the case of quantitative variables. The type I error rate (alpha) was set to 5% (two-sided).

3. Results

3.1. Study Population

The index case was a burn patient coming from Algeria. One hundred and seventy-one patients were admitted to the ICU during the first outbreak (from October 2022 to June 2023). Eighteen (10.52%) patients were infected by CRAB and seven (4%) became colonized. The second outbreak was triggered in October 2023, with two patients also burned and coming from another institution. No new patients were infected by CRAB and only one patient became colonized (Figure 1).

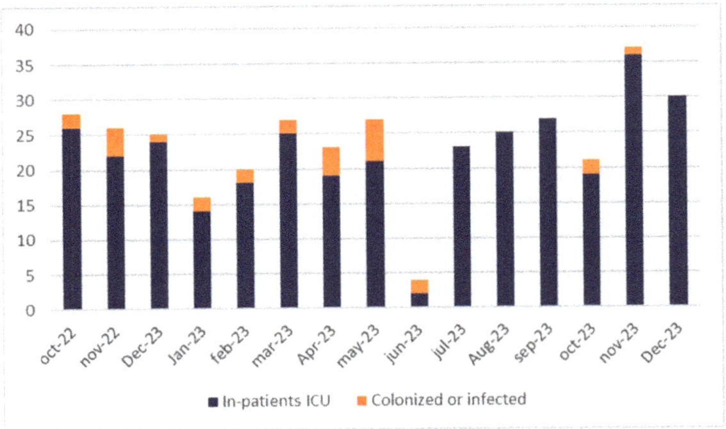

Figure 1. Epidemic curve of two CRAB outbreaks. Patients admitted to the ICU and not affected during the outbreaks are shown in blue. Orange represents patients colonized or infected by CRAB. First outbreak from October 2022 to June 2023. Second outbreak from October to November 2023.

Both outbreaks affected 28 critically ill patients with APACHE II: 14.1 (SD 5.4) points, who had long hospital stays, underwent mostly invasive procedures, and half required hemodynamic support. The reason for admission was burn patients (60.71%) and medical disease (21.42%). Immunosuppressed patients accounted for 21.42%. The most relevant characteristics of patients are described below (Table 1).

Table 1. Demographics, reason for admission, baseline characteristics, life-supporting therapies, and prognosis of patients colonized or infected by CRAB in ICU during both outbreaks (from October 2022 to November 2023).

Variable	All Patients n = 28
Age in years, median (IQR)	45.5 (30.7–64.25)
Male sex	18 (64.28%)
Reason for admission Medical Trauma Burn TEN	 6 (21.42%) 1 (3.57%) 17 (60.71%) 4 (14.28%)
APACHE II, mean (SD)	14.1 (5.4)
Age-adjusted Charlson index, median (IQR)	1 (1–4)
Underlying conditions Diabetes mellitus Chronic pulmonary disease Chronic renal insufficiency Liver cirrhosis HIV Solid cancer Hematologic cancer Immunosuppressive drugs Immunocompromised (all causes)	 3 (10.71%) 2 (7.14%) 0 1 (3.57%) 1 (3.57%) 3 (10.71%) 0 3 (10.71%) 6 (21.42%)
Length of hospital stay, median (IQR)	56.5 (37.25–92.70)
Length of ICU stay, median (IQR)	37 (19.50–66.75)
Invasive procedures Mechanical ventilation CRRT ECMO Vasopressor drugs Tracheostomy	 18 (64.28%) 4 (14.28%) 2 (7.14%) 15 (53.6%) 13 (46.4%)
Colonized Infected	8 (28.57%) 20 (71.42%)
First invasive infection VAP BSI	 10 (35.7%) 10 (35.7%)
ICU mortality	6 (21.42%)
Hospital mortality	7 (25%)
Early and related infection mortality (≤7 days)	0

TEN: Toxic epidermal necrolysis; HIV: human immunodeficiency virus; CRRT: continuous renal replacement therapy; ECMO: extracorporeal membrane oxygenation; VAP: ventilator-associated pneumonia. BSI: bloodstream infection.

Overall, 20 patients (71.42%) were infected, and 8 were colonized by CRAB (28.57%). Most of the infected patients had severe burns (70%) with greater and depth skin damage. Abbreviated Burn Severity Index (ABSI) and Total Body Surface Area (TBSA) affected were higher in burned patients with a nosocomial CRAB infection. All burn patients requiring urgent escharotomy became infected.

All patients with continuous renal replacement therapy (CRRT) developed an invasive infection. In one patient, ECMO was previously implanted for acute respiratory distress syndrome due to *Staphylococcus aureus* nosocomial pneumonia, and the other case was because of a VAP caused by CRAB. The differences observed between colonized and infected patients are described below (Table 2).

Table 2. Univariate analysis between colonized and infected patients by CRAB in ICU during both outbreaks (from October 2022 to November 2023).

	Colonized (n = 8)	Infected (n = 20)	*p*
Age in years, median (IQR)	29 (22–29)	33.5 (28.2–55.2)	0.258
Male sex	6 (75%)	12 (60%)	0.669
Reason for admission			*
Medical	3 (37.5%)	3 (15%)	
Trauma	0	1 (5%)	
Burn	3 (37.5%)	14 (70%)	
- ABSI, mean (SD)	4.5 (3.5)	7.64 (2.09)	
- TBSA %, mean (SD)	22.2 (15.3)	36 (15.4)	
- Escharotomy	0	5 (25%)	
TEN	2 (25%)	2 (10%)	
APACHE II, mean (SD)	11.75 (5.6)	15.1 (5.14)	0.165
Charlson index, median (IQR)	3 (0.5–4)	0 (0–2.5)	0.150
Underlying conditions			*
Diabetes mellitus	2 (25%)	1 (5%)	
Chronic pulmonary disease	1 (12.7%)	1 (5%)	
Chronic renal insufficiency	0	0	
Liver cirrhosis	1 (12.7%)	0	
HIV	1 (12.5%)	0	
Solid cancer	1 (12.5%)	2 (10%)	
Hematological cancer	0	0	
Immunosuppressive drugs	1 (12.7%)	2 (10%)	
Immunocompromised (all causes)	3 (37.5%)	3 (15%)	
Length of ICU stay	22 (12.25–39.5)	37 (23–79.5)	0.199
Length of hospital stay	54 (43.5–150.75)	57 (31.75–98.25)	0.746
Invasive procedures			*
Mechanical ventilation	3 (37.5%)	15 (75%)	
CRRT	0	4 (20%)	
ECMO	0	2 (10%)	
Vasopressor drugs	2 (25%)	13 (65%)	
Tracheostomy	2 (25%)	11 (55%)	
ICU mortality	0	6 (30%)	*
Hospital mortality	0	7 (35%)	*

* Differences have not been assessed due to the small sample size. ABSI: Abbreviated Burn Severity Index. TBSA: Total Body Surface Area TEN: Toxic epidermal necrolysis; HIV: human immunodeficiency virus; CRRT: continuous renal replacement therapy; ECMO: extracorporeal membrane oxygenation.

All-cause ICU mortality was 21.4% (6/28 patients). In deceased patients, APACHE II was higher, and invasive procedures were more frequent. Mechanical ventilation was required in 80.3% of these patients, and 50% had to undergo CRRT. Fifty percent (3/6) were burn patients with a higher ABSI and TBSA affected. No colonized patient died during the study period (Table 3).

Table 3. Univariate analysis of all-cause ICU mortality in colonized and infected patients by CRAB during both outbreaks (from October 2022 to November 2023).

	ICU Mortality (n = 6)	Survivors (n = 22)	*p*
Age in years (IQR)	56.3 (37–75)	45.5 (19–83)	0.259
Male sex	3 (50%)	15 (68.2%)	0.634
Reason for admission			
Medical	2 (33.3%)	4 (18.2%)	
Trauma	0	1 (4.5%)	
Burn	3 (50%)	14 (63.6%)	
- ABSI, mean (SD)	10 (1)	6.62 (2.18)	
- TBSA %, mean (SD)	42.2 (19.3)	30.47 (15.1)	0.025
- Escharotomy	2 (33%)	3 (13.6%)	0.24
TEN	1 (16.7%)	3 (13.6%)	

Table 3. *Cont.*

	ICU Mortality (n = 6)	Survivors (n = 22)	*p*
APACHE II, mean (SD)	19.33 (4.55)	12.73 (4.77)	0.01
Charlson index, median (IQR)	1 (0–4.5)	0.5 (0–4)	0.72
Underlying conditions			*
DM	1 (16.7%)	2 (9.1%)	
Chronic pulmonary disease	0	2 (9.1%)	
Chronic renal insufficiency	0	0	
Liver cirrhosis	0	1 (4.5%)	
HIV	0	1 (4.5%)	
Solid cancer	1 (16.7%)	2 (9.1%)	
Hematological cancer	0	0	
Immunosuppressive drugs	1 (16.7%)	2 (9.1%)	
Immunocompromised (all causes)	1 (16.7%)	5 (22.7%)	
Length of ICU stay, median (IQR)	44.5 (16.25–91.5)	37 (20.25–53.25)	0.764
Length of hospital stay, median (IQR)	44.5 (16.25–91.5)	56 (41.75–103)	0.236
Colonized	0	8 (36.3%)	0.141
Infected	6 (100%)	14 (63.6%)	
Invasive procedures			*
Mechanical ventilation	5 (83.3%)	13 (59.1%)	
CRRT	3 (50%)	1 (4.5%)	
ECMO	0	2 (9.1%)	
Vasopressor drugs	5 (83.3%)	10 (45.5%)	
Tracheostomy	3 (50%)	10 (45.5%)	
AKI	2 (33.3%)	2 (9.1%)	*

* Differences have not been assessed due to the small sample size. ABSI: Abbreviated Burn Severity Index. TBSA: Total Body Surface Area TEN: Toxic epidermal necrolysis; HIV: human immunodeficiency virus; CRRT: continuous renal replacement therapy; ECMO: extracorporeal membrane oxygenation; AKI: acute kidney injury.

3.2. *Characteristics, Treatments, and Outcomes of Patients with CRAB Infections*

Overall, 20 patients were infected. Ten (50%) developed a VAP, and the other 50% had a BSI. Catheter infections were the cause of 40% (4/10) of bacteremia, and 20% (2/10) were bacteremia of unknown origin. In 40% (4/10) of episodes, the source was skin and soft tissue infections or related to surgical procedures in burn patients. Fifty percent of the first CRAB infections were polymicrobial, and *Pseudomonas aeruginosa* (4/10) and *S. aureus* (2/10) were the most frequently isolated microorganisms (details in Supplementary Material). Three patients developed candidemia and one had a probable invasive pulmonary aspergillosis.

All deceased patients developed septic shock during CRAB infection, five patients (83.33%) due to a VAP, and one (16.66%) had a bacteremia. The SOFA score was higher, and in 50% (3/6) of cases, the empirical treatment of CRAB infections was inappropriate.

As for targeted therapy, cefiderocol was administered as monotherapy 40% (8/20) and in combination 25% (5/20) with other antimicrobials, mainly colistin and sulbactam. Eighty percent (8/10) of tested strains were resistant to tigecycline following CLSI criteria. Treatment was tailored according to the microbiological report. The clinical success rate in BSI was 100% (10/10). Clinical success in VAP was 77.7% (7/9); one patient did not receive antibiotic treatment because it was decided to discontinue life support treatment due to the severity of the burn injury (details in Supplementary Material).

Three patients with septic shock in the course of CRAB infections who received colistin as part of antibiotic treatment developed acute kidney injury (AKI). Five patients had a recurrent CRAB infection; three were treated with cefiderocol, and two with colistin in monotherapy. In only two cases, death was considered related to infection (both patients with recurrent VAP). Targeted treatment is described below (Table 4).

Table 4. Characteristics and outcomes of patients with CRAB infections.

CRAB Infections (n = 20)	ICU Mortality (n = 6)	Survivors (n = 14)
Septic shock	6 (100%)	6 (30%)
SOFA score, median (IQR)	11 (7.5–14.25)	4.5 (3–7.25)
VAP (n = 10)	5 (83.33%)	5 (35.71%)
BSI (n = 10)	1 (16.66%)	9 (64.28%)
Inappropriate empirical treatment	3 (50%)	3 (21.42%)
Targeted therapy Cefiderocol monotherapy Cefiderocol-based regimen [a] Colistin monotherapy or based regimen [b]	 2 (16.66%) 1 (16.66%) 3 (50%)	 6 (42.85%) 4 (28.57%) 3 (21.42%)
Polymicrobial infection	3 (50%)	7 (50%)
Recurrent CRAB infection	4 (66.6%)	1 (7.14%)
Invasive mycosis	2 (33.33%)	2 (14.28%)
AKI (infection related)	1 (16.66%)	2 (14.28%)
Early mortality (≤7 days)	0	
ICU infection related mortality	2 (33.33%)	
ICU mortality due to severity of burn injuries or decision to withhold or withdraw life-sustaining treatment because underlying conditions.	6 (100%)	

No differences have been made due to the small sample size. VAP: ventilator-associated pneumonia; BSI: bloodstream infection; AKI: acute kidney injury; [a]: colistin or/and sulbactam; [b]: sulbactam.

3.3. Cefiderocol Susceptibility Test

Susceptibility testing for cefiderocol was performed in the first isolate from 20 infected patients by disc diffusion method. Of these, four (20%) were resistant to cefiderocol and ComASP® was performed: three strains were susceptible with MIC = 2 mg/L, and one was resistant with MIC = 16 mg/L. On this last strain, synergistic activity with ampicillin/sulbactam was found with a FICI = 0.019.

Five patients (25%) had a clinical and microbiological recurrence. The tests of susceptibility for cefiderocol were performed in three patients; two isolates were resistant to disc diffusion, and only one had a MIC = 4 mg/L (details in Supplementary Material).

3.4. Phylogenetic Analysis of the Outbreak

Twenty-four clinical isolates (one per patient) and eight environmental isolates were subjected to whole genome sequencing. During the first outbreak, the initial analysis discovered that the index patient was initially colonized by two different strains of *A. baumannii*. The first strain belonged to the ST85 and carried the $bla_{\text{NDM-1}}$ carbapenemase gene while the second belonged to the ST2 and carried $bla_{\text{OXA-23}}$, as well as $bla_{\text{OXA-66}}$ carbapenemase genes.

The phylogenetic analysis revealed that the ST85 NDM-1-producer strain was transmitted to a second patient who was only colonized, while the ST2 strain was the cause of the major outbreak. This strain was identified in all but one of the studied patients from the first outbreak and multiple inanimate objects. A single nucleotide polymorphisms (SNP) analysis of cefiderocol-resistant strains showed that all of them presented mutations in the AmpC gene, which was related to progressively increasing MIC, and to cefiderocol resistance in one strain. That mutation was not present in the cefiderocol-susceptible strain isolated from the index patient.

The three CRAB isolates from the second outbreak were also identified as ST2, but in this case, phylogenetic analysis showed that the three isolates were not part of the previous outbreak and were not related to each other.

4. Discussion

Acinetobacter baumannii has emerged as a major nosocomial pathogen exhibiting high rates of resistance to clinically relevant antibiotics. It frequently causes outbreaks in health-care institutions and hospitals. The index case was a critically burned patient with multi-focal colonization and a CRAB infection. Main infection control measures implemented throughout the first outbreak included hand hygiene, contact isolation precautions, environmental cleaning, an active surveillance program to identify asymptomatic carriage, and finally patient cohorting in a contained area and using dedicated staff [20]. Lessons learned from this complex scenario helped to contain the second outbreak in which only one patient ended up colonized.

In our study, 20 patients developed a CRAB infection, and 70% were patients with severe burn injuries. Burn patients are at particularly high risk for invasive infection due to the impairment of host immunity and loss of skin barrier function, and infection attributable mortality ranges from 50 to 75% [21]. In our research, half of nosocomial infections were polymicrobial, with *P. aeruginosa* and *S. aureus* being the most frequently isolated microorganisms. Therefore, it is difficult to attribute a prognostic impact to the isolation of CRAB. When CRAB is isolated from a non-sterile site, it may represent colonization or infection, and distinguishing between the two is often a challenge [22]. Data from large retrospective studies identifies BSI as a negative predictor of clinical outcomes in burn patients [23]. Risk factors associated with mortality include age, SOFA score at the onset of bacteremia, and TBSA [24]. This impact could not be assessed in our study given the small sample size. Only one patient with CRAB bacteremia died. All-cause mortality in the ICU was 21.4%, but there were no infection-related deaths within seven days of diagnosis. ICU mortality was due to the severity of burn injuries, or the decision to withhold or withdraw life-sustaining treatment in patients admitted with life-threatening conditions and the futility of invasive measures, and palliative care was offered [25,26].

Cefiderocol-resistant was found in one ST85 NDM-1 producer strain and was transmitted to a second patient who was only colonized. ST2 strains carrying $bla_{\mathrm{OXA\text{-}23}}$, as well as $bla_{\mathrm{OXA\text{-}66}}$ carbapenemase genes, were the cause of the major outbreak; in addition, mutations in the AmpC gene were detected. Multidrug-resistant strains of this sequence type have been the cause of numerous ICU outbreaks worldwide [27–29]. The temporal and genomic relationship between the cases suggests that cefiderocol-resistant CRAB (MIC increased to 4 mg/L in one isolated) was selected, probably by increasing the use of cefiderocol in the ICU. In this context, it is possible that a subtherapeutic concentration of the antibiotic in the skin and soft tissue facilitated the progressive emergence of resistance. Some inoculum effects cannot be ruled out, especially in cases of a high bacterial inoculum infection such as VAP, leading to the selection of resistant bacteria [30]. In the second outbreak, two different CRAB ST2 strains were found, though in this case, the transmission was contained. Furthermore, the genomic analysis allowed for ruling out a possible reemergence of the previous outbreak.

Resistance to cefiderocol has been reported. In a systematic review, cefiderocol non-susceptibility was especially higher among NDM-producing *A. baumannii* isolates [31]. With regard to AmpC, in vitro studies with mutational analysis have found important amino acid changes in strains not susceptible to cefiderocol [32]. For *Enterobacterales*-producing class C β-lactamases, the selection of co-resistance to cefiderocol and other antimicrobials following cefepime treatment highlights the potential impact of mutational resistance in AmpC [33]. A recent study found treatment-emergent resistance and interpatient transmission of cefiderocol-resistant *A. baumannii* harbored disrupted *pir*A and *piu*A genes that were not disrupted among susceptible isolates. In this report of 11 critically ill burn patients, all isolates were identified as *A. baumannii* sequence type ST2, one of the major clones widely distributed in the United States. Each isolate harbored $bla_{\mathrm{oxa\text{-}23}}$, $bla_{\mathrm{oxa\text{-}66}}$, and $bla_{\mathrm{ADC\text{-}73}}$ [34]. OXA-$_{23}$-producing *A. baumannii* isolates have been reported in several countries, suggesting a wide distribution as well as from Spain [35,36].

In our study, treatment was tailored according to susceptibility testing for cefiderocol by disc diffusion method, and six isolates were resistant. However, using BMD ComASP® test, resistance was only confirmed in two strains with MIC $\geq$ 4 mg/L, and four strains were susceptible with high MIC = 2 mg/L. This circumstance may raise the need for a higher dose of antibiotics in certain common clinical scenarios in critically ill patients.

For *Acinetobacter* spp., there is as yet insufficient evidence to determine clinical breakpoints for cefiderocol. For these, EUCAST has determined a zone diameter that will exclude isolates with MIC values clearly above the PK-PD breakpoint (https://www.eucast.org/fileadmin/src/media/PDFs/EUCAST_files/Disk_criteria/Validation_2024/Acinetobacter_v_5.0_January_2024.pdf, accessed on 14 July 2024). Furthermore, the accuracy and reproducibility of cefiderocol testing results by disk diffusion and broth microdilution are markedly impacted by iron concentration and inoculum preparation, and may vary by disk and media manufacturer. Depending on the type of variance observed, false resistant or false susceptible results may occur (https://clsi.org/media/a5ndfge2/ast_newsletter23_final-24.pdf, accessed on 14 July 2024)

The reference method for cefiderocol antimicrobial susceptibility testing is BMD with iron-depleted Mueller–Hinton medium (ID-MH), whereas breakpoints recommended for disk diffusion are based on MH-agar plates. Recent research comparing the performance of different methods for testing in vitro activity of cefiderocol in 100 CRAB isolates found that disk diffusion and E-test on ID-MH agar plates exhibit higher diagnostic performance than on MH-agar plates and the commercial BMD methods. ComASP® showed 76% essential agreement with the standard BMD method [37]. On a limited number of isolates, the ComASP® microdilution panel was a valid method to determine cefiderocol MIC on isolates for which the disk diffusion results were uninterpretable, and the combination of both tests was an optimal approach to overcome the challenge of cefiderocol susceptibility testing in routine microbiology laboratories [38]. In terms of suggesting a strategy, disc diffusion could be useful for screening, and for resistant or uninterpretable isolates, a BMD test should be performed for definitive categorization [38–40].

The lack of harmonization between different committees with respect to cefiderocol breakpoints can lead to discrepant results [41]. The EUCAST breakpoints are generally more restrictive than those by the CLSI and allow us to detect the presence of strains with low levels of resistance. This aspect is particularly relevant when dealing with infections caused by microorganisms with very few therapeutic options, and even more so when therapeutic alternatives are considered suboptimal or associated with significant side effects, such as colistin and nephrotoxicity [42].

Cefiderocol is the first approved siderophore cephalosporin for the treatment of CRAB infections. The latest ESCMID guidelines recommend against cefiderocol for the treatment of infections caused by CRAB (conditional strength of recommendation, low level of evidence) [43]. The IDSA guidance document recommended that cefiderocol should be limited to the treatment of CRAB infections refractory to other antibiotics or when intolerance to other agents precludes their use [44]. Both documents agree to the treatment of severe CRAB infections using the combination of two in vitro active agents [43,44]. Data coming from the CREDIBLE-CR phase 3 study with survival rates higher with the best available therapy at the end of the study compared with cefiderocol were limited to making a different recommendation. However, it should be noted that patients assigned to the cefiderocol arm were more likely to be in the ICU at the time of randomization and have ongoing septic shock than those in the best available therapy arm, which may explain these results [45]. Data coming from real-world experience have yielded mixed results regarding the clinical effectiveness of cefiderocol for CRAB infections, especially in critically ill patients [46–48]. An interesting approach emerges from this study done by Dalfino et al. evaluating the effectiveness of first-line therapy with old and novel CRAB active antibiotics in VAP. Clinical failure was lower in the cefiderocol group. Timely targeted antibiotic treatment and cefiderocol-based first-line regimens strongly reduced failure risk [49]. This fact is especially relevant when treating severe infections in critically ill patients. Initial failure to choose the right antibiotic treatment often results in a worse outcome. Furthermore, a recent meta-analysis in observational studies providing proper adjustment for confounders showed that cefiderocol-based regimens were associated with a significantly lower risk of mortality in patients with CRAB infections [50].

In our study, for targeted therapy, cefiderocol was administered as monotherapy or in combination, mainly colistin and sulbactam in 64% of CRAB infections, and colistin monotherapy or in combination with 32%. The efficacy of combination treatment compared to cefiderocol monotherapy remains unresolved. Onorato et al. evaluated cefiderocol monotherapy and combination therapy among seven studies in a meta-analysis. They found a significantly lower mortality rate among patients receiving cefiderocol in monotherapy as compared to those treated with combination regimens. However, these findings were not confirmed in the sub-analysis including only patients with bloodstream infections, nor in the analysis including patients with pneumonia [51]. A recent review also found no significant difference in terms of mortality, microbiological eradication, and clinical cure between monotherapy and combination therapy [52].

In addition, the emergence of in vivo resistance to cefiderocol in the setting of CRAB infections has been reported [53]. In the Falcone et al. study, microbiological failure occurred in 17.4% of patients receiving cefiderocol versus 6.8% of those receiving colistin. The eight patients of the cefiderocol group with microbiological failure all had a BSI, and six received cefiderocol monotherapy. All relapsing *A. baumannii* strains isolated from patients receiving cefiderocol were re-tested, and four strains demonstrated resistance (MIC values range from 4 to $\geq$32 mg/L) [46]. In contrast, the Dalfino et al. study found lower microbiological failure in the cefiderocol group [49]. In post-hoc analysis of CREDIBLE-CR of MICs, in the cefiderocol group, 12 isolates (from 12 patients [15%]) had at least a four-fold increase in cefiderocol MIC from baseline (i.e., five for *A. baumannii*, one for *Stenotrophomonas maltophilia*, three for *Klebsiella pneumoniae*, and three for *P. aeruginosa*). Only four isolates had an MIC that increased to more than 2 µg/mL, of which three isolates had an MIC of more than 4 µg/mL [45]. In our study, we observed a temporal and genomic relationship between the strains with a progressively increasing MIC to 4 mg/L, but only in one isolate.

An interesting approach to reduce the risk of in vivo emergence of cefiderocol-resistant strains or restore susceptibility in cefiderocol-resistant *A. baumannii* strains could be the combination with β-lactamases-inhibitor, although this hypothesis has not been confirmed by clinical trials. High-dose ampicillin-sulbactam, as a component of combination therapy, is suggested as an alternative agent for CRAB infections. Sulbactam is a competitive, irreversible β-lactamase inhibitor that, in high doses, saturates PBP1a/1b and PBP3 of *A. baumannii* isolates. Although a high proportion of isolates are currently resistant to ampicillin-sulbactam, administration is recommended even in these circumstances [5,12,44]. Human-simulated exposure of cefiderocol in combination with ceftazidime/avibactam or sulbactam (with ampicillin) resulted in potent in vivo activity against 15 carbapenem-non-susceptible *A. baumannii* including cefiderocol-non-susceptible isolates [54]. In our research, we found a synergistic effect using ampicillin-sulbactam in one patient with a cefiderocol-resistant CRAB bacteremia. The potential role of β-lactamases-inhibitors such as avibactam or sulbactam has been evaluated. Avibactam showed synergistic activity and restored in vitro cefiderocol susceptibility in some *A. baumannii* strains with non-producing MBL-carbapenemases [37]. Avibactam and durlobactam could inhibit cefiderocol hydrolysis by PER-1 [55]. However, although data about the role of β-lactamases-inhibitors in restoring available treatment for CRAB are encouraging, antagonism has also been described depending on underlying resistance mechanisms or species involved [56,57].

The main limitation of this study is that it is a single-center observational and retrospective study with a small sample size. Despite this, we have been able to assess the most relevant aspects of the strategy to be followed in terms of prevention, diagnosis, and treatment in a very complex clinical scenario such as infections caused by CRAB.

We would also like to highlight that this is one of the few studies in which a phylogenetic analysis of a CRAB outbreak in critically ill patients has been performed. This has allowed us to monitor the behavior of CRAB strains over time, and to detect the underlying mechanisms related to resistance to a new antibiotic. In addition, we advise on the use of different cefiderocol susceptibility tests in order to avoid problems of accuracy in definitive categorization.

5. Conclusions

Infections caused by CRAB represent a major challenge in daily clinical practice due to the limited therapeutic options available and the potential impact on the prognosis of these patients. In our experience, cefiderocol could be considered a therapeutic option against CRAB infections with a better safety profile compared to other older antibiotics. Susceptibility testing to cefiderocol can be carried out by disk diffusion for screening, and for resistant or uninterpretable isolates, we suggest performing a BMD test for definitive categorization. The management of infections caused by CRAB should be approached from a global institutional perspective and requires the participation of a multidisciplinary team to design a prevention, diagnosis, and treatment strategy.

Supplementary Materials: The following supporting information can be downloaded at: https://www.mdpi.com/article/10.3390/antibiotics13080784/s1, Table S1: Source of infection, etiology, cefiderocol susceptibility test according to EUCAST criteria, targeted treatment, and outcomes in patients infected by CRAB during both outbreaks (from October 2022 to November 2023).

Author Contributions: Conceptualization, M.R.-A. and M.J.A.-M.; Data curation, M.R.-A., M.S.A.-S. and M.D.-A.; Investigation, M.R.-A., F.L.-P., J.B.C.-C. and E.R.-M.; Methodology, M.R.-A., M.J.A.-M., F.L.-P., J.B.C.-C., E.R.-M. and M.D.-A. Supervision, M.R.-A., F.L.-P., J.B.C.-C., J.C.R.-R. and M.J.A.-M.; Writing—original draft, M.R.-A., F.L.-P., J.B.C.-C., E.R.-M. and M.J.A.-M.; Writing—review and editing, M.R.-A., F.L.-P., J.B.C.-C., M.S.A.-S., J.C.R.-R. and M.J.A.-M. All authors made substantial contributions to the final manuscript. All authors agreed to be accountable for all aspects of the work. All authors have read and agreed to the published version of the manuscript.

Funding: This research received no external funding.

Institutional Review Board Statement: The study was conducted according to the principles stated in the Declaration of Helsinki. The local ethics committee approved the study protocol (PI-5933, 22 November 2023).

Informed Consent Statement: Not applicable.

Data Availability Statement: The dataset analyzed during the current study is available from the corresponding author upon reasonable request.

Conflicts of Interest: M.R.-A. has conducted consulting work for Viatris and Shionogi. M.R.-A. has served as a speaker for Pfizer, Gilead Sciences, and Shionogi. Mª.J.A.-M. has served as a speaker for Pfizer, MSD, and Shionogi. J.C.R.-R has served as a speaker for Shionogi. The remaining authors declare no conflict of interest.

References

1. Kollef, M.; Dupont, H.; Greenberg, D.E.; Viale, P.; Echols, R.; Yamano, Y.; Nicolau, D.P. Prospective role of cefiderocol in the management of carbapenem-resistant *Acinetobacter baumannii* infections: Review of the evidence. *Int. J. Antimicrob. Agents* **2023**, *62*, 106882. [CrossRef]
2. O'Donnell, J.N.; Putra, V.; Lodise, T.P. Treatment of patients with serious infections due to carbapenem-resistant *Acinetobacter baumannii*: How viable are the current options? *Pharmacotherapy* **2021**, *41*, 762–780. [CrossRef]
3. Cavallo, I.; Oliva, A.; Pages, R.; Sivori, F.; Truglio, M.; Fabrizio, G.; Pasqua, M.; Pimpinelli, F.; Di Domenico, E.G. *Acinetobacter baumannii* in the critically ill: Complex infections get complicated. *Front. Microbiol.* **2023**, *22*, 1196774. [CrossRef]
4. Borges Duarte, D.F.; Gonçalves Rodrigues, A. *Acinetobacter baumannii*: Insights towards a comprehensive approach for the prevention of outbreaks in health-care facilities. *APMIS* **2022**, *130*, 330–337. [CrossRef]
5. Shields, R.K.; Paterson, D.L.; Tamma, P.D. Navigating Available Treatment Options for Carbapenem-Resistant *Acinetobacter baumannii*-calcoaceticus Complex Infections. *Clin. Infect. Dis.* **2023**, *76* (Suppl. S2), S179–S193. [CrossRef]

6. Kyriakidis, I.; Vasileiou, E.; Pana, Z.D.; Tragiannidis, A. *Acinetobacter baumannii* Antibiotic Resistance Mechanisms. *Pathogens* **2021**, *10*, 373. [CrossRef]
7. Bassetti, M.; Castaldo, N.; Fantin, A.; Giacobbe, D.R.; Vena, A. Antibiotic therapy for nonfermenting Gram-negative bacilli infections: Future perspectives. *Curr. Opin. Infect. Dis.* **2023**, *36*, 615–622. [CrossRef]
8. Garnacho-Montero, J.; Gutiérrez-Pizarraya, A.; Díaz-Martín, A.; Cisneros-Herreros, J.M.; Cano, M.E.; Gato, E.; Ruiz de Alegría, C.; Fernández-Cuenca, F.; Vila, J.; Martínez-Martínez, L.; et al. *Acinetobacter baumannii* in critically ill patients: Molecular epidemiology, clinical features and predictors of mortality. *Enfermedades Infecc. Microbiol. Clin.* **2016**, *34*, 551–558. [CrossRef]
9. Tabah, A.; Buetti, N.; Staiquly, Q.; Ruckly, S.; Akova, M.; Aslan, A.T.; Leone, M.; Conway Morris, A.; Bassetti, M.; Arvaniti, K.; et al. Epidemiology and outcomes of hospital-acquired bloodstream infections in intensive care unit patients: The EUROBACT-2 international cohort study. *Intensive Care Med.* **2023**, *49*, 178–190. [CrossRef] [PubMed]
10. Falcone, M.; Tiseo, G.; Carbonara, S.; Marino, A.; Di Caprio, G.; Carretta, A.; Mularoni, A.; Mariani, M.F.; Maraolo, A.E.; Scotto, R.; et al. Mortality Attributable to Bloodstream Infections Caused by Different Carbapenem-Resistant Gram-Negative Bacilli: Results from a Nationwide Study in Italy (ALARICO Network). *Clin. Infect. Dis.* **2023**, *76*, 2059–2069. [CrossRef]
11. Luna, C.M.; Aruj, P.K. Nosocomial *Acinetobacter* pneumonia. *Respirology* **2007**, *12*, 787–791. [CrossRef]
12. Bouza, E.; Muñoz, P.; Burillo, A. How to treat severe *Acinetobacter baumannii* infections. *Curr. Opin. Infect. Dis.* **2023**, *36*, 596–608. [CrossRef]
13. Bassetti, M.; Vena, A.; Castaldo, N.; Giacobbe, D.R.; Peghin, M.; Grossi, P.A. Clinical evidence supporting cefiderocol for serious *Acinetobacter baumannii* infections. *Curr. Opin. Infect. Dis.* **2022**, *35*, 545–551. [CrossRef]
14. Bellomo, R.; Ronco, C.; Kellum, J.A.; Mehta, R.L.; Palevsky, P.; Acute Dialysis Quality Initiative Workgroup. Acute renal failure—Definition, outcome measures, animal models, fluid therapy and information technology needs: The Second International Consensus Conference of the Acute Dialysis Quality Initiative (ADQI) Group. *Crit. Care* **2004**, *8*, R204. [CrossRef]
15. CDC. CDC/NHSN Surveillance Definitions for Specific Types of Infections. 2024. Available online: https://www.cdc.gov/nhsn/pdfs/pscmanual/17pscnosinfdef_current.pdf (accessed on 1 January 2024).
16. Singer, M.; Deutschman, C.S.; Seymour, C.W.; Shankar-Hari, M.; Annane, D.; Bauer, M.; Bellomo, R.; Bernard, G.R.; Chiche, J.D.; Coopersmith, C.M.; et al. The Third International Consensus Definitions for Sepsis and Septic Shock (Sepsis-3). *JAMA* **2016**, *315*, 801–810. [CrossRef]
17. Zhou, S.; Zhang, X.H.; Zhang, Y.; Gong, G.; Yang, X.; Wan, W.H. The Age-Adjusted Charlson Comorbidity Index Predicts Prognosis in Elderly Cancer Patients. *Cancer Manag. Res.* **2022**, *14*, 1683–1691. [CrossRef]
18. Santos, R.P.; Mayo, T.W.; Siegel, J.D. Healthcare epidemiology: Active surveillance cultures and contact precautions for control of multidrug-resistant organisms: Ethical considerations. *Clin. Infect. Dis.* **2008**, *47*, 110–116. [CrossRef]
19. Palombo, M.; Bovo, F.; Amadesi, S.; Gaibani, P. Synergistic Activity of Cefiderocol in Combination with Piperacillin-Tazobactam, Fosfomycin, Ampicillin-Sulbactam, Imipenem-Relebactam and Ceftazidime-Avibactam against Carbapenem-Resistant Gram-Negative Bacteria. *Antibiotics* **2023**, *12*, 858. [CrossRef]
20. Mills, J.P.; Marchaim, D. Multidrug-Resistant Gram-Negative Bacteria: Infection Prevention and Control Update. *Infect. Dis. Clin. N. Am.* **2021**, *35*, 969–994. [CrossRef]
21. Corcione, S.; Lupia, T.; De Rosa, F.G.; Host and Microbiota Interaction Study Group (ESGHAMI) of the European Society of Clinical Microbiology and Infectious Diseases (ESCMID). Microbiome in the setting of burn patients: Implications for infections and clinical outcomes. *Burns Trauma* **2020**, *8*, tkaa033. [CrossRef]
22. Bartal, C.; Rolston, K.V.I.; Nesher, L. Carbapenem-resistant *Acinetobacter baumannii*: Colonization, Infection and Current Treatment Options. *Infect. Dis. Ther.* **2022**, *11*, 683–694. [CrossRef]
23. Patel, B.M.; Paratz, J.D.; Mallet, A.; Lipman, J.; Rudd, M.; Muller, M.J.; Paterson, D.L.; Roberts, J.A. Characteristics of bloodstream infections in burn patients: An 11-year retrospective study. *Burns* **2012**, *38*, 685–690. [CrossRef] [PubMed]
24. Ceniceros, A.; Pértega, S.; Galeiras, R.; Mourelo, M.; López, E.; Broullón, J.; Sousa, D.; Freire, D. Predicting mortality in burn patients with bacteraemia. *Infection* **2016**, *44*, 215–222. [CrossRef] [PubMed]
25. Tanaka Gutiez, M.; Efstathiou, N.; Innes, R.; Metaxa, V. End-of-life care in the intensive care unit. *Anaesthesia* **2023**, *78*, 636–643. [CrossRef] [PubMed]
26. Feldman, C.; Sprung, C.L.; Mentzelopoulos, S.D.; Pohrt, A.; Hartog, C.S.; Danbury, C.; Weiss, M.; Avidan, A.; Estella, A.; Joynt, G.M.; et al. Global Comparison of Communication of End-of-Life Decisions in the ICU. *Chest* **2022**, *162*, 1074–1085. [CrossRef]
27. Raddaoui, A.; Mabrouk, A.; Chebbi, Y.; Frigui, S.; Al-Gallas, N.; Abbassi, M.S.; Achour, W. Outbreak caused by pandrug-resistant blaOXA-69/blaOXA-23/blaGES harboring *Acinetobacter baumannii* ST2 in an intensive care unit. *Acta Microbiol. Immunol. Hung.* **2024**, *71*, 37–42. [CrossRef]
28. Osman, M.; Halimeh, F.B.; Rafei, R.; Mallat, H.; Tom, J.E.; Raad, E.B.; Diene, S.M.; Jamal, S.; Atrouni, A.A.; Dabboussi, F.; et al. Investigation of an XDR-*Acinetobacter baumannii* ST2 outbreak in an intensive care unit of a Lebanese tertiary care hospital. *Future Microbiol.* **2020**, *15*, 1535–1542. [CrossRef]
29. Baleivanualala, S.C.; Isaia, L.; Devi, S.V.; Howden, B.; Gorrie, C.L.; Matanitobua, S.; Sharma, S.; Wilson, D.; Kumar, S.; Maharaj, K.; et al. Molecular and clinical epidemiology of carbapenem resistant *Acinetobacter baumannii* ST2 in Oceania: A multicountry cohort study. *Lancet Reg. Health West. Pac.* **2023**, *40*, 100896. [CrossRef]
30. Danjean, M.; Hobson, C.A.; Gits-Muselli, M.; Courroux, C.; Monjault, A.; Bonacorsi, S.; Birgy, A. Evaluation of the inoculum effect of new antibiotics against carbapenem-resistant enterobacterales. *Clin. Microbiol. Infect.* **2022**, *28*, 1503.e1–1503.e3. [CrossRef]

31. Karakonstantis, S.; Rousaki, M.; Vassilopoulou, L.; Kritsotakis, E.I. Global prevalence of cefiderocol non-susceptibility in Enterobacterales, *Pseudomonas aeruginosa*, *Acinetobacter baumannii*, and *Stenotrophomonas maltophilia*: A systematic review and meta-analysis. *Clin. Microbiol. Infect.* **2024**, *30*, 178–188. [CrossRef]
32. Stracquadanio, S.; Nicolosi, A.; Privitera, G.F.; Massimino, M.; Marino, A.; Bongiorno, D.; Stefani, S. Role of transcriptomic and genomic analyses in improving the comprehension of cefiderocol activity in *Acinetobacter baumannii*. *mSphere* **2024**, *9*, e0061723. [CrossRef]
33. Shields, R.K.; Iovleva, A.; Kline, E.G.; Kawai, A.; McElheny, C.L.; Doi, Y. Clinical Evolution of AmpC-Mediated Ceftazidime-Avibactam and Cefiderocol Resistance in *Enterobacter cloacae* Complex Following Exposure to Cefepime. *Clin. Infect. Dis.* **2020**, *71*, 2713–2716. [CrossRef]
34. Smoke, S.M.; Brophy, A.; Reveron, S.; Iovleva, A.; Kline, E.G.; Marano, M.; Miller, L.P.; Shields, R.K. Evolution and Transmission of Cefiderocol-Resistant *Acinetobacter baumannii* During an Outbreak in the Burn Intensive Care Unit. *Clin. Infect. Dis.* **2023**, *76*, e1261–e1265. [CrossRef]
35. Merino, M.; Poza, M.; Roca, I.; Barba, M.J.; Sousa, M.D.; Vila, J.; Bou, G. Nosocomial outbreak of a multiresistant *Acinetobacter baumannii* expressing OXA-23 carbapenemase in Spain. *Microb. Drug Resist.* **2014**, *20*, 259–263. [CrossRef]
36. Gagnaire, J.; Gagneux-Brunon, A.; Pouvaret, A.; Grattard, F.; Carricajo, A.; Favier, H.; Mattei, A.; Pozzetto, B.; Nuti, C.; Lucht, F.; et al. Carbapenemase-producing *Acinetobacter baumannii*: An outbreak report with special highlights on economic burden. *Med. Mal. Infect.* **2017**, *47*, 279–285. [CrossRef]
37. Kolesnik-Goldmann, N.; Seth-Smith, H.M.B.; Haldimann, K.; Imkamp, F.; Roloff, T.; Zbinden, R.; Hobbie, S.N.; Egli, A.; Mancini, S. Com parison of Disk Diffusion, E-Test, and Broth Microdilution Methods for Testing In Vitro Activity of Cefiderocol in Acinetobacter baumannii. *Antibiotics* **2023**, *12*, 1212. [CrossRef]
38. Bianco, G.; Boattini, M.; Comini, S.; Banche, G.; Cavallo, R.; Costa, C. Disc Diffusion and ComASP® Cefiderocol Microdilution Panel to Overcome the Challenge of Cefiderocol Susceptibility Testing in Clinical Laboratory Routine. *Antibiotics* **2023**, *12*, 604. [CrossRef] [PubMed]
39. Matuschek, E.; Longshaw, C.; Takemura, M.; Yamano, Y.; Kahlmeter, G. Cefiderocol: EUCAST criteria for disc diffusion and broth microdilution for antimicrobial susceptibility testing. *J. Antimicrob. Chemother.* **2022**, *77*, 1662–1669. [CrossRef] [PubMed]
40. Dortet, L.; Niccolai, C.; Pfennigwerth, N.; Frisch, S.; Gonzalez, C.; Antonelli, A.; Giani, T.; Hoenings, R.; Gatermann, S.; Rossolini, G.M.; et al. Performance evaluation of the UMIC® Cefiderocol to determine MIC in Gram-negative bacteria. *J. Antimicrob. Chemother.* **2023**, *78*, 1672–1676. [CrossRef]
41. Delgado-Valverde, M.; Portillo-Calderón, I.; Recacha, E.; Pérez-Palacios, P.; Pascual, A. In Vitro Activity of Cefiderocol Compared to Other Antimicrobials against a Collection of Metallo-Beta-Lactamase-Producing Gram-Negative Bacilli from Southern Spain. *Microbiol. Spectr.* **2023**, *11*, e0493622. [CrossRef] [PubMed]
42. Lodise, T.P.; Yucel, E.; Obi, E.N.; Watanabe, A.H.; Nathanson, B.H. Incidence of acute kidney injury (AKI) and its impact on patient outcomes among adult hospitalized patients with carbapenem-resistant Gram-negative infections who received targeted treatment with a newer β-lactam or β-lactam/β-lactamase inhibitor-, polymyxin- or aminoglycoside-containing regimen. *J. Antimicrob. Chemother.* **2024**, *79*, 82–95.
43. Paul, M.; Carrara, E.; Retamar, P.; Tängdén, T.; Bitterman, R.; Bonomo, R.A.; de Waele, J.; Daikos, G.L.; Akova, M.; Harbarth, S.; et al. European Society of Clinical Microbiology and Infectious Diseases (ESCMID) guidelines for the treatment of infections caused by multidrug-resistant Gram-negative bacilli (endorsed by European society of intensive care medicine). *Clin. Microbiol. Infect.* **2022**, *28*, 521–547. [CrossRef]
44. Tamma, P.D.; Heil, E.L.; Justo, J.A.; Mathers, A.J.; Satlin, M.J.; Bonomo, R.A. Infectious Diseases Society of America Antimicrobial-Resistant Treatment Guidance: Gram-Negative Bacterial Infections. Infectious Diseases Society of America 2024; Version 4.0. Available online: https://www.idsociety.org/practice-guideline/amr-guidance/ (accessed on 14 July 2024).
45. Bassetti, M.; Echols, R.; Matsunaga, Y.; Ariyasu, M.; Doi, Y.; Ferrer, R.; Lodise, T.P.; Naas, T.; Niki, Y.; Paterson, D.L.; et al. Efficacy and safety of cefiderocol or best available therapy for the treatment of serious infections caused by carbapenem-resistant Gram-negative bacteria (CREDIBLE-CR): A randomised, open-label, multicentre, pathogen-focused, descriptive, phase 3 trial. *Lancet Infect. Dis.* **2021**, *21*, 226–240. [CrossRef] [PubMed]
46. Falcone, M.; Tiseo, G.; Leonildi, A.; Della Sala, L.; Vecchione, A.; Barnini, S.; Farcomeni, A.; Menichetti, F. Cefiderocol- Compared to Colistin-Based Regimens for the Treatment of Severe Infections Caused by Carbapenem-Resistant *Acinetobacter baumannii*. *Antimicrob. Agents Chemother.* **2022**, *66*, e0214221. [CrossRef]
47. Russo, A.; Bruni, A.; Gullì, S.; Borrazzo, C.; Quirino, A.; Lionello, R.; Serapide, F.; Garofalo, E.; Serraino, R.; Romeo, F.; et al. Efficacy of cefiderocol- vs colistin-containing regimen for treatment of bacteraemic ventilator-associated pneumonia caused by carbapenem-resistant *Acinetobacter baumannii* in patients with COVID-19. *Int. J. Antimicrob. Agents* **2023**, *62*, 106825. [CrossRef]
48. Pascale, R.; Pasquini, Z.; Bartoletti, M.; Caiazzo, L.; Fornaro, G.; Bussini, L.; Volpato, F.; Marchionni, E.; Rinaldi, M.; Trapani, F.; et al. Cefiderocol treatment for carbapenem-resistant *Acinetobacter baumannii* infection in the ICU during the COVID-19 pandemic: A multicentre cohort study. *JAC Antimicrob. Resist.* **2021**, *3*, dlab174. [CrossRef]
49. Dalfino, L.; Stufano, M.; Bavaro, D.F.; Diella, L.; Belati, A.; Stolfa, S.; Romanelli, F.; Ronga, L.; Di Mussi, R.; Murgolo, F.; et al. Effectiveness of First-Line Therapy with Old and Novel Antibiotics in Ventilator-Associated Pneumonia Caused by Carbapenem-Resistant *Acinetobacter baumannii*: A Real Life, Prospective, Observational, Single-Center Study. *Antibiotics* **2023**, *12*, 1048. [CrossRef] [PubMed]

50. Gatti, M.; Cosentino, F.; Giannella, M.; Viale, P.; Pea, F. Clinical efficacy of cefiderocol-based regimens in patients with carbapenem-resistant *Acinetobacter baumannii* infections: A systematic review with meta-analysis. *Int. J. Antimicrob. Agents* **2024**, *63*, 107047. [CrossRef] [PubMed]
51. Onorato, L.; de Luca, I.; Monari, C.; Coppola, N. Cefiderocol either in monotherapy or combination versus best available therapy in the treatment of carbapenem-resistant *Acinetobacter baumannii* infections: A systematic review and meta-analysis. *J. Infect.* **2024**, *88*, 106113. [CrossRef]
52. Karruli, A.; Migliaccio, A.; Pournaras, S.; Durante-Mangoni, E.; Zarrilli, R. Cefiderocol and Sulbactam-Durlobactam against Carbapenem-Resistant *Acinetobacter baumannii*. *Antibiotics* **2023**, *12*, 1729. [CrossRef]
53. Bassetti, M.; Vena, A.; Giacobbe, D.R. Management of nonfermenting gram-negative infections: A critique of the guidelines. *Curr. Opin. Infect. Dis.* **2023**, *36*, 609–614. [CrossRef]
54. Gill, C.M.; Santini, D.; Takemura, M.; Longshaw, C.; Yamano, Y.; Echols, R.; Nicolau, D.P. In vivo efficacy & resistance prevention of cefiderocol in combination with ceftazidime/avibactam, ampicillin/sulbactam or meropenem using human-simulated regimens versus *Acinetobacter baumannii*. *J. Antimicrob. Chemother.* **2023**, *78*, 983–990. [PubMed]
55. Liu, X.; Lei, T.; Yang, Y.; Zhang, L.; Liu, H.; Leptihn, S.; Yu, Y.; Hua, X. Structural Basis of PER-1-Mediated Cefiderocol Resistance and Synergistic Inhibition of PER-1 by Cefiderocol in Combination with Avibactam or Durlobactam in *Acinetobacter baumannii*. *Antimicrob. Agents Chemother.* **2022**, *66*, e0082822. [CrossRef] [PubMed]
56. Mezcord, V.; Wong, O.; Pasteran, F.; Corso, A.; Tolmasky, M.E.; Bonomo, R.A.; Ramirez, M.S. Role of β-lactamase inhibitors on cefiderocol activity against carbapenem-resistant *Acinetobacter* species. *Int. J. Antimicrob. Agents* **2023**, *61*, 106700. [CrossRef] [PubMed]
57. Wong, O.; Mezcord, V.; Lopez, C.; Traglia, G.M.; Pasteran, F.; Tuttobene, M.R.; Corso, A.; Tolmasky, M.E.; Bonomo, R.A.; Ramirez, M.S. Hetero-antagonism of avibactam and sulbactam with cefiderocol in carbapenem-resistant *Acinetobacter* spp. *bioRxiv* **2024**. [CrossRef]

antibiotics MDPI

Article

Catastrophic *Streptococcus pyogenes* Disease: A Personalized Approach Based on Phenotypes and Treatable Traits

Juan Carlos Ruiz-Rodríguez [1,2,3], Luis Chiscano-Camón [1,2,3,*], Carolina Maldonado [1,2], Adolf Ruiz-Sanmartin [1,2], Laura Martin [1,2], Ivan Bajaña [1,2], Juliana Bastidas [1,2], Rocio Lopez-Martinez [4], Clara Franco-Jarava [4], Juan José González-López [5], Vicent Ribas [6], Nieves Larrosa [5], Jordi Riera [1,2], Xavier Nuvials-Casals [1,2] and Ricard Ferrer [1,2,3]

1 Intensive Care Department, Vall d'Hebron University Hospital, Vall d'Hebron Barcelona Hospital Campus, 08035 Barcelona, Spain; juancarlos.ruiz@vallhebron.cat (J.C.R.-R.); carolina.maldonado@vallhebron.cat (C.M.); adolfo.ruiz@vallhebron.cat (A.R.-S.); laura.martinsanchez@vallhebron.cat (L.M.); ivanrene.bajana@vallhebron.cat (I.B.); juliana.bastidas@vallhebron.cat (J.B.); jordi.rieradelbrio@vallhebron.cat (J.R.); xavier.nuvials@vallhebron.cat (X.N.-C.)

2 Shock, Organ Dysfunction and Resuscitation Research Group, Vall d'Hebron Research Institute (VHIR), Vall d'Hebron University Hospital, Vall d'Hebron Barcelona Hospital Campus, 08035 Barcelona, Spain

3 Departament of Medicine, Universitat Autonoma de Barcelona, 08193 Barcelona, Spain

4 Immunology Department, Vall d'Hebron University Hospital, Vall d'Hebron Barcelona Hospital Campus, 08035 Barcelona, Spain; rocio.lopez@vallhebron.cat (R.L.-M.); clfranco.hj23.ics@gencat.cat (C.F.-J.)

5 Microbiology Department, Vall d'Hebron University Hospital, Vall d'Hebron Barcelona Hospital Campus, 08035 Barcelona, Spain; juanjo.gonzalez@vallhebron.cat (J.J.G.-L.); nieves.larrosa@vallhebron.cat (N.L.)

6 Eurecat, Centre Tecnològic de Catalunya, EHealth Unit, 08005 Barcelona, Spain; vicent.ribas@eurecat.org

* Correspondence: luissilvestre.chiscano@vallhebron.cat; Tel.: +34-6595-84804

Abstract: Streptococcal toxic shock syndrome (STTS) is a critical medical emergency marked by high morbidity and mortality, necessitating swift awareness, targeted treatment, and early source control due to its rapid symptom manifestation. This report focuses on a cohort of 13 patients admitted to Vall d'Hebron University Hospital Intensive Care Unit, Barcelona, from November 2022 to March 2023, exhibiting invasive *Streptococcus pyogenes* infections and meeting institutional sepsis code activation criteria. The primary infections were community-acquired pneumonia (61.5%) and skin/soft tissue infection (30.8%). All patients received prompt antibiotic treatment, with clinical source control through thoracic drainage (30.8%) or surgical means (23.1%). Organ support involved invasive mechanical ventilation, vasopressors, and continuous renal replacement therapy as per guidelines. Of note, 76.9% of patients experienced septic cardiomyopathy, and 53.8% required extracorporeal membrane oxygenation (ECMO). The study identified three distinct phenotypic profiles—hyperinflammatory, low perfusion, and hypogammaglobulinemic—which could guide personalized therapeutic approaches. STTS, with a mean SOFA score of 17 (5.7) and a 53.8% requiring ECMO, underscores the need for precision medicine-based rescue therapies and sepsis phenotype identification. Integrating these strategies with prompt antibiotics and efficient source control offers a potential avenue to mitigate organ failure, enhancing patient survival and recovery in the face of this severe clinical condition.

Keywords: severe sepsis; septic shock; multiorgan dysfunction; precision medicine; hemoadsorption; *S. pyogenes*; sepsis phenotypes; streptococcal toxic shock syndrome

1. Introduction

A significant increase in invasive group A streptococcal (GAS) infections has been observed since September 2022 [1,2] in several European countries and the USA. In our geographical area different series have already been published, showing an increase in their incidence [3]. Streptococcal toxic shock syndrome (STSS) is a critical life-threatening condition, including invasive infections principally by group A streptococcus (GAS, *S. pyogenes*) [4].

1.1. Streptococcal Pathophysiology

Streptococcal infections are quite prevalent and can result in a range of conditions, varying from self-limiting to severe disease, including bacteremia, pneumonia, meningitis, endocarditis, arthritis, sinusitis, and infections of soft tissues such as necrotizing fasciitis and myositis [5]. The precise mechanism of STSS is not fully understood. However, it is linked to a cascade of effects involving streptococcal toxins, including enterotoxins with superantigenic properties and other streptococcal enzymes and toxins. These elements interact with the host immune system in a particular manner [6].

One commonly accepted premise is that bacterial pathogens must initially establish close contact with extracellular matrix proteins (ECM) in host cells to establish a successful infection. Highly specific adhesins facilitate this initial interaction with ECM proteins or cells. These adhesins and other macromolecules that provoke the internalization of bacteria or the invasion of host cells are collectively called "invasins". Streptococci, in particular, is characterized by an extensive and highly variable array of adhesins and invaders. The expression of these proteins is subject to differential regulation and is influenced by signals from various environments within the human host [7,8]. Given the diverse repertoire of adhesins and invasins in streptococci, these pathogens have developed multiple strategies to achieve internalization and survival within host cells, including evading antibiotic actions and host immune responses [9,10].

Recognization and attachment to diverse ECM proteins are crucial steps in the streptococcal colonization of human tissues. Firstly, lipoteichoic acid (LTA) is thought to mediate the first step of adhesion with low cellular specificity [11]. Then, the expression of the hyaluronic acid (HyA) capsule protects against phagocytosis by immune system cells. The HyA capsule can act as a non-protein adhesin by binding to the HyA receptor CD44 on skin keratinocytes [12]. Most importantly, the interaction between HyA and CD44 receptors leads to cytoskeletal rearrangements in human epithelial cells. These rearrangements disrupt intracellular junctions and allow the dissemination of streptococci into deeper, underlying sterile tissue [13]. Models of human skin indicated that cell signaling triggered by the interaction of the GAS capsule with CD44 opened intercellular junctions and promoted tissue penetration by GAS through a paracellular route with no evident portal of entry on many occasions [14]. M protein [15] and the C5a peptidase [16] also contribute to skin invasion, granting bacterial aggregation, which may also be crucial for colonization, resistance to phagocytosis, and the subsequent invasion of cells. Next, in a stationary phase, once the invasion has occurred, the production of exotoxins, such as streptolysin, streptokinase, or hyaluronidase, triggers platelet and leukocyte aggregation, and, more importantly, the production of superantigens leading to the polyclonal activation of lymphocytes, the inflammatory cytokine storm cascade, and the state of shock, the third phase of GAS infection.

Classically, the clinical presentation of STSS is described in three phases. The third one, which is the one we will focus on, is characterized by a severe distributive shock associated with multiple organ dysfunction. Despite aggressive therapy, many patients will die within 24 to 48 h of admission.

1.2. Streptococcal Pathophysiology Related to Septic Shock Management

The latest edition of the Surviving Sepsis Campaign (SSC) guidelines underscores the necessity for precise and protocolized care in managing septic shock [17]. Implementing such measures is linked to a significant decrease in mortality [18]. However, mortality from infection in its sepsis version remains high [19]. Certain patient subsets unresponsive to standard treatments might find relief in alternative therapies, viewed as rescue interventions. The existing consensus description of sepsis, encompassing "life-threatening organ dysfunction resulting from a dysregulated host response to infection", is expansive, capturing the inherent diversity of the ailment [20]. The diversity in this situation stems from multiple factors: varying infection causes, unique comorbidities and genetics in individual hosts, and differences in the timing of diagnosis and treatment among patients.

These elements influence the progression of sepsis at the individual patient level and their reactions to therapeutic interventions.

Seymour et al. [21], utilizing an extensive database, characterized four distinct sepsis phenotypes based on varied demographics, laboratory parameters, and patterns of organ dysfunction. These were found to correlate with biomarker concentrations and mortality rates. The identification of these phenotypes suggests the potential benefit of more targeted and personalized therapeutic approaches for patients at a heightened risk of clinical deterioration [22]. The emergence of these challenges underscores the importance of precision medicine. Precision medicine enables the customization of healthcare interventions for specific patient groups, taking into account factors such as disease susceptibility, diagnosis, prognosis, and treatment response.

1.3. Objectives of This Study

In this report, the objective is to describe a population of patients who are mostly in severe septic shock and multiorganic dysfunction due to STSS, highlighting certain aspects of the inflammatory and immunological response that can determine the application of precision medicine.

2. Results

Our study includes a population of 13 patients (demographic and clinical characteristics are described in Table 1, and analytical characteristics during the first 24 h are described in Table 2) without any significant comorbidity. The predominant infection source was community-acquired pneumonia (61.5%) and skin and soft tissue infections (30.8%). Regarding microbiology, positive peripheral blood cultures were identified in five (38.5%) cases. Notably, there were seven viral coinfections mainly due to the Influenza B virus (FLUBV) (38.5%). No previous use of NSAIDs was reported.

Table 1. Characteristics of the study population. The data have been expressed as "n" (%) if they are categorical and as median (interquartile range) or mean (standard deviation) if they are quantitative.

		n = 13
Age [years, m (SD)]		42 (13.8)
Gender [n (%)]	Female	7 (53.8)
	Male	6 (46.2)
Comorbidities [n (%)]	Hypertension	3 (23.1)
	Obesity	1 (7.7)
	Cardiac	1 (7.7)
	Inmunosuppression	2 (15.4)
	Peripheral Vascular Disease	1 (7.7)
APACHE II [m (SD)]		29 (15)
SOFA [m (SD)]		17 ± 5.7
Infection source [n (%)]	Respiratory	8 (61.5)
	SSTIs	4 (30.8)
	PID	1 (7.7)
Source control [n (%)]	Thorax Drainage	4 (30.8)
	Surgery	3 (23.1)
Coinfection [n (%)]	FLUB-V	5 (38.5)
	Metapneumovirus	2 (15.4)

Table 1. *Cont.*

		n = 13
Microbiologic culture-positive tests	Isolated PBC [n (%)]	5 (38.5)
	PBC + BAL [n (%)]	2 (15.4)
	Bronchoalveolar lavage [n (%)]	4 (31)
	Skin/soft tissue [n (%)]	1 (7.7)
	PBC + Ascitic fluid [n (%)]	1 (7.7)
Septic Shock [n (%)]		13 (100)
Septic Cardiomyopathy [n (%)]		10 (76.9)
Cardiovascular SOFA [m (SD)]		4 (0.6)
Dobutamine use [n (%)]		10 (76.9)
Hydrocortisone [n (%)]		13 (100)
IMV [n (%)]		9 (69.2)
ECMO (VA. VV) [n (%)]	Total [n(%)]	7 (53.8)
	VA [n(%)] Low perfusion phenotype	5 (38.4)
CRRT [n (%)]		10 (76.9)
HA [n (%)]	(total)	10 (76.9)
	Cytosorb®	9 (69.2)
	Toraymixin®	6 (46.2)
	Oxiris®	2 (15.4)
Sequential hemoadsorption [n (%)]	Cytosorb® + Toraymixin®	6 (46.2)
Low IgG [n (%)]		9 (69.2)
Cytokine HA duration [hours, m (SD)]		50 (34)
Length of ICU stay [days, m (SD)]		33 (40)
Length of hospital stay [days, m (SD)]		54.85 (42)
ICU mortality [n (%)]		3 (23.1%)
In hospital mortality [n (%)]		3 (23.1%)

APACHE—Acute Physiology And Chronic Health Evaluation; BAL—Bronchoalveolar lavage; CRRT—continuous renal replacement therapy; ECMO—extracorporeal membrane oxygenation (VA—venoarterial, VV—venovenous); FLUB-V—Influenza-B virus; HA—hemoadsorption; ICU—intensive care unit; IMV—invasive mechanical ventilation; m—mean; n—number of population; PBC—peripheral blood culture; PID—Pelvic Inflammatory Disease; SD—standard deviation; SOFA—sequential organ failure assessment; SSTIs—Skin and Soft Tissue Infections.

Table 2. Analytical characteristics of the study population. The data have been expressed as "n" (%) if they are categorical and as median (interquartile range) or mean (standard deviation) if they are quantitative.

Analytical Characteristics of the Study Population	
Leukocyte count [(/mm^3) m (SD)]	6670 (6868)
Lymphocyte count [(/mm^3) m (SD)]	261 (180)
Neutrophil count [(/mm^3) m (SD)]	5863 (6546)

Table 2. *Cont.*

Analytical Characteristics of the Study Population	
CRP [(mg/dL) m (SD)]	25.83 (11)
PCT [(ng/mL) m (SD)]	167.33 (203)
IL-6 [(pg/mL) m (SD)]	108,110.45 (104,325)
IgG [(mg/dL) m (SD)]	402 (230)
IgM [(mg/dL) m (SD)]	61.5 (29)
IgA [(mg/dL) m (SD)]	130 (77)
EAA [m (SD)]	0.93 (0.33)
Platelet count [($\times 10^9$/L) m (SD)]	105,000 (61,000)
Ferritin [(ng/mL) m (SD)]	2495 (3155)

CRP—C-reactive protein; EAA—Endotoxin Activity Assay; Ig—immunoglobulin, IL—interleukin; m—mean; n—number of population; PCT—procalcitonin; SD—standard deviation;.

2.1. General Management and Conventional Organ Support

All patients received early antibiotic treatment with Penicillin G and Clindamycin, in addition to empirical Meropenem, within the first 72 h of disease onset. Meropenem was withdrawn after other sources of infection were ruled out. Clindamycin [23] was used for 3 days in all cases, and Penicillin G was employed until resolution of the source of infection (extended regimens were administered in cases of necrotizing pneumonia or skin wounds until clinical or radiological resolution). Thus, individualized regimens were prescribed. Source control was performed by thoracic drainage (30.8%) or other measures for surgical control (23.1%). Organ support was provided through invasive mechanical ventilation (IMV) [24]. Vasopressors and continuous renal replacement therapy (CRRT) [25] were also administered in compliance with clinical guidelines. Corticosteroid therapy, in the form of hydrocortisone administered at 50 mg intervals every six hours, was incorporated as a component of septic shock management. Hydrocortisone has been used until withdrawal of vasoactive drugs or resolution of shock, with tapering if administered for more than seven days.

2.2. Personalized Treatment

Our study focused on a subgroup of patients with severe septic shock who met the criteria for STSS, as indicated by a mean SOFA score of 17 (with a standard deviation of 5.7) points. We describe different phenotypes that may result in a personalized approach based on treatable traits: hyperinflammatory, low perfusion, or hypogammaglobulinemic profile.

Implementing this multi-faceted approach was based on phenotypic considerations; regardless of an anticipated high mortality risk predicted to exceed 50% according to SOFA or APACHE II criteria [26–28], the survival rate was 77%.

2.2.1. Hyperinflammatory Phenotype

Personalized therapies were employed utilizing cytokine hemoadsorption (HA) (Cytosorb® (CytoSorbents (Corporation, Monmouth Junction, NJ, USA)) and endotoxin HA (Toraymixin® (Toray, Tokyo, Japan)) (76.9%), guided by biomarker assessment. Specifically, patients treated with Cytosorb® or Toraymixin® exhibited plasmatic concentrations of IL-6 of 108, 110.45 (104,325) pg/mL and Endotoxin Activity (EAA) of 0.93 (0.33), respectively. A sequential HA (cytokine HA followed by endotoxin HA) was implemented in six (46.2%) cases.

2.2.2. Low Perfusion Phenotype

Notably, 76.9% of cases exhibited septic cardiomyopathy coupled with severe multiorgan dysfunction. Moreover, 53.8% of patients were supported by extracorporeal membrane oxygenation (ECMO) therapy, either as a response to distributive shock (specifically, five (38.4%) patients required venoarterial ECMO] or in the face of refractory hypoxemia.

2.2.3. Low Immunoglobulin Phenotype

Hypogammaglobulinemia was defined by gammaglobulins (IgG) levels falling below 500 mg/dL or two standard deviations below reference values for age [29]. The administration of 2 g/kg of polyclonal gammaglobulin was promptly initiated upon clinical suspicion of STSS. Furthermore, patients showing plasma IgG concentrations below 500 mg/dL received 250 mg/kg/d administered via a 10 h infusion over three consecutive days. Nine (69.2%) patients exhibited low immunoglobulin phenotype.

3. Discussion

Sepsis and septic shock should be considered diverse diseases encompassing various clinical trajectories and distinct phenotypic expressions. Given its association with heightened mortality risk, patients afflicted with this condition necessitate a meticulously structured and protocol-driven therapeutic approach. The fundamental sepsis management principles, including infection control, initial resuscitation, and comprehensive organ support, form the cornerstones of treatment. Yet, personalized interventions targeting specific pathophysiological mechanisms can significantly benefit specific patient phenotypes. In the context of STSS, combining immunoglobulin and hemoperfusion may benefit severe cases with septic shock and multiple organ failure admitted to the ICU [30,31], complementing the core management bundles. Within our studied population, we identified three distinct phenotypic profiles that merit discussion: the hyperinflammatory profile characterized by elevated cytokine levels or pronounced endotoxemia, the low perfusion phenotype, and the low immunoglobulin (Ig) phenotype (Table 3).

Table 3. Distinguishing between phenotypes in patients with severe septic shock due, based on identifiable treatable traits.

Precision Medicine Strategies		Target (s)	Clinical Application
Hyperinflammatory profile	High endotoxinemia	Endotoxinemia	Rescue therapy Hemoadsorption
	Severe hypercytokinemia	Cytokine levels	
	Sequential hemoadsorption	Endotoxin and cytokine hemoadsorption	
Low perfusion phenotype	Patients with septic cardiomyopathy		ECMO venoarterial
Low immunoglobulin phenotype	Sepsis-associated hypogammaglobulinemia250 mg/kg/d by a 10 h infusion for 3 consecutive days		

In the current body of literature, a range of terms have been used to describe presentations of septic shock, particularly those indicating a poor prognosis. In critically ill adult patients, commonly used terms include "refractory septic shock", "catecholamine resistance", or "high dose norepinephrine". However, it is essential to highlight that there is no universally agreed-upon consensus regarding exact definitions for these medical situations [32]. Distinguishing between phenotypes of patients with severe septic shock due to STSS based on identifiable treatable features has the potential to improve patient outcomes.

3.1. Hyperinflammation with High Cytokine Phenotype

The use of HA therapy as a rescue therapy may be considered in a situation of septic shock and multiorgan dysfunction refractory to standard treatment. Cytokine HA may have a role as rescue therapy in a particular subgroup of patients with severe septic shock, hyperlactatemia, multiorgan failure, and very high hypercytokinemia. There is no threshold of plasma cytokine levels for initiating or withholding the therapy. In this context, blood purification techniques have the potential to attenuate the inflammatory process, exerting a swiftly substantial, non-selective impact on the cytokine storm. Using adsorption cartridges in STSS may introduce a novel therapeutic approach for severe cases. Their effectiveness in regulating proinflammatory mediators, which play a significant role in cellular toxicity and organ dysfunction, could prove pivotal in lowering the mortality rate [33]. Plasmapheresis has been proposed to manage STSS, but the evidence for its use is still low, based on isolated case reports [34]. Still, certain pharmacokinetic drawbacks of HA cannot be overlooked, such as variations in antibiotic plasmatic concentrations [35]. In any case, it is important to monitor antibiotic levels, specifically when the periods of HA are long. Cytokine HA is a safe procedure without relevant associated adverse effects [36]. In our case, no adverse effects were observed.

3.2. *Hyperinflammatory with High Endotoxemic Phenotype*

Endotoxin has been identified as one of the therapeutic targets for sepsis and septic shock. The elimination of endotoxin through blood purification techniques, specifically via HA, has been proposed [37]. Endotoxemia and the excessive production of inflammatory mediators, manifested as a cytokine storm, are linked to the severity of sepsis and septic shock, influencing patient prognosis [38]. Klein et al. [39] performed a post-hoc analysis on the Euphrates trial [40] on 194 patients with EAA between 0.6–0.89. A survival benefit was observed in patients who received polymyxin (PMX) hemofilter therapy. In a review of recent studies, Shoji et al. [41] demonstrated a survival benefit of PMX hemoperfusion. Lately, in a multicenter, prospective, and observational study, it was reported that the baseline EAA may predict the outcome of critically ill septic patients receiving PMX-HA [42]. It is thus justifiable to consider patients experiencing septic shock and severe multiorgan dysfunction, with well-managed control of the infectious source and an EAA of 0.6–0.9, as potential candidates for endotoxin HA.

3.3. *Sequential Approach*

Current practice has shown that HA helps in the recovery of immune homeostasis. However, for certain patients, endotoxin-only adsorption may be insufficient [43]. Sequential HA (endotoxin HA with PMX, Toraymixin®, and subsequent cytokine HA with Cytosorb®) has been implemented in highly selected patients [44]. Sequential HA is intended to remove the primary stimulus that induces the dysregulated inflammatory response. Candidates for sequential HA include patients experiencing septic shock, multi-organ dysfunction, elevated endotoxemia, and hypercytokinemia (particularly extremely high levels of IL-6). Continuous monitoring of plasma cytokines (IL-6, IL-10) can provide guidance to clinicians for therapy management.

3.4. *Low Perfusion Phenotype*

We introduced the term "low perfusion" to categorize patients experiencing septic cardiomyopathy, characterized by insufficient perfusion even when on vasoactive agents and receiving supportive treatment tailored to other phenotypes. The use of mechanical circulatory support continues to be a subject of debate in the management of refractory septic shock among adult patients [45]. The venoarterial (VA) configuration of ECMO support presents an appealing choice for shock management, particularly in patients experiencing severe concurrent cardiac and pulmonary failure. However, high-quality evidence supporting its use in adults is still limited. Riera et al. [46] conducted a review highlighting extracorporeal membrane oxygenation (ECMO) as a supportive method rather than a treatment. The authors pointed out that with an appropriate configuration and well-defined management, this method may rescue specific adult septic patients with no other survival options.

3.5. Low Immunoglobulin Phenotype

The supplemental utilization of intravenous immunoglobulin (IVIG) in STSS is theoretically justified by its anti-inflammatory and immunomodulatory properties. Additionally, supporting evidence comes from observational studies and one historically controlled trial [47]. The INSTINCT trial found no significant distinction between the placebo and intervention groups in relation to the primary outcome, which involved evaluating functional status through the Physical Component Summary (PCS) score of the 36-item short-form health survey (SF-36) six months after randomization. In addition, mortality and multiple organ failure did not show differences. However, it is important to note that patients with confirmed STSS accounted for less than 10% of the study population, making it challenging to draw definitive conclusions for this subgroup. In line with guidelines from the Infectious Diseases Society of America (IDSA), there is an emphasis on the necessity for further studies to assess the efficacy of IVIG for this particular indication [48]. Hence, recommending the routine use of IVIG in STSS is not feasible, and decisions should be made case-by-case. SSC guidelines provide a weak recommendation for the use of immunoglobulins (Ig) as a treatment for septic patients due to the low certainty of evidence in the main studies [49] and meta-analyses [50]. This SSC recommendation should be limited only to patients with normoglobulinemia since the studies have not assessed the status of immunoglobulins as an inclusion criterion. However, it is reasonable that in septic shock and multiorgan failure, IVIG could be beneficial in the presence of hypogammaglobulinemia. Polyvalent intravenous immunoglobulins represent a promising approach to modulating pro- and anti-inflammatory responses [51]. The optimal dosing and timing of administration of IVIG in STSS is uncertain. The treatment with polyclonal gammaglobulin of 1 or 2 g/kg is accepted (level of evidence 2C) [52]. In another study, projecting information beyond the existing data, RCTs in Kawasaki disease were recommended for early treatment with a high dose (2 g/kg) [53]. Other strategies proposed IgM- and IgA-enriched polyclonal IVIG doses of 250 mg/kg/d using a 10 h infusion for 3 consecutive days [54].

3.6. STSS and Its Relation to Precision Medicine Guided by Phenotypes

There is considerable variability in sepsis features among patients due to differences in age, causative microorganisms, focus type, and patient comorbidities. At the pathophysiological level, the inflammatory response manifests in two stages: the proinflammatory response and the anti-inflammatory response, which can differ among individuals or even within the same individual based on the severity continuum they are experiencing.

The emergence of initiatives aimed at enhancing sepsis diagnosis and treatment has been observed in recent years. Precision medicine introduces a novel approach to patient management, allowing specific subgroups to benefit from therapeutic strategies that may not be suitable for the general sepsis patient population. Sepsis management involves well-structured, protocolized interventions subject to continuous revision, as emphasized throughout the manuscript. While all patients should undergo the fundamental pillars of sepsis treatment—infection control, initial resuscitation, and multiorgan support—certain subpopulations may benefit more from tailored therapies.

Due to the diverse nature of sepsis, clinical progression varies among patients. Low-risk patients may undergo conventional management to ensure a favorable prognosis. In contrast, high-risk patients, prone to organ dysfunction and mortality, may necessitate adjuvant-specific therapies aligned with their pathophysiological characteristics. This diversity underscores the emergence of precision medicine in sepsis, aiming to individualize the management of septic patients by identifying distinct endotypes or subgroups based on genetic or biological dissimilarities. Precision medicine facilitates the characterization of homogeneous patient subgroups exhibiting similar evolutionary patterns and responses to specific treatments.

Certainly, we acknowledge that treatments based on these phenotypes are not yet supported by evidence in the form of randomized clinical trials. Therefore, they are not recommended by the SSC guidelines. We want to emphasize this point conscientiously.

However, subgroups of patients refractory to conventional treatments could benefit from specific treatments based on phenotype characterization. These are patients with a high risk of mortality and are often not included in randomized studies. Their accurate identification and selection could lead to an improvement in survival rates.

In our series, it is imperative to underscore the timely initiation of antibiotic therapy and source control and the integration of precision medicine tailored to sepsis phenotypes, incorporating gammaglobulin supplementation. The application of hemoadsorptive treatments, guided by real-time monitoring of cytokine levels and endotoxemia, along with the strategic utilization of ECMO in its various configurations, has culminated in a survival rate of 77%. This outcome notably surpasses the mortality rates anticipated by the SOFA and APACHE II scoring classification systems.

In the realm of precision medicine, focusing on STSS, interventions for modulation of the inflammatory cascade can include the use of antibodies to inhibit lymphocyte activation and subsequently mitigate the cytokine storm. For instance, Reltecimob, a CD28 T-lymphocyte receptor mimetic designed to suppress T-cell stimulation, has been developed. Bulger et al. [55] administered this treatment within six hours of diagnosing necrotizing soft tissue infections via surgical methods in patients with a SOFA score of $\geq$3. The study involved 290 patients, with an average screening SOFA score of 5.5 $\pm$ 2.4, and the results demonstrated improved resolution of organ dysfunction and time to hospital discharge.

In approaching refractory patients, a multidisciplinary approach is imperative, from the comprehensive perspective of the intensivist to the data evaluated by the immunologist and microbiologist to adjust the treatment in real-time.

Although our study included a small sample, implementing this multi-faceted approach was based on phenotypic considerations. Despite the anticipated high predicted mortality risk exceeding 50% according to SOFA or APACHE II criteria, the survival rate was 77%.

3.7. Limitations

This study has some limitations. First, this single-center study includes a small number of patients with no control group. Thus, the findings of these observations should be confirmed in larger comparative studies and cannot be extrapolated to other ICU settings. We described a very selected profile of patients in septic shock and multiorgan dysfunction with real-time monitoring of cytokines and high endotoxemia. Therefore, our conclusions should not be applied to all types of patients.

4. Materials and Methods

4.1. Study Design and Setting, Inclusion Criteria and Analyzed Data and Scores

The present retrospective study included all patients admitted to the Intensive Care Unit (ICU) of Vall d'Hebron University Hospital, Barcelona, Spain, with invasive infection by *Streptococcus pyogenes* during the period between November 2022 and March 2023.

Patients met the criteria for activating the Vall d'Hebron University Hospital in-hospital sepsis code (ISC). The Centers for Disease Control and Prevention's (CDC's) definition of STSS was followed [30,56]. The data collected included demographic variables, past medical history and clinical and analytical variables. The severity of the disease was evaluated through the Acute Physiology and Chronic Health Disease Classification System (APACHE II) [57] and Sequential Organ Failure Assessment (SOFA) scores [58]. Both scores were calculated using the worst parameters measured during the first 24 h of ICU admission. The presence of septic shock or sepsis was assessed according to the Sepsis 3 criteria [20]. ARDS was assessed in accordance with the Berlin definition criteria [59]. Data on the incidence of acute kidney injury (AKI) or failure and the need for continuous renal replacement therapy (CRRT), were collected in line with the latest Kidney Disease: Improving Global Outcomes (KDIGO) Clinical Practice Guideline criteria [25]. Length of ICU stay and ICU and in-hospital mortality were also registered.

Using clinical evaluation and biomarker determination, we identified different phenotypes that may result in a personalized approach based on treatable traits: hyperinflammatory profile, low perfusion profile, and hypogammaglobulinemic profile. Patients were treated accordingly as previously described.

4.2. Statistical Analysis

We used the Statistical Package for the Social Sciences SPSS Statistics 18.0 software (SPSS Inc., Chicago, IL, USA) for statistical analyses. Continuous variables were tested with the Kolmogorov–Smirnov test. Qualitative or categorical variables were described as numbers and percentages. Quantitative or continuous variables were described as means, standard deviations, medians, and interquartile ranges depending on their probabilistic distributions.

4.3. Ethics Statement

The data collection of the study is supported by the local Clinical Research Ethics Committee (PR (AG) 336/2016). The study complied with the General Data Protection Regulation (GDPR) (Regulation (EU) 2016/679), and was performed in accordance with the ethical standards in the 1964 Declaration of Helsinki and its later amendments. The committee complies both in its composition and in the Standard Work Procedure (SWP) with the Best Clinical Practice (BCP) standards (CPMP/ICH/135/95) and with Royal Decree 1090/2015. The datasets used and analyzed during the current study are available from the corresponding author upon reasonable request.

5. Conclusions

Streptococcal Toxic Shock Syndrome (STSS) constitutes a profoundly severe clinical condition associated with a notably high mortality rate. Prospective therapeutic approaches that integrate targeted interventions rooted in precision medicine and discerning sepsis phenotypes, in conjunction with early administration of antibiotics and proficient source control, could improve patient outcomes by mitigating the rapid progression towards multiorgan failure. The multidisciplinary approach involving diverse medical disciplines plays a pivotal role in discerning distinctive characteristics, commonly referred to as phenotypes, in septic patients.

Author Contributions: J.C.R.-R.: Substantial contributions to the conception or design of the work; or the acquisition, analysis, or interpretation of data for the work. Drafting the work or reviewing it critically for important intellectual content. L.C.-C.: Substantial contributions to the conception or design of the work; or the acquisition, analysis, or interpretation of data for the work. Drafting the work or reviewing it critically for important intellectual content. C.M.: Drafting the work or reviewing it critically for important intellectual content. Final approval of the version to be published. A.R.-S.: Drafting the work or reviewing it critically for important intellectual content. Final approval of the version to be published. L.M.: Drafting the work or reviewing it critically for important intellectual content. Final approval of the version to be published. I.B.: Substantial contributions to the conception or design of the work; or the acquisition, analysis, or interpretation of data for the work. J.B.: Substantial contributions to the conception or design of the work; or the acquisition, analysis, or interpretation of data for the work. R.L.-M.: Substantial contributions to the conception or design of the work; or the acquisition, analysis, or interpretation of data for the work. C.F.-J.: Substantial contributions to the conception or design of the work; or the acquisition, analysis, or interpretation of data for the work. J.J.G.-L.: Substantial contributions to the conception or design of the work; or the acquisition, analysis, or interpretation of data for the work. V.R.: Substantial contributions to the conception or design of the work; or the acquisition, analysis, or interpretation of data for the work. N.L.: Substantial contributions to the conception or design of the work; or the acquisition, analysis, or interpretation of data for the work. J.R.: Substantial contributions to the conception or design of the work; or the acquisition, analysis, or interpretation of data for the work. Final approval of the version to be published. X.N.-C.: Substantial contributions to the conception or design of the work; or the acquisition, analysis, or interpretation of data for the work. Final approval of the version to be published. R.F.: Final approval of the version to be published, Agreement to be accountable for all aspects of the work in ensuring that questions related to the accuracy or integrity of any part of the work are appropriately investigated and resolved. All authors have read and agreed to the published version of the manuscript.

Funding: This research received no external funding.

Institutional Review Board Statement: We complied with the guidelines for human studies and our research was conducted ethically in accordance with the World Medical Association Declaration of Helsinki. Information revealing the subject's identity is to be avoided. The study was approved by the local Clinical Research Ethics Committee (PR (AG) 336/2016) with exemption from informed consent.

Informed Consent Statement: The study was approved by the local Clinical Research Ethics Committee (PR (AG) 336/2016) with an exemption for informed consent.

Data Availability Statement: The datasets used and analyzed during the current study are available from the corresponding author upon reasonable request. The data are not publicly available due to preserve as much as possible the identity of the patients described.

Acknowledgments: We would like to thank Erika-Paola Plata-Menchaca for reviewing the manuscript and their final corrections.

Conflicts of Interest: The authors declare no conflicts of interest. Author V.R. was employed by the company Eurecat, Centre Tecnològic de Catalunya, EHealth Unit.

References

1. Holdstock, V.; Twynam-Perkins, J.; Bradnock, T.; Dickson, E.M.; Harvey-Wood, K.; Kalima, P.; King, J.; Olver, W.J.; Osman, M.; Sabharwal, A.; et al. National case series of group A streptococcus pleural empyema in children: Clinical and microbiological features. *Lancet Infect. Dis.* **2023**, *23*, 154–156. [CrossRef] [PubMed]
2. van Kempen, E.B.; Bruijning-Verhagen, P.C.J.; Borensztajn, D.; Vermont, C.L.; Quaak, M.S.W.; Janson, J.A.; Maat, I.; Stol, K.; Vlaminckx, B.J.M.; Wieringa, J.W.; et al. Increase in Invasive Group a Streptococcal Infections in Children in the Netherlands, A Survey Among 7 Hospitals in 2022. *Pediatr. Infect. Dis. J.* **2023**, *42*, e122–e124. [CrossRef] [PubMed]
3. Talavera, M.; Martínez, A.; Vicent, C.; Frasquet, J.; Orera, Á.; Ramírez, P. Four cases of unexpected severe community-acquired pneumonia aetiology: Group A Streptococcus pyogenes disruption. *Med. Intensiv.* **2023**, *47*, 475–477. [CrossRef]
4. Stevens, D. Reappearance of scarlet fever toxin A among streptococci in the Rocky Mountain West: Severe group A streptococcal infections associated with a toxic shock-like syndrome. *N. Engl. J. Med.* **1989**, *321*, 1–7. [CrossRef] [PubMed]
5. Stevens, D.L.; Bryant, A.E. Severe group A streptococcal infections. In *Streptococcus Pyogenes: Basic Biology to Clinical Manifestations*; Ferretti, J.J., Stevens, D.L., Fischetti, V.A., Eds.; University of Oklahoma Health Sciences Center: Oklahoma City, OK, USA, 2016; pp. 661–665.
6. Proft, T.; Fraser, J.D. Streptococcal superantigens: Biological properties and potential role in disease. In *Streptococcus Pyogenes: Basic Biology to Clinical Manifestations*; Ferretti, J.J., Stevens, D.L., Fischetti, V.A., Eds.; University of Oklahoma Health Sciences Center: Oklahoma City, OK, USA, 2016.
7. Nobbs, A.H.; Lamont, R.J.; Jenkinson, H.F. Streptococcus adherence and colonization. *Microbiol. Mol. Biol. Rev.* **2009**, *73*, 407–450. [CrossRef] [PubMed]
8. Courtney, H.S.; Hasty, D.L.; Dale, J.B. Molecular mechanisms of adhesion, colonization, and invasion of group A streptococci. *Ann. Med.* **2002**, *34*, 77–87. [CrossRef] [PubMed]
9. Rohde, M.; Chhatwal, G.S. Adherence and invasion of streptococci to eukaryotic cells and their role in disease pathogenesis. *Curr. Top. Microbiol. Immunol.* **2013**, *368*, 83–110.
10. Brouwer, S.; Barnett, T.C.; Rivera-Hernandez, T.; Rohde, M.; Walker, M.J. Streptococcus pyogenes adhesion and colonization. *FEBS Lett.* **2016**, *590*, 3739–3757. [CrossRef]
11. Courtney, H.S.; von Hunolstein, C.; Dale, J.B.; Bronze, M.S.; Beachey, E.H.; Hasty, D.L. Lipoteichoic acid and M protein: Dual adhesins of group A streptococci. *Microb. Pathog.* **1992**, *12*, 199–208. [CrossRef]
12. Cywes, C.; Stamenkovic, I.; Wessels, M.R. CD44 as a receptor for colonization of the pharynx by group A Streptococcus. *J. Clin. Investig.* **2000**, *106*, 995–1002. [CrossRef]
13. Wessels, M.R. Cell Wall and Surface Molecules: Capsule. In *Streptococcus Pyogenes: Basic Biology to Clinical Manifestations*; Ferretti, J.J., Stevens, D.L., Fischetti, V.A., Eds.; University of Oklahoma Health Sciences Center: Oklahoma City, OK, USA, 2016. Available online: https://www.ncbi.nlm.nih.gov/sites/books/NBK333410/ (accessed on 2 January 2024).
14. Cywes, C.; Wessels, M. Group A Streptococcus tissue invasion by CD44-mediated cell signalling. *Nature* **2001**, *414*, 648–652. [CrossRef]
15. Cue, D.; Lam, H.; Cleary, P.P. Genetic dissection of the Streptococcus pyogenes M1 protein: Regions involved in fibronectin-bindingand intracellular invasion. *Microb. Pathog.* **2001**, *31*, 231–242. [CrossRef]
16. Purushothaman, S.S.; Wang, B.; Cleary, P.P. M1 protein triggers a phosphoinositide cascade for group A Streptococcus invasion of epithelial cells. *Infect. Immun.* **2003**, *71*, 5823–5830. [CrossRef]

17. Evans, L.; Rhodes, A.; Alhazzani, W.; Antonelli, M.; Coopersmith, C.M.; French, C.; Machado, F.R.; Mcintyre, L.; Ostermann, M.; Prescott, H.C.; et al. Surviving sepsis campaign: International guidelines for management of sepsis and septic shock 2021. *Intensive Care Med.* **2021**, *47*, e1063–e1143. [CrossRef] [PubMed]
18. Levy, M.M.; Rhodes, A.; Phillips, G.S.; Townsend, S.R.; Schorr, C.A.; Beale, R.; Osborn, T.; Lemeshow, S.; Chiche, J.D.; Artigas, A.; et al. Surviving Sepsis Campaign: Association between performance metrics and outcomes in a 7.5-year study. *Crit. Care Med.* **2015**, *43*, 3–12. [CrossRef] [PubMed]
19. Yébenes, J.C.; Ruiz-Rodriguez, J.C.; Ferrer, R.; Clèries, M.; Bosch, A.; Lorencio, C.; Rodriguez, A.; Nuvials, X.; Martin-Loeches, I.; Artigas, A. Epidemiology of sepsis in Catalonia: Analysis of incidence and outcomes in a European setting. *Ann. Intensive Care* **2017**, *7*, 19. [CrossRef]
20. Singer, M.; Deutschman, C.S.; Seymour, C.W.; Shankar-Hari, M.; Annane, D.; Bauer, M.; Bellomo, R.; Bernard, G.R.; Chiche, J.D.; Coopersmith, C.M.; et al. The Third International Consensus Definitions for Sepsis and Septic Shock (Sepsis-3). *JAMA* **2016**, *315*, 801–810. [CrossRef] [PubMed]
21. Seymour, C.W.; Kennedy, J.N.; Wang, S.; Chang, C.C.H.; Elliott, C.F.; Xu, Z.; Berry, S.; Clermont, G.; Cooper, G.; Gomez, H.; et al. Derivation, Validation, and Potential Treatment Implications of Novel Clinical Phenotypes for Sepsis. *JAMA* **2019**, *321*, 2003–2017. [CrossRef]
22. Ruiz-Rodriguez, J.C.; Plata-Menchaca, E.P.; Chiscano-Camón, L.; Ruiz-Sanmartin, A.; Pérez-Carrasco, M.; Palmada, C.; Ribas, V.; Martínez-Gallo, M.; Hernández-González, M.; Gonzalez-Lopez, J.J.; et al. Precision medicine in sepsis and septic shock: From omics to clinical tools. *World J. Crit. Care Med.* **2022**, *11*, 1–21. [CrossRef]
23. Babiker, A.; Li, X.; Lai, Y.L.; Strich, J.R.; Warner, S.; Sarzynski, S.; Dekker, J.P.; Danner, R.L.; Kadri, S.S. Effectiveness of adjunctive clindamycin in β-lactam antibiotic-treated patients with invasive β-haemolytic streptococcal infections in US hospitals: A retrospective multicentre cohort study. *Lancet Infect. Dis.* **2021**, *21*, 697–710. [CrossRef]
24. Grasselli, G.; Calfee, C.S.; Camporota, L.; Poole, D.; Amato, M.B.; Antonelli, M.; Arabi, Y.M.; Baroncelli, F.; Beitler, J.R.; Bellani, G.; et al. ESICM guidelines on acute respiratory distress syndrome: Definition, phenotyping and respiratory support strategies. *Intensive Care Med.* **2023**, *49*, 727–759. [CrossRef]
25. Khwaja, A. KDIGO clinical practice guidelines for acute kidney injury. *Nephron Clin. Pract.* **2012**, *120*, c179–c184. [CrossRef]
26. Ribas Ripoll, V.J.; Vellido, A.; Romero, E.; Ruiz-Rodríguez, J.C. Sepsis mortality prediction with the Quotient Basis Kernel. *Artif. Intell. Med.* **2014**, *61*, 45–52. [CrossRef]
27. Ribas, V.J.; López, J.C.; Ruiz-Sanmartin, A.; Ruiz-Rodríguez, J.C.; Rello, J.; Wojdel, A.; Vellido, A. Severe sepsis mortality prediction with relevance vector machines. In Proceedings of the 2011 Annual International Conference of the IEEE Engineering in Medicine and Biology Society, Boston, MA, USA, 30 August 2011–3 September 2011.
28. Knaus, W.A.; Zimmerman, J.E.; Wagner, D.P.; Draper, E.A.; Lawrence, D.E. APACHE-acute physiology and chronic health evaluation: A physiologically based classification system. *Crit. Care Med.* **1981**, *9*, 591–597. [CrossRef]
29. Bermejo-Martín, J.F.; Rodriguez-Fernandez, A.; Herrán-Monge, R.; Andaluz-Ojeda, D.; Muriel-Bombín, A.; Merino, P.; García-García, M.M.; Citores, R.; Gandía, F.; Almansa, R.; et al. Immunoglobulins IgG1, IgM and IgA: A synergistic team influencing survival in sepsis. *J. Intern. Med.* **2014**, *276*, 404–412. [CrossRef]
30. Schmitz, M.; Roux, X.; Huttner, B.; Pugin, J. Streptococcal toxic shock syndrome in the intensive care unit. *Ann. Intensive Care* **2018**, *8*, 88. [CrossRef] [PubMed]
31. Hellman, T.; Uusalo, P.; Järvisalo, M.J. Renal Replacement Techniques in Septic Shock. *Int. J. Mol. Sci.* **2021**, *22*, 10238. [CrossRef] [PubMed]
32. Antonucci, E.; Polo, T.; Giovini, M.; Girardis, M.; Martin-Loeches, I.; Nielsen, N.D.; Lozsán, F.J.C.; Ferrer, R.; Lakbar, I.; Leone, M. Refractory septic shock and alternative wordings: A systematic review of literature. *J. Crit. Care* **2023**, *75*, 154258. [CrossRef] [PubMed]
33. Kawaguchi, T.; Igaki, N.; Kinoshita, S.; Matsuda, T.; Kida, A.; Moriguchi, R.; Sakai, M.; Tamada, F.; Oimomi, M.; Goto, T. A new therapeutic strategy for streptococcal toxic shock syndrome: A key target for cytokines. *Intern. Med.* **2003**, *42*, 211–218. [CrossRef] [PubMed]
34. Hoeper, M.M.; Abou-Rebyeh, F.; Athman, C.; Schwarz, A. Plasmapheresis in streptococcal toxic shock syndrome. *Crit. Care Med.* **2001**, *29*, 2399. [CrossRef] [PubMed]
35. Scheier, J.; Nelson, P.J.; Schneider, A.; Colombier, S.; Kindgen-Milles, D.; Deliargyris, E.N.; Nolin, T.D. Mechanistic Considerations and Pharmacokinetic Implications on Concomitant Drug Administration During CytoSorb Therapy. *Crit. Care Explor.* **2022**, *4*, e0688. [CrossRef]
36. Honore, P.; Hoste, E.; Molnár, Z.; Jacobs, R.; Joannes-Boyau, O.; Malbrain, M.; Forni, L. Cytokine removal in human septic shock: Where are we and where are we going. *Ann. Intensive Care* **2019**, *9*, 56. [CrossRef]
37. Ricci, Z.; Romagnoli, S.; Reis, T.; Bellomo, R.; Ronco, C. Hemoperfusion in the intensive care unit. *Intensive Care Med.* **2022**, *48*, 1397–1408. [CrossRef]
38. Chousterman, B.G.; Swirski, F.K.; Weber, G.F. Cytokine storm and sepsis disease pathogenesis. *Semin. Immunopathol.* **2017**, *39*, 517–528. [CrossRef] [PubMed]
39. Klein, D.J.; Foster, D.; Walker, P.M.; Bagshaw, S.M.; Mekonnen, H.; Antonelli, M. Polymyxin B hemoperfusion in endotoxemic septic shock patients without extreme endotoxemia: A post hoc analysis of the EUPHRATES trial. *Intensive Care Med.* **2018**, *44*, 2205–2212. [CrossRef] [PubMed]

40. Dellinger, R.P.; Bagshaw, S.M.; Antonelli, M.; Foster, D.M.; Klein, D.J.; Marshall, J.C.; Palevsky, P.M.; Weisberg, L.S.; Schorr, C.A.; Trzeciak, S.; et al. Effect of Targeted Polymyxin B Hemoperfusion on 28-Day Mortality in Patients With Septic Shock and Elevated Endotoxin Level: The EUPHRATES Randomized Clinical Trial. *JAMA* **2018**, *320*, 1455–1463. [CrossRef] [PubMed]
41. Shoji, H.; Ferrer, R. Potential survival benefit and early recovery from organ dysfunction with polymyxin B hemoperfusion: Perspectives from a real-world big data analysis and the supporting mechanisms of action. *J. Anesth. Analg. Crit. Care* **2022**, *2*, 27. [CrossRef] [PubMed]
42. Cutuli, S.L.; De Rosa, S.; Ferrer, R.; Ruiz-Rodriguez, J.C.; Forfori, F.; Ronco, C.; Antonelli, M.; EUPHAS2-G50 Collaborative Study Group; Cutuli, S.L.; De Rosa, S.; et al. Endotoxin activity trend and multi-organ dysfunction in critically ill patients with septic shock, who received Polymyxin-B hemadsorption: A multicenter, prospective, observational study. *Artif. Organs* **2023**, *47*, 1361–1370. [CrossRef] [PubMed]
43. Malard, B.; Lambert, C.; Kellum, J.A. In vitro comparison of the adsorption of inflammatory mediators by blood purification devices. *Intensive Care Med. Exp.* **2018**, *6*, 12. [CrossRef] [PubMed]
44. Ruiz-Rodríguez, J.C.; Chiscano-Camón, L.; Palmada, C.; Ruiz-Sanmartin, A.; Pérez-Carrasco, M.; Larrosa, N.; González, J.J.; Hernández-González, M.; Ferrer, R. Endotoxin and Cytokine Sequential Hemoadsorption in Septic Shock and Multi-Organ Failure. *Blood Purif.* **2022**, *51*, 630–633. [CrossRef]
45. Cheng, A.; Sun, H.Y.; Tsai, M.S.; Ko, W.J.; Tsai, P.R.; Hu, F.C.; Chen, Y.C.; Chang, S.C. Predictors of survival in adults undergoing extracorporeal membrane oxygenation with severe infections. *J. Thorac. Cardiovasc. Surg.* **2016**, *152*, 1526–1536.e1. [CrossRef]
46. Riera, J.; Argudo, E.; Ruiz-Rodríguez, J.C.; Ferrer, R. Extracorporeal Membrane Oxygenation for Adults With Refractory Septic Shock. *ASAIO J.* **2019**, *65*, 760–768. [CrossRef] [PubMed]
47. Sriskandan, S.; Ferguson, M.; Elliot, V.; Faulkner, L.; Cohen, J. Human intravenous immunoglobulin for experimental streptococcal toxic shock: Bacterial clearance and modulation of inflammation. *J. Antimicrob. Chemother.* **2006**, *58*, 117–124. [CrossRef]
48. Madsen, M.B.; Hjortrup, P.B.; Hansen, M.B.; Lange, T.; Norrby-Teglund, A.; Hyldegaard, O.; Perner, A. Immunoglobulin G for patients with necrotising soft tissue infection (INSTINCT): A randomised, blinded, placebo-controlled trial. *Intensive Care Med.* **2017**, *43*, 1585–1593. [CrossRef] [PubMed]
49. Werdan, K.; Pilz, G.; Bujdoso, O.; Fraunberger, P.; Neeser, G.; Schmieder, R.E.; Viell, B.; Marget, W.; Seewald, M.; Walger, P.; et al. Score-based immunoglobulin G therapy of patients with sepsis: The SBITS study. *Crit. Care Med.* **2007**, *35*, 2693–2701.
50. Alejandria, M.M.; Lansang, M.A.D.; Dans, L.F.; Mantaring, J.B., 3rd. Intravenous immunoglobulin for treating sepsis, severe sepsis and septic shock. *Cochrane Database Syst. Rev.* **2013**, *9*, CD001090. [CrossRef]
51. Busani, S.; Damiani, E.; Cavazzuti, I.; Donati, A.; Girardis, M. Intravenous immunoglobulin in septic shock: Review of the mechanisms of action and meta-analysis of the clinical effectiveness. *Minerva Anestesiol.* **2016**, *82*, 559–572.
52. Olivares, M.M.; Olmos, C.E.; Álvarez, M.I.; Fajardo, A.M.; Zea-Vera, A.F.; Ortega, M.C.; Medina, D.; Pérez, P.M.; Beltrán, D.G.; Duque, B.; et al. Colombian Guidelines of clinical practice for the use of immunoglobulins in the treatment of replacement and immunomodulation. *Rev. Alerg. Mex.* **2017**, *64* (Suppl. S2), s5–s65. [CrossRef] [PubMed]
53. Newburger, J.W.; Takahashi, M.; Beiser, A.S.; Burns, J.C.; Bastian, J.; Chung, K.J.; Colan, S.D.; Duffy, C.E.; Fulton, D.R.; Glode, M.P.; et al. A single intravenous infusion of gamma globulin as compared with four infusions in the treatment of acute Kawasaki syndrome. *N. Engl. J. Med.* **1991**, *324*, 1633–1639. [CrossRef]
54. Berlot, G.; Vassallo, M.C.; Busetto, N.; Nieto Yabar, M.; Istrati, T.; Baronio, S.; Quarantotto, G.; Bixio, M.; Barbati, G.; Dattola, R.; et al. Effects of the timing of administration of IgM- and IgA-enriched intravenous polyclonal immunoglobulins on the outcome of septic shock patients. *Ann. Intensive Care* **2018**, *8*, 122. [CrossRef]
55. Bulger, E.M.; May, A.K.; Robinson, B.R.; Evans, D.C.; Henry, S.; Green, J.M.; Toschlog, E.; Sperry, J.L.; Fagenholz, P.; Martin, N.D.; et al. A Novel Immune Modulator for Patients With Necrotizing Soft Tissue Infections (NSTI): Results of a Multicenter, Phase 3 Randomized Controlled Trial of Reltecimod (AB 103). *Ann. Surg.* **2020**, *272*, 469–478. [CrossRef] [PubMed]
56. Lappin, E.; Ferguson, A.J. Gram-positive toxic shock syndromes. *Lancet Infect. Dis.* **2009**, *9*, 281–290. [CrossRef] [PubMed]
57. Knaus, W.A.; Draper, E.A.; Wagner, D.P.; Zimmerman, J.E. APACHE II: A severity of disease classification system. *Crit. Care Med.* **1985**, *13*, 818–829. [CrossRef] [PubMed]
58. Vincent, J.L.; Moreno, R.; Takala, J.; Willatts, S.; De Mendonça, A.; Bruining, H.; Reinhart, C.K.; Suter, P.; Thijs, L.G. The SOFA (Sepsis-related Organ Failure Assessment) score to describe organ dysfunction/failure. On behalf of the Working Group on Sepsis-Related Problems of the European Society of Intensive Care Medicine. *Intensive Care Med.* **1996**, *22*, 707–710. [CrossRef]
59. Ranieri, V.I.T.O.; Rubenfeld, G.D.; Thompson, B.T.; Ferguson, N.D.; Caldwell, E.; Fan, E.; Camporota, L. Acute respiratory distress syndrome: The Berlin Definition. *JAMA* **2012**, *307*, 2526–2533.

antibiotics

MDPI

Article

Antimicrobial Efficacy of Impregnated Human Acellular Dermal Substitutes in Burn Wound Models

Marianna Hajská [1,†], Elena Kurin [2,†], Silvia Bittner Fialová [2,*], Marian Vidiščák [1] and Arpád Panyko [1]

[1] 4th Department of Surgery, Faculty of Medicine and University Hospital Bratislava, Comenius University Bratislava, Ružinovská 6, 82606 Bratislava, Slovakia; marianna.hajska@fmed.uniba.sk (M.H.); marian.vidiscak@fmed.uniba.sk (M.V.); arpad.panyko@fmed.uniba.sk (A.P.)

[2] Department of Pharmacognosy and Botany, Faculty of Pharmacy, Comenius University Bratislava, Odbojárov 10, 83232 Bratislava, Slovakia; elena.kurin@uniba.sk

[*] Correspondence: fialova@fpharm.uniba.sk; Tel.: +421-2-9016-9206

[†] These authors contributed equally to this work.

Abstract

Burn wound infections remain a major clinical challenge due to delayed healing, scarring, and the risk of sepsis, especially when complicated by multidrug-resistant (MDR) Gram-negative pathogens and biofilm formation. Acellular dermal matrices (ADMs) are widely used in reconstructive and burn surgery, yet they lack intrinsic antimicrobial activity, necessitating their combination with topical agents. **Background/Objectives**: This study investigates the antimicrobial and cytocompatibility profiles of ADMs impregnated with various antimicrobial agents, using in vitro planktonic and biofilm burn wound models. While the incorporation of antimicrobials into scaffolds has been previously explored, this study is, to our knowledge, the first to directly compare seven clinically relevant antimicrobial agents after they were impregnated into an ADM in a standardized in vitro model. **Methods:** Seven topical antimicrobials were tested against MDR *Pseudomonas aeruginosa* and *Acinetobacter baumannii* from burn patients. **Results**: The ADM with 1% acetic acid (AA) showed superior antimicrobial activity, achieving > 7 $\log_{10}$ reductions in planktonic assays and complete inhibition of *P. aeruginosa* biofilms. In NIH 3T3 fibroblast cytotoxicity assays, the 1% AA ADM maintained cell viability at control levels, indicating excellent biocompatibility. Compared with agents such as Betadine®, Octenilin®, and colistin, which showed cytotoxicity, and Prontosan®, which showed low efficacy, 1% AA uniquely combined potent antibacterial effects with minimal toxicity. **Conclusions**: Among the seven antimicrobial agents impregnated into ADMs, 1% AA demonstrated a unique efficacy and safety profile, supporting its potential for clinical application in integrated wound dressings and implantable biomaterials for infection control in burn care.

Keywords: wound infections; acellular dermal matrices; antimicrobial agents; *Pseudomonas aeruginosa*; *Acinetobacter baumannii*; 1% acetic acid

1. Introduction

Acellular dermal matrices (ADMs) are widely utilized in burn and reconstructive surgery, as well as in plastic surgery and orthopedics, due to their ability to support tissue regeneration [1–3]. Additionally, ADMs have applications in the management of chronic wounds and in tissue reconstruction [4,5]. These dermal allografts, completely devoid of cellular components, serve as scaffolds for in vitro cell cultivation, including dermal fibroblasts and keratinocytes [6]. An ADM is derived from cadaveric allografts through various decellularization techniques, like physical, chemical, or biological, often used in combination to preserve the extracellular matrix structure while removing immunogenic elements [7]. Despite being non-toxic and non-antigenic, a standard ADM lacks inherent antimicrobial properties, necessitating the application of topical antimicrobial agents to reduce the risk of infection.

Burn wound infections represent a major complication in the acute phase of burn disease. Factors such as extensive wound contamination, burn-induced immunosuppression, prolonged hospitalization, and invasive procedures facilitate infections by multidrug-resistant nosocomial pathogens [8]. The most common isolated bacteria from burn wounds include *Pseudomonas aeruginosa, Staphylococcus aureus, Acinetobacter baumannii, Enterococcus faecalis, Escherichia coli, Klebsiella pneumoniae*, and *Enterobacter* spp. [9]. Infections significantly prolong wound healing, impair dermal maturation, and contribute to pathological scarring. Additionally, bacterial invasion of deeper tissues can lead to disseminated infection and sepsis [10,11].

A key challenge in burn wound management is the increasing prevalence of antimicrobial resistance, driven in part by biofilm formation. Bacterial biofilms consist of structured microbial communities encased in an extracellular polymeric substance, which enhances resistance to antibiotics, disinfectants, and host immune responses [12]. Biofilms are commonly detected in burn wounds, further complicating treatment [13].

Scientific evidence suggests that the application of topical antimicrobial agents can significantly reduce morbidity and mortality in burn patients by preventing and controlling wound infections [10]. These agents can be applied at all stages of wound management, providing both prophylactic and therapeutic benefits. Importantly, systemic antibiotic therapy often fails in burn wounds due to compromised vascularization, further emphasizing the necessity of localized antimicrobial interventions [11]. Topical antimicrobial agents are widely recommended in clinical practice guidelines for burn wound care, primarily to prevent infections that can lead to delayed healing, sepsis, or death. Notably, some topical preparations remain a commonly used agent in deeper burns and low-resource settings due to their broad-spectrum activity and low resistance profile, particularly against *Staphylococcus aureus* and *Pseudomonas aeruginosa*. In contrast, the use of topical antibiotics is typically limited to superficial or facial wounds, as evidence indicates that topical antibiotic application may contribute more significantly to antimicrobial resistance [14]. Therefore, in the context of rising antimicrobial resistance, selecting effective topical agents while minimizing the risk of resistance transmission remains a critical priority [15].

The aim of this study was to enhance the antimicrobial properties of ADMs by impregnating them with selected antimicrobial agents and evaluating its efficacy in in vitro burn wound models contaminated with multidrug-resistant *Pseudomonas aeruginosa* and *Acinetobacter baumannii*.

2. Results

2.1. Antibacterial and Antibiofilm Activity of Antiseptic Agents Impregnated on ADMs

The ADMs impregnated with 1% AA, vancomycin, colistin, and Betadine® were significantly effective against the growth of the planktonic form of *P. aeruginosa*, as shown in Figure 1.

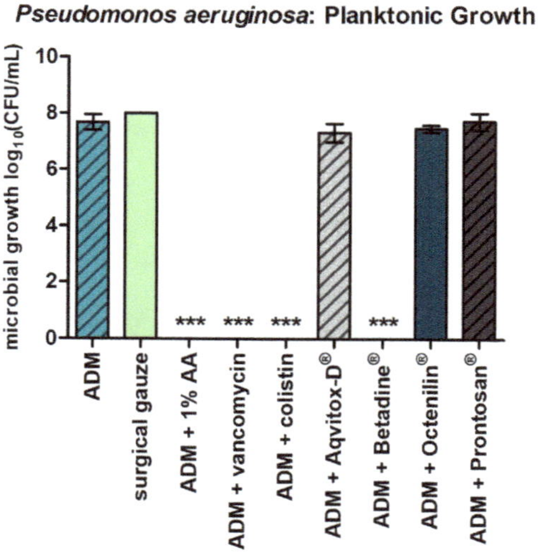

Figure 1. *P. aeruginosa* in planktonic form and ADMs with the tested agents. The bars represent the mean ± SD, n = 3. *** $p < 0.001$ for comparisons among the samples (ANOVA/Turkey).

These treatments resulted in a $\log_{10}$ reduction of >7 CFU/mL in bacterial counts, indicating a strong inhibitory effect according to internationally recognized standards (Table 1). This substantial reduction reflects a marked decrease in viable bacterial cells compared with the untreated control, indicating a powerful inhibitory effect. According to standardized interpretation criteria, a reduction greater than 3 $\log_{10}$ CFU/mL is classified as strong antimicrobial activity, further underscoring the effectiveness of these treatments in suppressing bacterial growth. In contrast, ADMs treated with Aqvitox-D®, Octenilin®, and Prontosan® showed no measurable antimicrobial activity.

Table 1. The bacterial growth-inhibitory activity expressed as $\log_{10}$ colony-forming units per milliliter ($\Delta\log_{10}$ CFU/mL) of the various agents impregnated on an ADM against the planktonic form and biofilms of *P. aeruginosa* and *A. baumannii*. The limit of detection (LOD) for the plating method was 1 CFU/mL, meaning that counting below this value could not be reliably detected. For these samples, a value of >7 $\log_{10}$ is reported as the maximum detectable reduction based on the LOD.

	$\Delta\log_{10}$(CFU/mL)						
	1% AA	**Vancomycin**	**Colistin**	**Aqvitox-D®**	**Betadine®**	**Octenilin®**	**Prontosan®**
Pseudomonas aeruginosa: Planktonic Growth	>7	>7	>7	0.37	>7	0.22	−0.04
antimicrobial activity	strong	strong	strong	no	strong	no	no
Pseudomonas aeruginosa: Biofilm Growth	>7	0.22	2.26	0.74	0.10	0.75	0.16
antimicrobial activity	strong	no	significant	slight	no	slight	no
Acinetobacter baumannii: Planktonic Growth	>7	>7	>7	>7	>7	>7	−0.47
antimicrobial activity	strong	strong	strong	strong	strong	strong	no
Acinetobacter baumannii: Biofilm Growth	>7	4.26	>7	−0.33	>7	−0.70	0.76
antimicrobial activity	strong	strong	strong	no	strong	no	slight

Based on the standard interpretation, a reduction of >3 $\log_{10}$ was classified as strong antibacterial activity, 1–3 $\log_{10}$ as significant antibacterial activity, 0.5–1 $\log_{10}$ as slight antibacterial activity, and <0.5 $\log_{10}$ as no activity.

In the 24 h biofilm model of *P. aeruginosa*, only the ADM impregnated with 1% AA completely inhibited the biofilm growth (Figure 2), achieving a $\log_{10}$ reduction of >7, which qualifies as strong antimicrobial activity (Table 1). The ADM impregnated with colistin also significantly reduced biofilm formation, with a $\log_{10}$ reduction of 2.26, corresponding to significant antimicrobial activity. In contrast, the remaining agents showed no measurable effect on biofilm growth, with slight or no log reduction observed.

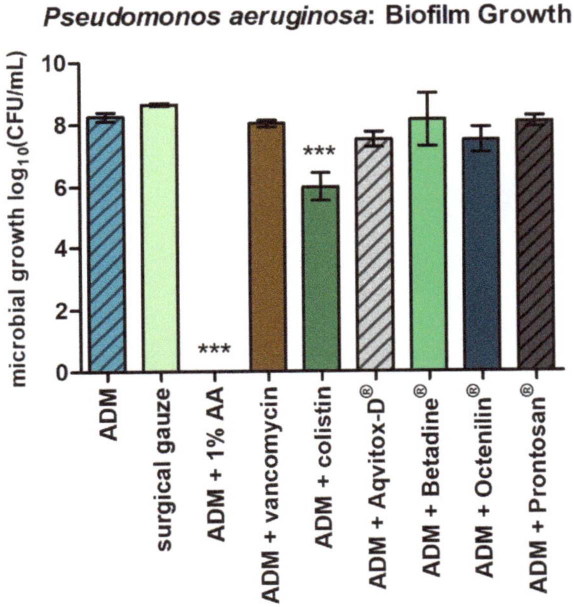

Figure 2. *P. aeruginosa* in a 24 h biofilm and the ADMs with the tested agents. The bars represent the mean ± SD, n = 3. *** $p < 0.001$ for comparisons among the samples (ANOVA/Turkey).

For *A. baumannii* in planktonic form (Figure 3), the ADMs impregnated with all tested agents, except Prontosan®, resulted in a significant reduction in bacterial growth. The overall $\log_{10}$ reduction reached >7, indicating a strong antimicrobial effect according to the standardized classification (Table 1).

In the 24 h biofilm model of *A. baumannii* (Figure 4), the ADMs impregnated with 1% AA, Betadine®, colistin, and vancomycin demonstrated strong antimicrobial activity, with $\log_{10}$ reductions of >7 for 1% AA, colistin, and Betadine® and 4.26 for vancomycin, all classified as strong effects according to Table 1. Prontosan® showed slight antibacterial activity, with a $\log_{10}$ reduction of 0.76. In contrast, the ADMs treated with Aqvitox-D® and Octenilin® showed no measurable antimicrobial effect, indicating a lack of efficacy against biofilm growth.

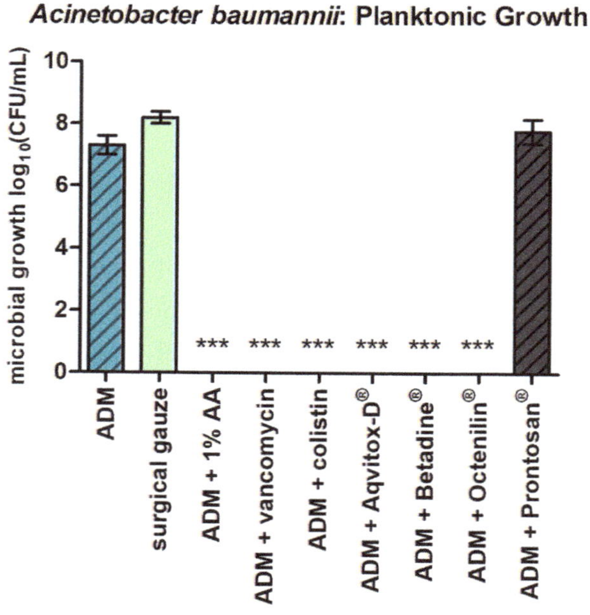

Figure 3. *A. baumannii* in planktonic form and the ADMs with the tested agents. The bars represent the mean ± SD, n = 3. *** $p < 0.001$ for comparisons among the samples (ANOVA/Turkey).

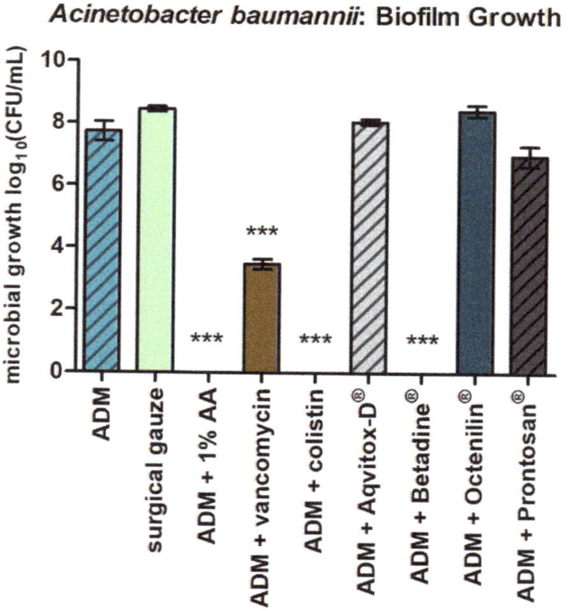

Figure 4. *A. baumannii* in a 24 h biofilm and the ADMs with the tested agents. The bars represent the mean ± SD, n = 3. *** $p < 0.001$ for comparisons among the samples (ANOVA/Turkey).

2.2. Cell Viability: Cytotoxicity of Antimicrobial Agents Combined with ADMs

The cytotoxic effects of various antibacterial agents in combination with an acellular dermal matrix (ADM) were evaluated on 3T3 fibroblast cells over a 5-day period (Figure 5). Cell viability is expressed as the percentage relative to untreated 3T3 control cells.

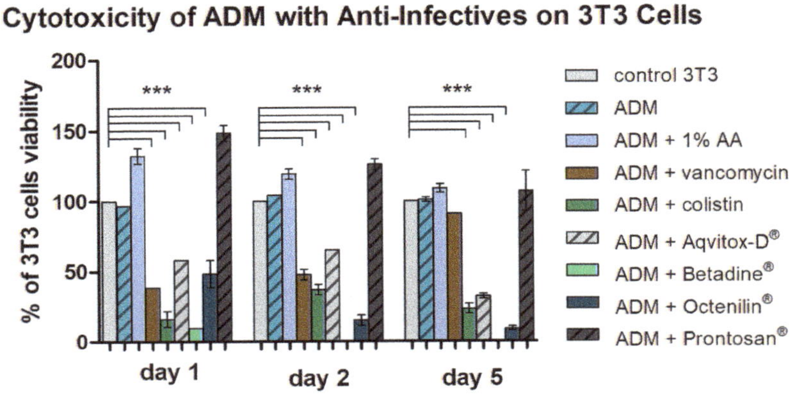

Figure 5. Evaluation of the cytotoxic effects of ADMs combined with various antibacterial agents on 3T3 fibroblasts, based on cell viability testing. Cell viability was assessed on days 1, 2, and 5 to capture both early and late responses. Viable adherent cells were detached by trypsinization and counted using a Bürker chamber; values are expressed as the percentage relative to untreated controls. The results represent the mean ±SD from three independent experiments (n = 3). *** $p < 0.001$ for comparisons among the samples (ANOVA/Tukey).

On the first day, both the ADM alone and ADMs combined with 1% AA and Prontosan® maintained high levels of cell viability, with significant increases observed comparable with or exceeding the control. These conditions showed no signs of cytotoxicity and maintained cell viability comparable with the control. The ADMs combined with vancomycin, Aqvitox-D®, or Octenilin® showed moderate cytotoxicity (viability below 70%), while ADMs combined with colistin and, especially, Betadine® demonstrated high cytotoxicity (viability below 30%) and reduced viability of fibroblasts, with all reductions being statistically significant.

On day two, the ADM combined with 1% AA and the ADM combined with Prontosan® showed the lowest cytotoxicity, maintaining cell viability above normal levels, with a statistically significant increase. Next, the ADM combined with vancomycin and the ADM combined with Aqvitox-D® demonstrated statistically significant moderate cytotoxicity, with cell viability dropping below 70%. Similarly, the ADM combined with colistin also showed statistically significant moderate cytotoxicity, with a viability around 40%. The ADMs combined with Octenilin® and Betadine® exhibited high cytotoxicity (viability below 30%), with Betadine® showing the most pronounced effect, reducing cell viability to nearly 0%.

On day five, the highest cell viability was observed in treatments with ADMs combined with 1% AA and Prontosan®, both maintaining levels above the control, indicating no cytotoxicity. Notably, the ADM combined with vancomycin showed improved cell viability, reaching approximately 90%, suggesting a possible delayed protective or adaptive response. In contrast, the ADMs combined with colistin and Aqvitox-D® exhibited statistically significantly high cytotoxicity, with cell viability dropping below 30%. Similarly, the ADMs combined with Octenilin® and Betadine® also demonstrated statistically significant severe cytotoxic effects, with Betadine® reducing viability to nearly 0%.

Overall, the ADM in combination with 1% AA consistently demonstrated the most favorable biocompatibility, maintaining or even enhancing 3T3 cell viability at all observed time points, with levels exceeding the control baseline. In contrast, combinations with Betadine®, Octenilin®, colistin, and Aqvitox-D® exhibited marked and, in most cases, statistically significant cytotoxicity, particularly after prolonged exposure, with Betadine® showing the most severe effect.

3. Discussion

Infectious complications of burn wounds represent a significant medical challenge, contributing to delayed healing, the formation of deep burn scars, and, in cases where microorganisms infiltrate the systemic circulation, life-threatening conditions such as sepsis [10,11]. One of the major factors complicating the treatment of burn wound infections is the increasing bacterial resistance to antimicrobial agents. A key mechanism of this resistance is the formation of microbial biofilms [11].

ADMs are widely utilized across various surgical specialties, with their most common application in burn surgery. However, in clinical practice, it is currently employed only in combination with topically applied antimicrobial agents. Scientific studies have demonstrated that the use of topical antimicrobial agents reduces morbidity and mortality in patients with extensive burns [10]. A recent multicenter study reported excellent clinical outcomes with the use of an antimicrobial-coated acellular porcine dermal matrix in hernia repair [16]. Additionally, Yang et al. [17] demonstrated the beneficial effect of impregnated acellular dermal matrices (ADMs) in infection treatment by developing a levofloxacin-loaded porcine acellular dermal matrix hydrogel for urinary infection management.

In this study, we investigated the antimicrobial efficacy of impregnated acellular dermal replacements in in vitro models of burn wounds contaminated or infected with multidrug-resistant Gram-negative bacteria, which are among the most frequently isolated pathogens in such wounds. Unlike previous studies available in the literature [9,18], our work focused on ADMs impregnated with antimicrobial agents rather than a combination of ADMs with topically applied agents. According to the current literature, the concept of impregnated ADMs has not yet been introduced into clinical practice, nor has their efficacy against bacterial strains been studied in in vitro models.

Using a modified methodology based on Hammond et al. [19], we developed the following two in vitro burn wound models: a planktonic growth model and a biofilm model. We tested two multidrug-resistant Gram-negative bacterial strains, *P. aeruginosa* and *A. baumannii*, both isolated from burn patients. Seven topical antimicrobial agents were evaluated, as follows: 1% AA, vancomycin, colistin, Aqvitox-D® (hypochlorous acid and sodium hypochlorite), Betadine® (povidone-iodine), Octenilin® (octenidine dihydrochloride), and Prontosan® (polyhexamethylene biguanide hydrochloride). ADMs were prepared following the method described by Dragúňová et al. [6], impregnated with the respective antimicrobial substances, and subsequently applied to the in vitro burn wound models.

Our findings demonstrate that the ADM impregnated with 1% AA exhibited exceptional antimicrobial efficacy against the tested multidrug-resistant Gram-negative bacterial strains. This agent showed the strongest inhibitory effect against both planktonic bacteria and biofilm formation after 24 h. The strong antibacterial performance of 1% AA, characterized by $\log_{10}$ reductions exceeding > 7 in all planktonic assays, clearly surpasses the threshold for "strong" antimicrobial activity as defined by standard classification criteria. Moreover, 1% AA was the only agent that completely inhibited biofilm formation of *P. aeruginosa* and was one of the most effective agents against biofilm-forming *A. baumannii*, alongside colistin and Betadine®.

This is especially notable given the high tolerance of biofilms to conventional antibiotics and antiseptics [20,21]. AA, a weak organic acid, has historically been used in medicine; for example, Hippocrates recommended it for wound care. It is present in vinegar at a 3–5% concentration. It can be produced inexpensively via fermentation or synthesis, is stable upon autoclaving, and has favorable storage properties [22]. Moreover, AA biodegrades into CO_2 and H_2O, making it environmentally friendly and sustainable. Unlike antibiotics, it does not pollute soil and water or contribute to antimicrobial resistance. The antibacterial effect of AA is primarily attributed to its ability to penetrate bacterial cell membranes in its protonated form, leading to cytoplasmic acidification and disruption of vital cellular functions. This uncoupling effect dissipates the proton-motive force and inhibits bacterial respiration, ultimately compromising cell viability. Such a mechanism is particularly effective against planktonic bacterial forms [23]. Moreover, by lowering the wound bed pH, which is typically elevated in chronic wounds [24], AA can inhibit bacterial proliferation, suppress biofilm formation, and modulate the local environment to favor tissue regeneration. This acidification not only reduces the toxicity of bacterial by-products like ammonia but also helps restore physiological pH levels that support collagen synthesis, angiogenesis, and immune cell function, further enhancing its therapeutic potential [25]. Acidification of the wound environment, particularly in burns and chronic wounds, can reduce elevated alkaline pH levels toward a more physiological range, thereby supporting keratinocyte proliferation and tissue repair. It was shown that maintaining a wound pH of 4 significantly enhanced re-epithelialization, collagen synthesis, and overall healing compared with more neutral conditions [26]. Similarly, it was demonstrated that burn wounds treated with a pH 3.5 buffer exhibited significantly faster epithelialization than those treated with neutral or alkaline solutions [27]. Notably, this concentration of acetic acid has been used in our clinical practice for an extended period, particularly for the management of burn wounds, donor sites, and grafted areas, with very good local tolerance and without reports of irritation, supporting its potential applicability.

While other agents such as vancomycin and colistin showed similar antimicrobial potency in the planktonic phase, they failed to match the broad-spectrum and biofilm-targeting capacity of 1% AA. The fact that some commonly used antiseptics (e.g., Octenilin®, Aqvitox-D®, and Prontosan®) lacked significant efficacy further underscores the therapeutic potential of 1% AA in wound care and implant-associated infections. Cytotoxicity testing on NIH 3T3 fibroblast cells revealed substantial differences in the biocompatibility of the tested combinations. Once again, the ADM combined with 1% AA demonstrated outstanding results, consistently maintaining cell viability above 100% at all observed time points. These values not only reflect non-cytotoxic behavior but also confirm the biocompatibility of the material with fibroblasts. This may be partly attributed to the acidifying effect of AA, which helps restore the naturally acidic pH of intact skin, maintained by organic acid secretion from keratinocytes. In contrast, chronic wounds become alkaline, which promotes protease activity and the accumulation of toxic by-products, impairing the healing process [28]. Similarly, the ADM combined with Prontosan® showed a non-toxic profile with a high cell viability comparable to the control; however, its antimicrobial activity was markedly limited, reducing its overall therapeutic value in infected-wound settings.

In contrast, Betadine® and Octenilin® showed severe and persistent cytotoxic effects, with Betadine® reducing cell viability to nearly zero across all time points. This may be attributed to povidone-iodine's ability to significantly reduce fibroblast proliferation, increase apoptosis and necrosis, and impair wound closure during early healing stages [29]. Although octenidine is considered safe for superficial use, its application in deeper wounds has been associated with tissue necrosis, chronic inflammation, and delayed healing, which may explain the observed in vitro cytotoxicity and suggests limited suitability for tissue-integrated therapies [30].

Similarly, Aqvitox-D® led to a progressive decline in cell viability, likely due to the concentration-dependent cytotoxicity of hypochlorite, which at ≥0.01% impairs fibroblast adhesion and mitochondrial function. In addition, even diluted NaOCl solutions (0.025–0.0025%) have been shown to cause sublethal cellular damage [31]. Likewise, colistin led to a progressive decline in fibroblast cell viability, confirming its high cytotoxic potential, particularly with prolonged exposure; this is consistent with its known neurotoxicity in clinical use, which results in oxidative stress and apoptosis [32]. Additionally, colistin is nephrotoxic, inducing apoptosis and autophagy, leading to colistin-induced nephrotoxicity [33]. Even vancomycin, though showing recovery on day 5, initially exhibited moderate cytotoxicity. It has been shown to affect fibroblasts at higher concentrations, indicating a dose-dependent cytotoxic response [34].

While the direct comparison of these specific agents, particularly the focus on 1% AA, is novel, it should be noted that the broader concept of loading antimicrobial agents into scaffolds is not entirely new. However, to our knowledge, this is the first study to directly compare seven different antimicrobial agents post-impregnation in a standardized in vitro ADM model, thereby providing comparative insights into their respective antimicrobial, antibiofilm, and cytocompatibility profiles. This approach revealed the distinct advantages of 1% AA. From a clinical standpoint, the combination of robust antimicrobial and antibiofilm activity and excellent cytocompatibility makes 1% AA an ideal candidate for use in tissue-integrated wound dressings or implant coatings. This dual advantage is critical in managing infected wounds where both bacterial clearance and tissue regeneration are essential, making it especially promising for applications in regenerative medicine and chronic wound management.

4. Materials and Methods

4.1. Acellular Allodermis—Acellular Dermal Matrix (ADM)

A human ADM (Figure S1) was prepared using a novel decellularization method developed by Dragúňová [6]. The process involved enzymatic separation of the epidermis from cadaveric skin allografts using a trypsin (Sigma-Aldrich, Merck KGaA, Darmstadt, Germany) and ethylenediaminetetraacetic acid (EDTA) solution (Sigma-Aldrich, Merck KGaA, Darmstadt, Germany), followed by mechanical removal and dermal lavage in hypotonic injection water to induce cell lysis. Histological analysis and cytotoxicity assays confirmed the complete removal of cellular components and the non-toxicity of the final product. The decellularized ADM was subsequently cryopreserved in the Cell and Tissue Bank. Before experimentation, the ADM was meshed at a 3:1 ratio, cut into 5 × 5 cm pieces, and impregnated for 24 h in antimicrobial solutions (1 mL), with each 25 cm^2 piece submerged in 100 mL of the respective solution.

4.2. Bacterial Strains

Two multidrug-resistant Gram-negative bacterial strains, *Pseudomonas aeruginosa* and *Acinetobacter baumannii*, were selected for testing. These strains were isolated from burn patients hospitalized in the Burn ICU and characterized by their resistance profiles at the University Microbiology Institute, CU Bratislava.

4.3. *Antimicrobial Agents*

Seven antimicrobial agents, including five topical antimicrobials and two antibiotics, were used for the ADM impregnation (1 mL for each), as follows: 1% AA solution (Sigma-Aldrich, Merck KGaA, Darmstadt, Germany); Aqvitox-D® = mixture of hypochlorous acid and sodium hypochlorite < 0.05% (Aqvitox Technology s.r.o., Bratislava, Slovakia); Betadine® solution = 10% povidone-iodine (EGIS Pharmaceuticals PLC, Budapest, Hungary); Octenilin® solution = octenidine dihydrochloride (Schülke & Mayr GmbH, Vienna, Austria); Prontosan® solution = 0.1% polyhexamethylene biguanide hydrochloride (B.Braun Konzern Medical, Melsungen, Germany); 0.3 mg colistin (1 MIU in 100 mL physiological saline, KOLOMYCÍN 1 MIU TEVA Pharmaceuticals, Tel Aviv, Israel); and 50 mg vancomycin (1 MIU in 20 mL physiological saline, EDICIN 1 g, Sandoz Group AG, Basel, Switzerland). The comparison of antibacterial agents in this study was based on clinically relevant doses corresponding to commonly used concentrations in practice rather than on equipotent antimicrobial units. Control samples consisted of the ADM immersed in physiological saline (B.Braun Konzern Medical, Melsungen, Germany) and sterile gauze (5 × 5 cm, Sterilux® ES, Heidenheim an der Brenz, Germany).

4.4. *In Vitro Burn Wound Models*

Two distinct in vitro burn wound models were created based on a modified method by Hammond et al. [19], as follows:

Model A—simulated planktonic bacterial growth:

For model preparation [9,19], sterile cellulose disks (6 mm in diameter, Thermo Scientific™ Oxoid™ Disc, Waltham, MA, USA) were placed onto Luria-Bertani agar (LBA, Sigma-Aldrich, Merck KGaA, Darmstadt, Germany) plates. A bacterial suspension containing 10^2 CFU was applied to each disk. The impregnated ADM (1 mL of antimicrobial agent), non-impregnated ADM, or sterile gauze (5 × 5 cm, Sterilux® ES, Heidenheim an der Brenz, Germany) was placed over the contaminated disks immediately after inoculation to simulate planktonic bacterial growth. To ensure uniform contact between the ADM and bacterial disks, sterile Petri dishes (60 mm in diameter) were placed over the ADM surface.

Model B—simulated biofilm formation:

Sterile cellulose disks were prepared as in Model A. However, the disks were incubated for 24 h at 37 °C to promote biofilm formation prior to ADM application. Before placing the ADM, the disks were gently rinsed with sterile phosphate-buffered saline (PBS, Sigma-Aldrich, Merck KGaA, Darmstadt, Germany) to remove non-adherent planktonic bacteria, leaving only the biofilm intact. The impregnated ADM, non-impregnated ADM, or sterile gauze was then placed on top of the disks. To ensure uniform contact between the ADM and bacterial disks, sterile Petri dishes (60 mm in diameter) were placed on top of the ADM surface.

For both models, following 24 h of incubation at 37 °C, each cellulose disk was transferred into a sterile test tube containing 1 mL of PBS. Bacteria were released by vigorous shaking at 2200 rpm for three consecutive cycles of two minutes each. The bacterial suspension was serially diluted in PBS using decimal dilutions, and 10 µL from each dilution was plated onto LBA plates. The plates were incubated for 20 h at 37 °C, after which bacterial colonies were enumerated and calculated as the CFU per disk to assess the antimicrobial efficacy.

4.5. *Determination of Microbial Growth Reduction*

The antimicrobial efficacy was quantified as the difference in $\log_{10}$ colony-forming units per milliliter ($\Delta\log_{10}$ CFU/mL) between the untreated controls and treated samples

(Table 1). The number of viable microorganisms in the samples was assessed by calculating both the colony-forming units per milliliter (CFU/mL) and the total microbial count (expressed as CFU). To evaluate the antimicrobial efficacy, the reduction in microbial growth was determined by comparing the microbial load after 24 h of incubation to the initial value, in accordance with Wiegand et al. [35]. The antimicrobial efficacy was indicated by a reduction in bacterial counts in $\log_{10}$ CFU/mL compared with the baseline control and classified according to internationally recognized standards. The reduction in growth was calculated using Equation (1), as follows:

$$\Delta \text{logCFU/mL} = \log_{10}(\text{CFUc/mL}) - \log_{10}(\text{CFUs/mL}) \quad (1)$$

where CFUc is the control, and CFU is the sample.

The extent of antimicrobial activity was interpreted based on the magnitude of the log reduction, as in Table 2.

Table 2. The interpretation of antibacterial activity.

<0.5-log growth reduction	no antimicrobial activity
0.5–1.0-log growth reduction	slight antimicrobial activity
>1.0–3.0-log growth reduction	significant antimicrobial activity
>3.0-log growth reduction	strong antimicrobial activity

The limit of detection (LOD) for the plating method was 1 CFU/mL ($\log_{10}$ = 0), meaning that counts below this value could not be reliably detected. For these samples, reductions greater than 7 $\log_{10}$ are reported as >7 $\log_{10}$ to reflect the maximum detectable reduction based on the LOD.

4.6. Cytotoxicity Tests

3T3 NIH murine fibroblasts (3T3) were purchased from the ECCACC collection (Lambda Life, Petržalka, Slovakia, ECCACC number: 850 22,108) and cultivated in Dulbecco-modified medium (Pan Biotech, Aidenbach, Germany) supplemented with 10% fetal calf serum (Pan Biotech, Aidenbach, Germany). The 3T3 cells were routinely cultured according to standard procedures (incubated in humidified air at 37 °C with 7.0% CO_2) and passaged at least once a week.

Cytotoxicity was assessed using a modified method based on [36]. The murine fibroblast cell line NIH 3T3 was cultured as described above until reaching confluence. At time 0 h, 60,000 cells were seeded into 6 cm diameter Petri dishes, followed by incubation at 37 °C in a humidified atmosphere with 7% CO_2. Three experimental groups were established, as follows:

Untreated 3T3 cells (negative control);

3T3 cells with acellular dermal matrix;

3T3 cells with ADM impregnated with 100 µL of one of the tested antibacterial agents, including 1% AA, Aqvitox-D®, Betadine®, Octenilin®, Prontosan®, colistin, and vancomycin.

Each sample was tested in triplicate. The antibacterial agents were applied by directly placing ADM fragments pre-impregnated with the respective agent onto the 3T3 monolayers. Cell morphology was monitored microscopically before and after treatment. After 24 h (Figures S2 and S3), 48 h, and 5 days, the ADM was removed, and the wells were washed with PBS and EDTA. Cells were detached using trypsin and counted using a Bürker's counting chamber. The number of adherent cells at each time point was compared with the untreated control. The percentage of viable, adherent cells was calculated to reflect the cytotoxicity, with lower percentages indicating higher cytotoxic effects. All procedures were performed under sterile conditions.

4.7. Statistical Analysis

All measurements were performed in triplicate (n = 3), and the results are expressed as the mean ± standard deviation (SD). The statistical analysis was carried out using one-way ANOVA, followed by Tukey's post hoc test for multiple comparisons. Analyses were conducted using GraphPad Prism version 5.01 software (GraphPad Software, Boston, MA, USA). Differences were considered statistically significant at the following thresholds: $p < 0.05$ (*), $p < 0.01$ (**), and $p < 0.001$ (***).

5. Conclusions

This study highlights the potential of ADM impregnated with antimicrobial agents as a promising approach for the treatment of burn wound infections, particularly those caused by multidrug-resistant Gram-negative bacteria. Our in vitro models demonstrated that the ADM impregnated with 1% AA exhibited superior antimicrobial activity against both planktonic and biofilm-associated forms of Pseudomonas aeruginosa and Acinetobacter baumannii. Among all tested agents, 1% AA was the only compound capable of completely inhibiting biofilm formation by *P. aeruginosa*, while also showing strong efficacy against *A. baumannii*. These results position AA as a highly effective antimicrobial agent with robust antibiofilm properties. In addition to its antimicrobial efficacy, 1% AA demonstrated excellent biocompatibility, maintaining high fibroblast viability throughout the observation period. This contrasts with the cytotoxic profiles observed for several commonly used antiseptics and antibiotics, such as Betadine®, Octenilin®, and colistin. The combination of strong antibacterial effect and cytocompatibility is particularly important for applications where both infection control and tissue regeneration are essential. Given its low cost, environmental safety, and lack of contribution to antimicrobial resistance, AA represents a sustainable and clinically relevant solution for infected-wound management. While the concept of loading antimicrobial agents into scaffolds is not entirely new, our study is, to our knowledge, the first to directly compare seven different antimicrobial agents post-impregnation into an ADM using a standardized in vitro model. This allowed us to identify the unique performance of 1% acetic acid, particularly its ability to inhibit biofilm formation by *P. aeruginosa*, while maintaining high cytocompatibility. The use of an impregnated ADM, rather than topical application alone, offers the advantage of prolonged local release, enhanced tissue integration, and potential use in implantable devices. Further preclinical and clinical studies are warranted to validate these findings and to explore the translational potential of AA-based ADM dressings in burn care and regenerative medicine.

Supplementary Materials: The following supporting information can be downloaded at: https://www.mdpi.com/article/10.3390/antibiotics14070707/s1, Figure S1: Histological image of acellular dermal matrix (ADM) showing preserved extracellular matrix and absence of cells, confirming scaffold integrity; Figure S2: Morphology of NIH 3T3 fibroblasts after 24-h incubation with (A) sterile gauze (control) and (B) with acellular dermal matrix (ADM) without antibacterial agents; Figure S3: Morphology of NIH 3T3 fibroblasts after 24-h incubation with 1% acetic acid (A) and with Betadine® (B).

Author Contributions: M.H.: Conceptualization, Data curation, Formal analysis, Investigation, Methodology, Validation, Visualization, Writing—original draft, and Writing—review and editing; E.K.: Data curation, Formal analysis, Investigation, Visualization, and Writing—original draft; S.B.F.: Data Curation, Writing—Original Draft, Visualization, Project administration, Funding acquisition, and Writing—review and editing; M.V.: Investigation, Supervision, and Writing—review and editing; A.P.: Data curation, Investigation, and Writing—review and editing. All authors have read and agreed to the published version of the manuscript.

Funding: This research was funded by the Grant Agency VEGA 1/0170/24 and by the Slovak Research and Development Agency, under contract APVV-19-0056.

Institutional Review Board Statement: Not applicable.

Informed Consent Statement: Not applicable.

Data Availability Statement: All data generated or analyzed during this study are included in the article.

Acknowledgments: The authors would like to thank Lívia Slobodníková, for characterizing bacteria and their resistance profiles, and Janka Dragúňová, from the Cell and Tissue Bank, University Hospital Bratislava, for her valuable assistance in the preparation of cells and tissues.

Conflicts of Interest: The authors declare no conflicts of interest.

Abbreviations

The following abbreviations are used in this manuscript:

AA	Acetic Acid
ADMs	Acellular Dermal Matrices
CFU	Colony Forming Units
EDTA	Ethylenediaminetetraacetic Acid
NIH/3T3	Mouse Embryo Fibroblast Cell Line Clone 3T3
PBS	Phosphate-Buffered Saline

References

1. Li, X.; Meng, X.; Wang, X.; Li, Y.; Li, W.; Lv, X.; Xu, X.; Lei, Z.; Li, J. Human Acellular Dermal Matrix Allograft: A Randomized, Controlled Human Trial for the Long-Term Evaluation of Patients with Extensive Burns. *Burns* **2015**, *41*, 689–699. [CrossRef] [PubMed]
2. Spear, S.L.; Sher, S.R.; Al-Attar, A.; Pittman, T. Applications of Acellular Dermal Matrix in Revision Breast Reconstruction Surgery. *Plast. Reconstr. Surg.* **2014**, *133*, 1–10. [CrossRef] [PubMed]
3. Acevedo, D.C.; Shore, B.; Mirzayan, R. Orthopedic Applications of Acellular Human Dermal Allograft for Shoulder and Elbow Surgery. *Orthop. Clin. N. Am.* **2015**, *46*, 377–388. [CrossRef] [PubMed]
4. Winters, C.L.; Brigido, S.A.; Liden, B.A.; Simmons, M.; Hartman, J.F.; Wright, M.L. A Multicenter Study Involving the Use of a Human Acellular Dermal Regenerative Tissue Matrix for the Treatment of Diabetic Lower Extremity Wounds. *Adv. Skin Wound Care* **2008**, *21*, 375–381. [CrossRef]
5. Chien, P.N.; Zhang, X.R.; Nilsu, D.; Faruq, O.; Van Anh, L.T.; Nam, S.Y.; Heo, C.Y. In Vivo Comparison of Three Human Acellular Dermal Matrices for Breast Reconstruction. *In Vivo* **2021**, *35*, 2719–2728. [CrossRef]
6. Dragúňová, J.; Kabát, P.; Babál, P.; Mrázová, H.; Boháč, M.; Krajčíová; Koller, J. Development of a New Method for the Preparation of an Acellular Allodermis, Quality Control and Cytotoxicity Testing. *Cell Tissue Bank.* **2017**, *18*, 153–166. [CrossRef]
7. Koller, J.; Orság, M. Skin Grafting Options at the Burn and Reconstructive Surgery Department of the Faculty Hospital in Bratislava. *Acta Chir. Plast.* **2006**, *48*, 65–71.
8. Glasser, J.S.; Guymon, C.H.; Mende, K.; Wolf, S.E.; Hospenthal, D.R.; Murray, C.K. Activity of Topical Antimicrobial Agents against Multidrug-Resistant Bacteria Recovered from Burn Patients. *Burns* **2010**, *36*, 1172–1184. [CrossRef]
9. Hajská, M.; Slobodníková, L.; Hupková, H.; Koller, J. In Vitro Efficacy of Various Topical Antimicrobial Agents in Different Time Periods from Contamination to Application against 6 Multidrug-Resistant Bacterial Strains Isolated from Burn Patients. *Burns* **2014**, *40*, 713–718. [CrossRef]
10. Church, D.; Elsayed, S.; Reid, O.; Winston, B.; Lindsay, R. Burn Wound Infections. *Clin. Microbiol. Rev.* **2006**, *19*, 403–434. [CrossRef]

11. van Langeveld, I.; Gagnon, R.C.; Conrad, P.F.; Gamelli, R.L.; Martin, B.; Choudhry, M.A.; Mosier, M.J. Multiple-Drug Resistance in Burn Patients: A Retrospective Study on the Impact of Antibiotic Resistance on Survival and Length of Stay. *J. Burn. Care Res.* **2017**, *38*, 99–105. [CrossRef] [PubMed]
12. Thomas, R.E.; Thomas, B.C. Reducing Biofilm Infections in Burn Patients' Wounds and Biofilms on Surfaces in Hospitals, Medical Facilities and Medical Equipment to Improve Burn Care: A Systematic Review. *Int. J Environ. Res. Public Health* **2021**, *18*, 13195. [CrossRef] [PubMed]
13. Kennedy, P.; Brammah, S.; Wills, E. Burns, Biofilm and a New Appraisal of Burn Wound Sepsis. *Burns* **2010**, *36*, 49–56. [CrossRef]
14. Norman, G.; Christie, J.; Liu, Z.; Westby, M.J.; Jefferies, J.M.; Hudson, T.; Edwards, J.; Mohapatra, D.P.; Hassan, I.A.; Dumville, J.C. Antiseptics for Burns. *Cochrane Database Syst. Rev.* **2017**, *2017*, CD011821. [CrossRef]
15. Garcia, J.A.G.; Chavez, A.M.G.; Grados, J.D.J.O. Topical Antimicrobial Agents for the Prevention of Burn-Wound Infection. What Do International Guidelines Recommend? A Systematic Review. *World J. Plast. Surg.* **2022**, *11*, 3–12. [CrossRef]
16. Ilahi, O.N.; Velmahos, G.; Janis, J.E.; Kovach, S.J.; McLean, S.F.; Askari, R.; Sommer, C.A.; Agarwal, S.; Srinivasan, J.; Wong, A.K.; et al. Prospective, Multicenter Study of Antimicrobial-Coated, Noncrosslinked, Acellular Porcine Dermal Matrix (XenMatrix^{TM} AB Surgical Graft) for Hernia Repair in All Centers for Disease Control and Prevention Wound Classes: 24-Month Follow-up Cohort. *Ann. Med. Surg.* **2023**, *85*, 1571–1577. [CrossRef]
17. Yang, Y.; Yang, G.W.; Lu, J.J.; Chen, H.R.; Guo, Y.Q.; Yang, N.; Zhu, Y.Z.; Liu, X.Q.; Su, T.T.; Liu, Y.Y.; et al. Fabrication of Levofloxacin-Loaded Porcine Acellular Dermal Matrix Hydrogel and Functional Assessment in Urinary Tract Infection. *J. Nanobiotechnology* **2024**, *22*, 52. [CrossRef]
18. Dai, T.; Huang, Y.-Y.; Sharma, S.K.; Hashmi, J.T.; Kurup, D.B.; Hamblin, M.R. Topical Antimicrobials for Burn Wound Infections. *Recent Pat. Antiinfect. Drug Discov.* **2010**, *5*, 124–151. [CrossRef]
19. Hammond, A.A.; Miller, K.G.; Kruczek, C.J.; Dertien, J.; Colmer-Hamood, J.A.; Griswold, J.A.; Horswill, A.R.; Hamood, A.N. An in Vitro Biofilm Model to Examine the Effect of Antibiotic Ointments on Biofilms Produced by Burn Wound Bacterial Isolates. *Burns* **2011**, *37*, 312–321. [CrossRef]
20. Cooper, R.A.; Bjarnsholt, T.; Alhede, M. Biofilms in Wounds: A Review of Present Knowledge. *J. Woundcare* **2014**, *23*, 570–582. [CrossRef]
21. Omar, A.; Wright, J.B.; Schultz, G.; Burrell, R.; Nadworny, P. Microbial Biofilms and Chronic Wounds. *Microorganisms* **2017**, *5*, 9. [CrossRef] [PubMed]
22. Bjarnsholt, T.; Alhede, M.; Jensen, P.Ø.; Nielsen, A.K.; Johansen, H.K.; Homøe, P.; Høiby, N.; Givskov, M.; Kirketerp-Møller, K. Antibiofilm Properties of Acetic Acid. *Adv. Wound Care* **2015**, *4*, 363–372. [CrossRef] [PubMed]
23. Kundukad, B.; Schussman, M.; Yang, K.; Seviour, T.; Yang, L.; Rice, S.A.; Kjelleberg, S.; Doyle, P.S. Mechanistic Action of Weak Acid Drugs on Biofilms. *Sci. Rep.* **2017**, *7*, 4783. [CrossRef] [PubMed]
24. Goswami, A.G.; Basu, S.; Banerjee, T.; Shukla, V.K. Biofilm and Wound Healing: From Bench to Bedside. *Eur. J. Med. Res.* **2023**, *28*, 157. [CrossRef]
25. Thapa, R.K.; Kim, J.O.; Kim, J. Antimicrobial Strategies for Topical Biofilm-Based Wound Infections: Past, Present, and Future. *J. Pharm. Investig.* **2023**, *53*, 627–641. [CrossRef]
26. Sim, P.; Strudwick, X.L.; Song, Y.M.; Cowin, A.J.; Garg, S. Influence of Acidic PH on Wound Healing In Vivo: A Novel Perspective for Wound Treatment. *Int. J. Mol. Sci.* **2022**, *23*, 13655. [CrossRef]
27. Kaufman, T.; Eichenlaub, E.H.; Angel, M.F.; Levin, M.; Futrell, J.W. Topical Acidification Promotes Healing of Experimental Deep Partial Thickness Skin Burns: A Randomized Double-Blind Preliminary Study. *Burns* **1985**, *12*, 84–90. [CrossRef]
28. Kruse, C.R.; Singh, M.; Targosinski, S.; Sinha, I.; Sørensen, J.A.; Eriksson, E.; Nuutila, K. The Effect of PH on Cell Viability, Cell Migration, Cell Proliferation, Wound Closure, and Wound Reepithelialization: In Vitro and In Vivo Study. *Wound Repair. Regen.* **2017**, *25*, 260–269. [CrossRef]
29. Rueda-Fernández, M.; Melguizo-Rodríguez, L.; Costela-Ruiz, V.J.; de Luna-Bertos, E.; Ruiz, C.; Ramos-Torrecillas, J.; Illescas-Montes, R. Effect of the Most Common Wound Antiseptics on Human Skin Fibroblasts. *Clin. Exp. Dermatol.* **2022**, *47*, 1543–1549. [CrossRef]
30. Lachapelle, J.M. A Comparison of the Irritant and Allergenic Properties of Antiseptics. *Eur. J. Dermatol.* **2014**, *24*, 3–9. [CrossRef]
31. Hidalgo, E.; Dominguez, C. Growth-Altering Effects of Sodium Hypochlorite in Cultured Human Dermal Þbroblasts. *Life Sci.* **2000**, *67*, 1331–1344. [CrossRef]
32. Xie, B.; Liu, Y.; Chen, C.; Velkov, T.; Tang, S.; Shen, J.; Dai, C. Colistin Induces Oxidative Stress and Apoptotic Cell Death through the Activation of the AhR/CYP1A1 Pathway in PC12 Cells. *Antioxidants* **2024**, *13*, 827. [CrossRef] [PubMed]
33. Dai, C.; Li, J.; Tang, S.; Li, J.; Xiao, X. Colistin-Induced Nephrotoxicity in Mice Involves the Mitochondrial, Death Receptor, and Endoplasmic Reticulum Pathways. *Antimicrob. Agents Chemother.* **2014**, *58*, 4075–4085. [CrossRef] [PubMed]

34. Liu, J.X.; Bravo, D.; Buza, J.; Kirsch, T.; Kennedy, O.; Rokito, A.; Zuckerman, J.D.; Virk, M.S. Topical Vancomycin and Its Effect on Survival and Migration of Osteoblasts, Fibroblasts, and Myoblasts: An in Vitro Study. *J. Orthop.* **2018**, *15*, 53–58. [CrossRef] [PubMed]
35. Wiegand, C.; Heinze, T.; Hipler, U.C. Comparative in Vitro Study on Cytotoxicity, Antimicrobial Activity, and Binding Capacity for Pathophysiological Factors in Chronic Wounds of Alginate and Silver-Containing Alginate. *Wound Repair. Regen.* **2009**, *17*, 511–521. [CrossRef]
36. Vitteková, M.; Dragúňová, J.; Kabát, P.; Božiková, M.; Bakoš, D.; Koller, J. Cytotoxicity Testing of Scaffolds Potentially Suitable for the Preparation of Three-Dimensional Skin Substitutes. *Cell Tissue Bank.* **2014**, *15*, 345–355. [CrossRef]

MDPI AG
Grosspeteranlage 5
4052 Basel
Switzerland
Tel.: +41 61 683 77 34

Antibiotics Editorial Office
E-mail: antibiotics@mdpi.com
www.mdpi.com/journal/antibiotics

www.ingramcontent.com/pod-product-compliance
Lightning Source LLC
Chambersburg PA
CBHW061611210926
51850CB00009B/2292
* 9 7 8 3 7 2 5 8 6 3 1 0 5 *